A PHOTOGRAPHIC ATLAS OF
Histology
SECOND EDITION

Michael J. Leboffe, D.A.
San Diego City College

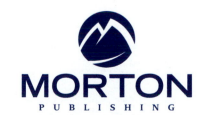

MORTON
PUBLISHING

925 W. Kenyon Avenue, Unit 12
Englewood, CO 80110

www.morton-pub.com

■ Book Team

Publisher:	Douglas Morton
President:	David Ferguson
Acquisitions Editor:	Marta Martins
Project Manager:	Melanie Stafford
Associate Project Manager:	Rayna Bailey
Production Manager:	Joanne Saliger
Production Assistant / Interior Design and Composition:	Will Kelley
Illustrations:	Imagineering Media Services, Inc.

To Selah Grace, Josiah Benjamin, and Teagan Elyse—
three of my favorite studies in tissue perfection.

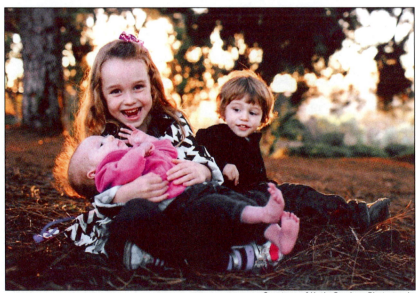

Courtesy of Katie Gardner Photography

Printed in the United States of America

10 9 8 7 6 5 4

ISBN-13: 978-161731-068-3

Library of Congress Control Number 2012951977

This book is the product of a lot of blood (Chapter 6), sweat (Chapter 11), and tears (Chapter 9). But enough about me…

I've included the preface to the first edition, written in 2003, because my goals haven't changed in writing this revision. I still intend for this to be a practical atlas of histology, one that you will find useful to have at your side as you look through the microscope trying to find all those assigned tissues and cells and layers and … well, you get the idea (or *will*). With that in mind, I have used commercially available slides to photograph. (Granted, some of these may no longer be in production, but they were at one time and your college may still have some!) Many are nonhuman mammalian specimens but still show what needs to be shown. After all, mammals are, in fact, more alike than different at the tissue level. And, as before, pathology specimens have not been included.

This is, in many ways, a new book. By unofficial count, there are 559 light micrographs in this edition, with 195 of them replacing images from the first edition and 101 images new to this edition. In other words, more than half the micrographs are new ones. Beyond these, due to the generosity of the folks at Morton Publishing, the entire art program has been redone, with the inclusion of nearly 40 original renderings, 10 of which replaced the ones in the first edition with the remainder being new to this edition. And while the main goal of this atlas is to help you while you are at the microscope, we have included 21 electron micrographs, most of which are new, where they will enhance your understanding of structure.

I truly hope that this atlas helps you in your histological studies (and you get the all-important grade!). But beyond that, I hope it contributes in some small way to your success in your chosen field and assists you in developing an appreciation of the fabric of the human body.

Mike
March 2013
La Mesa, California

:: Preface to the First Edition

The primary goal and overriding theme of *A Photographic Atlas of Histology* is practicality. And while I expect that it will get used during home study and test review, I wrote with the student sitting at the microscope with a box of slides to examine in mind. My hope is that the images in this book will assist that student in identifying what needs to be seen. Towards this end, I used commercially available microscope slides to photograph, so the images represent the quality and diversity of what a student is actually likely to encounter in the laboratory; pathological specimens have not been used. I also have minimized the inclusion of electron micrographs, because beginning histology students are not typically required (or even allowed) to use an electron microscope. Finally, I wrote captions for the images as if I was showing projected images to a class, so they tend to be lengthy and descriptive.

The textual material is intended to be a concise synopsis of histological basics, not an exhaustive treatise on the discipline. Further, it is assumed the student has a basic background in anatomy, so gross anatomy is not covered. Neither is physiology discussed beyond a general description of function. You may want to examine other references that cover these topics in detail.

Histology is a challenging, but exciting discipline–once you develop certain skills. Beginners often dread spending hours over a microscope and then have difficulty "seeing anything." With practice and experience come a sharpened eye and strategies for successful examination of microscopic preparations, which make the process more rewarding. I have made some suggestions in Chapter 1 to quicken your arrival at this point. I encourage you to give them a try.

By the way, if you begin to imagine the cells are looking back at you, you've been studying too hard. It's time for a break.

I wish you success on your upcoming adventure.

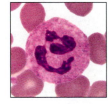

■ Acknowledgments

Rarely is a book the work of one person, even when there is a single author. This is certainly true of this book. I am deeply indebted to the following people for their contributions and support.

Right off the bat, I want to rectify an oversight that has nagged at me for the 10 years since the first edition. To my horror and embarrassment, I neglected to acknowledge the person most responsible for kick-starting my career in the direction of anatomy. Harry Plymale, DVM, of San Diego State University taught the Histology course I spoke of under the section heading, "Strategies for Studying Histology" (page 2). He modeled the discipline, attention to detail, and enthusiasm for the topic, and to the extent that I manifest these for my students, Harry is in large part responsible. He also provided me with my first teaching opportunity at SDSU as a graduate teaching assistant in Human Anatomy, which put me on a career path of teaching that subject long before I transitioned into teaching microbiology. So, Harry: for all you've done for my career, thank you from the bottom of my heart. And thank you again for so graciously understanding my oversight 10 years ago.

Thanks to the entire Morton Publishing Team, starting with Doug Morton, Founder and now CEO of the company. His vision and business model of producing high-quality textbooks at affordable prices has carried this "Little Engine That Could" publishing company from modest beginnings to a force to be reckoned with in their publication niche. Currently presiding over the company's expansion and success are the troika of David Ferguson, President; Chrissy DeMier, Vice President of Operations; and Carter Fenton, Vice President of Sales and Marketing. They are a capable, ambitious, young, and energetic team of leaders, and I see great things for Morton Publishing in the next couple of decades with them at the helm. One of the changes they have instituted is the amount of support provided to the authors. In my 18 years of writing for Morton, I have never worked with such a large project team. Marta Martins began the project as Associate Editor and compiled and organized the reviews in such a way that it made my job of using the reviews much easier. She did so well, in fact, that she was promoted off my project and is now Acquisitions Editor for Morton! Stepping in was Rayna Bailey, Associate Project Manager, who cheerfully took care of permissions, acquisitions, and other nuisance jobs so that I could focus on the writing and photography. Then, she just as cheerfully copyedited my manuscripts and elevated their quality immeasurably. She also acted as intermediary with Imagineering Media Services, Inc., of Toronto, Ontario, who produced all of the beautiful new artwork for this edition. Thanks also to Carolyn Acheson, who indexed the manuscript, and to Melanie Stafford, who proofread it. Finally, Joanne Saliger, Production Manager, and Will Kelley, Production Assistant, have designed a beautiful book, one that has artistic appeal and makes readers forget that they are studying "dull old anatomy!" By my count, this is the 16th project Joanne's team has designed for me and each one is better looking than the previous one. Outside of the immediate project team, I am also indebted to all the others at Morton who support authors' efforts in Sales, Marketing, and Customer Service. No matter how good the product is, the "word" has to get out to students and faculty and these people do an extraordinary job.

The reviewers of the first edition made many, many useful and thoughtful comments and suggestions, most of which I addressed and/or incorporated into this edition. Thanks to Ted Fleming, Bradley University; Sara Delozier, Delgado Community College; Danielle King, Santa Rosa Junior College; and Edith Robbins, Borough of Manhattan Community College, all of whom reviewed the entire text. Thanks also go to my colleagues at San Diego City College who used the book and informally offered their suggestions over the years: Luz Alvarez, Greg Brulte, Julie Haugness-White, Phil Osborne, Joe Penaflor, and Rosa Runcie. I especially want to acknowledge the two anatomists with whom I have most closely worked: Anita Hettena and Carla Sweet. Thank you, ladies, for your cheery smiles, insightful feedback, and friendship.

Micrographs require a microscope, and I want to thank my two representatives, Craig Rappaport and Shanan Miller, from Olympus America Inc., for their assistance and support over the years. Microscopes also require microscope slides. Thanks to the customer service representatives and histology technicians at Carolina Biological Supply Company, Ward's Science, and especially Catherine Conant at Triarch Incorporated for their help with specimens when I needed it. Thanks also to Marlene DeMers of San Diego State University for generously sharing her collection of blood smears.

As always, mistakes and oversights are my responsibility. If you have suggestions or see errors, please contact Morton Publishing (contact@morton-pub.com) and we will address them, if not in the next printing, then in the next edition.

Thanks to all!

Contents

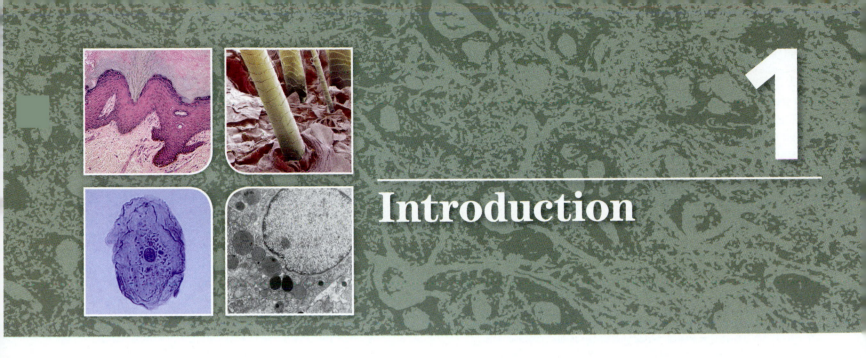

Introduction

What Is Histology?

Literally, histology is the study of tissues (*histos* = tissue; *logos* = treatise). Tissues are collections of cells that have a similar structure and function. In adults, there are four major tissues:

- Epithelial tissue (epithelium)
- Connective tissue
- Muscle tissue
- Nervous tissue

In modern usage, the term *histology* has come to include all levels of microscopic anatomy, from tissues down to cells and cell ultrastructure, as well as the ways in which the tissues are combined to form organs and organ systems.

Why Study Histology?

Histology is the bridge between structure and function. It is at the microscopic level that we begin to see how an organ actually performs its functions. It is virtually impossible to discuss organ function without first considering its microscopic structure.

Histological Techniques—Microscopy

The **light microscope** (Figure 1-1) is used to examine specimens by transillumination, that is, by shining light through them. The **mechanical components** include **focus adjustments**, a **mechanical stage**, and a **light source**. The **optical components** include a **condenser, objective lenses,** and **ocular lenses.** The condenser concentrates the light and uniformly illuminates the specimen. Light from the specimen is **refracted** (bent) by the objective lens to produce a magnified image, which is magnified again as it passes through the ocular lens

and is transmitted to the retina of the eye. Sample light micrographs are shown in Figure 1-2.

The amount of magnification produced is marked on each lens. Total specimen magnification is the product of the power of the objective lens and the ocular lens. Because typical microscopes have 4× (scanning power), 10× (low power), 40× (high dry power), and 100× (oil immersion) objectives and 10× oculars, the total magnifications are 40×, 100×, 400×, and 1000×, respectively.

Magnification is not the only important feature of a microscope. The ability to produce magnification with good **resolution** is what really matters. Basically, resolution is the ability of a lens to produce a clear image. Technically, it is the ability of a lens to reveal two individual points as being separate. The closer together two points are when they can be seen as separate, the better the resolution of the microscope. The limit of resolution for light microscopes is about 0.1 μm, which allows production of quality images magnified up to about 1500× (which will probably exceed the ability of your microscope).

The **electron microscope** uses an electron beam to create an image. The limit of resolution is improved by a factor of 1,000 (theoretically down to 0.1 nm, but more realistically down to 2 nm) over the light microscope, and the maximum magnification is about 150,000×. **Transmission electron microscopes (TEM)** (Figure 1-3) produce a two-dimensional image of an ultrathin section by capturing electrons that have passed through the specimen. The degree of interaction between the electrons and the heavy metal stain affects the kinetic energy of the electrons, which are collected by a fluorescent plate. The light of varying intensity produced is directly proportional to the electron's kinetic energy and is used to produce the image. Another sensor allows the image to be digitized and displayed on a computer monitor. The TEM is useful for studying a cell's interior—its

ultrastructure. A sample transmission electron micrograph is shown in Figure 1-4.

A **scanning electron microscope (SEM)** (Figure 1-5) is used to make a three-dimensional image of the specimen's surface. In this technique, a focused beam of electrons is passed over the gold-coated specimen's surface. Some electrons are reflected (*backscatter electrons*), whereas other electrons (*secondary electrons*) are emitted from the metallic coating. These electrons are captured and used to produce the three-dimensional image. A sample scanning electron micrograph is shown in Figure 1-6.

Histological Techniques— Specimen Preparation

In some cases, specimens may be examined immediately after removal from the body with staining as the only form of preparation. A blood smear is an example. However, in addition to staining, most specimens must be prepared prior to observation. Preparation involves various chemical treatments, embedding with a supporting medium, and slicing into thin sections. An overview of the specific steps follows.

- **Fixation** The specimen is treated with a chemical fixative, such as formalin, that alters its chemical composition and slows its deterioration. Chemical modification may include protein denaturation and cross-linking, and preservation of lipids and carbohydrates.

- **Dehydration** Beginning with a 50–70% alcohol solution, the specimen is bathed in successively more concentrated alcohol solutions (up to 100%) to remove water.

- **Clearing** Treatment with xylene makes the specimen transparent.

- **Embedding** In preparation for cutting the specimen into thin slices (sections), it is treated with a supporting medium, such as paraffin. (Paraffin is insoluble in water and alcohol but is soluble in xylene, thus making the dehydration and clearing steps necessary.) First, the specimen is infiltrated with liquid paraffin. The specimen is then embedded in paraffin, which is allowed to solidify into a block. Plastics are sometimes used for embedding because they allow thinner sections (1–2 μm) to be made and result in fewer distortions of the specimen.

- **Sectioning** The solidified block containing the specimen is mounted on an instrument called a **microtome** (Figure 1-7). The microtome has a steel or glass blade and a mechanism that moves the block a preset distance (usually 5–10 μm for paraffin) after each cut. Thus, each time a cut is made, the block is moved a distance equal to the thickness of the next slice. In this fashion, many slices of uniform thickness are made.

- **Mounting** Each section is applied to a glass slide.

- **Staining** To provide contrast, specimens are colorized with various stains. The colored portion of some staining solutions is acidic. Acidic stains colorize basic (alkaline, positively charged) cellular structures, which are said to be **acidophilic** (acid-loving). Basic stains are used to colorize acidic cellular structures, which are said to be **basophilic** (base-loving). Hematoxylin and eosin stain (H&E) is used for most routine preparations and consists of a basic and an acidic component. The basic stain hematoxylin and the acid stain eosin produce the purple and pink specimens frequently encountered in a histology laboratory. Table 1-1 lists some common stains and the structures they highlight. Because most stains are aqueous solutions, the paraffin must be removed and the section rehydrated prior to stain application. Following staining, the specimen is again dehydrated and a cover slip is permanently mounted over it for protection and improved image production by the microscope. The mounting medium not only glues the cover slip to the slide, it may include ingredients that preserve tissues and minimize fading of the stain(s).

This entire process may take 48 hours to complete. For specimens that need to be examined quickly (such as with surgical samples), the tissue may be sectioned using a freezing microtome. Freezing replaces the embedding process and makes dehydration and clearing unnecessary. Freezing microtomes are also used when lipids are to be examined in tissue because they are removed when treated with solvents such as xylene.

Preparation of specimens for electron microscopy is similar to the preparation described above. Glutaraldehyde and osmium tetroxide are commonly used as fixatives. The latter has the additional benefit of being electron dense, which provides contrast in the image and thereby acts as a stain when viewed with the transmission electron microscope. Uranyl acetate, lead citrate, and/or osmium tetroxide are also used as stains. Tissues are typically embedded in plastic prior to being cut into sections of the desired thickness (frequently in the 100 nm range).

Specimen preparation for use with the scanning electron microscope involves fixing and dehydration, followed by coating with a thin layer of gold, which interacts with the electron beam to produce the image.

Strategies for Studying Histology

I took my first histology class in 1975 as a graduate student. My professor told us of a supplemental atlas (diFiore's *Atlas of Human Histology*, then in its fourth edition) that was available as a "crutch" if we needed it. After one lab period, I set my grad student pride aside and gladly purchased my crutch. At the time, I thought I was alone in my struggles.

However, teaching anatomy and histology for more than 35 years has convinced me that this discipline is just plain difficult for most students to master. Nevertheless, "difficult" does not equate to "impossible" or "not worthwhile." Here are some tips that I hope will help you learn what you need to know.

- Read the slide's label. It will tell you what the specimen is, how it was sectioned (or if it is a "whole mount"), and often what stain was used.

- Realize that most slides have more tissues and/or organs on them than what is written on the label (Figure 1-8). One of the most difficult skills to acquire in histology is to find the "correct" part of the slide to examine.

- Examine the slide without the microscope to get an idea of what the section looks like. Often, you can see a lot without magnification. It also should help you "zero in" on the area of the slide you want to examine, because you can position the slide on the stage with the relevant part centered. (Remember, the specimen's image will be upside down and backward from its orientation on the stage.)

- Begin microscopic examination at scanning or low power. Get a feeling for what is on the slide and how the parts are related. When you see something of particular interest, center it and move to the higher powers.

- Do not overilluminate the specimen. Using too much light results in loss of detail in the image. Reduce the light with the iris diaphragm to a point where you can still see the specimen, but it is not too bright. (As a guide, close the iris diaphragm until the image starts to get darker. Then, open it up again just a tad.) You will need to increase the light at each higher magnification to get the same degree of illumination, because the field gets successively darker as higher power objectives are used.

- This one may be the hardest. Don't be satisfied with looking at a single example of each assigned specimen. Look at several, then look at some more—especially if they are from a different organism or manufacturer. It takes examination of many examples before you begin to recognize the common construction.

- Most specimens have been cut into thin slices and you will be expected (eventually) to convert the essentially two-dimensional image you see on the microscope into a fully functional, three-dimensional object. This is equivalent to asking a person who has never seen a loaf of bread to imagine what the loaf looks like after examining a single slice. This skill will come with practice and by looking at three-dimensional drawings of specimens as you examine them on the slides. Because so many structures are tubular, it will also be useful to examine Figure 1-9 to see the many ways a tube appears, depending on how it is cut. In most cases, the microscope slide's label will tell you how the specimen was sectioned or prepared (Table 1-2). Be forewarned, however, that parts within the specimen may have been sectioned differently than the whole specimen because of their different orientation.

- Don't overestimate slide quality. Photos in texts show good examples, but not every slide of an organ will show everything you need to see, and neither will slides necessarily be of uniform quality. In books such as this one, what you don't see are the dozens of slides, fields, and photographs that were discarded because of poor quality.

- Your microscope, like the one used to take the photomicrographs in this book, probably has objectives that produce total magnifications of 40×, 100×, 400×, and maybe 1000×. However, photomicrograph magnifications are changed during the production process when they are either enlarged or reduced in size. Those differences are reflected in the magnifications listed with each micrograph. This means you may not be able to re-create the magnifications of the images you see in this book with your microscope.

Table 1-1 Commonly Used Histological Stains

Stain	Comment
Azan	Stains nuclei, nucleoli, and RBCs red; muscle orange; and connective tissue blue
Azure B	Stains DNA blue-green and RNA purple
Cresyl violet	Typically a bacterial stain, it can be used to stain neuronal Nissl bodies purple
Da Fano silver method	Stains Golgi apparatus black
Feulgen stain	Stains DNA reddish violet
Giemsa-Wright stain	Used for staining blood and bone marrow smears; stains cytoplasm light blue; cytoplasmic granules pink, purple, or unstained; and nuclei dark purple
Hematoxylin and eosin (H&E)	H&E is a commonly used stain. Hematoxylin is a basic stain that colors acidic structures a purplish blue. These include the nucleus and regions with abundant ribosomes or rough endoplasmic reticulum, in addition to cartilage matrix. Eosin is an acidic stain and makes basic regions of the cell—that is, most of it—pink. It also stains collagen and elastic fibers pink.
Iron hematoxylin	Stains nuclei, chromosomes, mitochondria, centrioles, and muscle striations black
Masson's trichrome	Results in three colors: basophilic structures are stained dark blue; collagen is stained green or light blue; and cytoplasm, keratin, muscle, and erythrocytes are stained red
Methylene blue	Stains nuclear material and Nissl substance blue
Osmium	Stains lipids a dark brown
Periodic acid-Schiff (PAS)	Colors complex carbohydrates red (magenta). Cells or cellular structures that stain red are said to be PAS positive. Glycogen, brush borders, and the mucin in goblet cells are PAS positive.
Silver stain	Used for staining delicate structures, such as reticular fibers and neuronal processes
Sudan red	Stains fat cells red
Trypan blue	Phagocytic cells accumulate this blue dye in their phagolysosomes when they engulf it
Verhoeff stain	Stains elastic fibers dark blue to black; nuclei bluish-gray to black

Table 1-2 Microscope Slide Label Markings

Type of Preparation	Meaning	Label Marking
Cross section	The specimen was cut across its long axis	c.s. or x.s.
Longitudinal section	The specimen was cut along its long axis	l.s.
Section	The section was made in no particular orientation relative to the specimen	sec.
Smear	A type of whole mount in which the specimen was spread thinly on the slide (generally this is used with a liquid, such as with blood smears)	smear
Spread	A type of whole mount in which the specimen was stretched out across the slide (not commonly used)	spread
Teased preparation	A type of whole mount in which the specimen was picked apart	ts
Transverse section	The specimen was cut across its long axis	t.s.
Whole mount	The specimen was not sectioned	w.m.

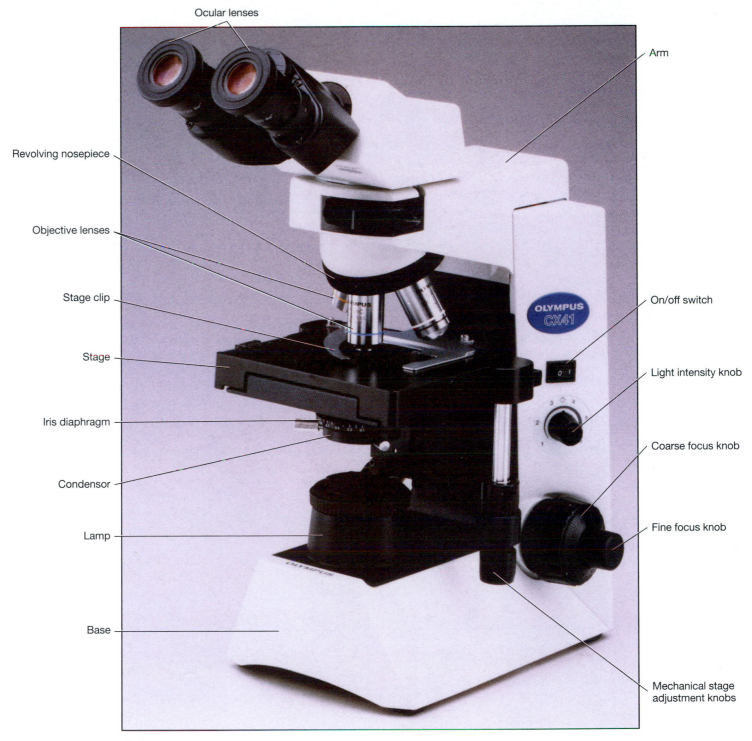

Ocular lenses

Arm

Revolving nosepiece

Objective lenses

On/off switch

Stage clip

Light intensity knob

Stage

Iris diaphragm

Coarse focus knob

Condensor

Fine focus knob

Lamp

Base

Mechanical stage adjustment knobs

1-1 **Light Microscope** ◖ The light microscope uses visible light and lenses to produce a magnified image of a specimen. (Photograph courtesy of Olympus America Inc.)

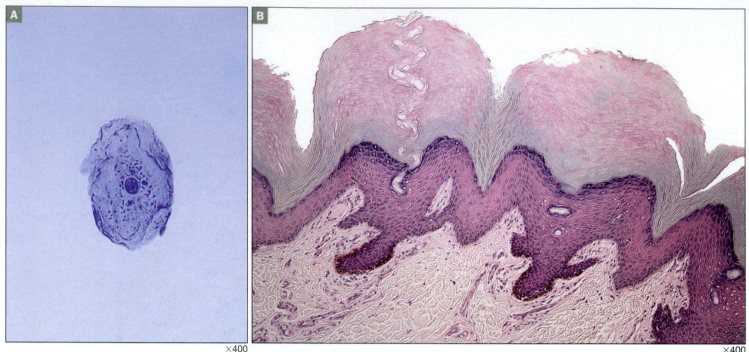

×400

×400

1-2 Light Micrographs ■ A photograph of a microscopic image is a micrograph. These images were made with a light microscope and are called light micrographs. Most of the images in this book are light micrographs. (**A**) This is a wet-mount preparation of cells gently scraped from inside the oral cavity and stained with methylene blue. In a wet mount, the specimen is placed directly in a drop of water and stain on the microscope slide and viewed with no additional preparation. This is the only micrograph of a wet mount in the book, but you may have the opportunity to make your own. (×400) (**B**) This light micrograph of a skin specimen has been sectioned and stained with H&E. Most specimens in this book have been sectioned. (×400)

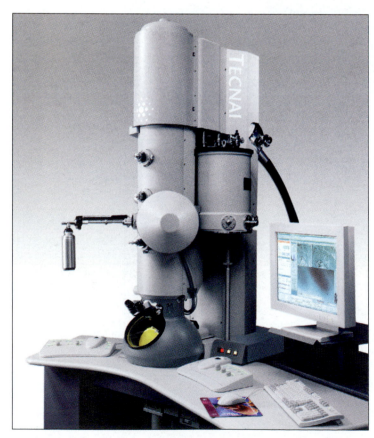

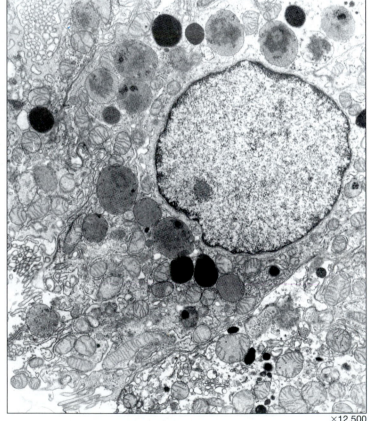

×12,500

1-3 Transmission Electron Microscope ■ The transmission electron microscope produces an image using electrons that pass through the specimen. The image is then viewed on the monitor. This particular model magnifies from 8× up to 630,000×. (Photograph courtesy of FEI Worldwide)

1-4 Transmission Electron Micrograph ■ The TEM produces images of sectioned specimens. Since light is not used, the image is not in color. This cell was magnified ×12,500. (Photograph courtesy of UCSD Medical Center)

A Photographic Atlas of Histology

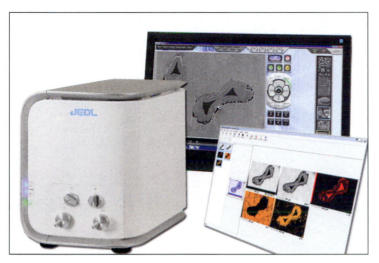

1-5 **Scanning Electron Microscope** ◾ Shown is a research grade scanning benchtop electron microscope. Notice the three-dimensional images on the computer. (Photograph courtesy of JEOL, USA)

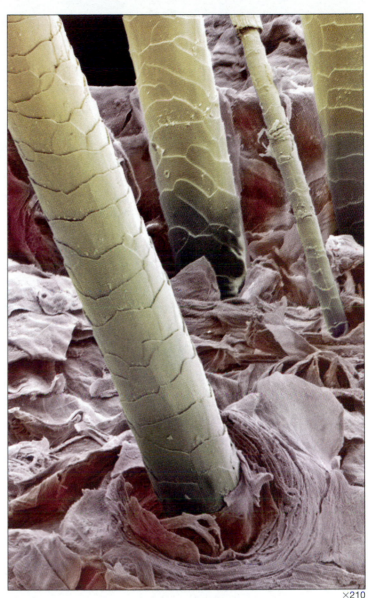

×210

1-6 **Scanning Electron Micrograph** ◾ The SEM produces three-dimensional images and can make even the most ordinary specimens spectacular. Shown are human hairs emerging from the "smooth" skin. Like the TEM, SEM images are black and white, but this one has been colorized to make it look pretty. (×210)

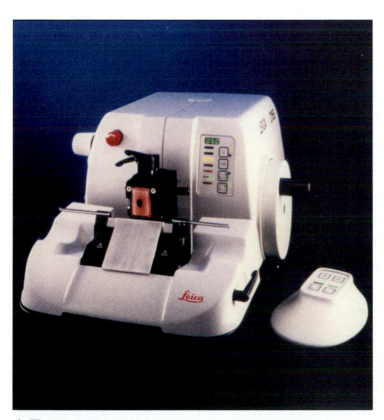

1-7 **Microtome** ◾ A microtome is used to make thin sections of specimens to be mounted on a microscope slide. (Photograph courtesy of Leica Microsystems Inc.)

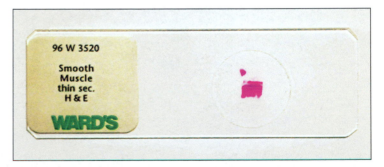

96 W 3520

Smooth
Muscle
thin sec.
H & E

WARD'S

1-8 **Microscope Slide Label** ◾ The label of this slide tells you that it has a thin section of smooth muscle stained with H&E. What it doesn't tell you is that the specimen is actually of the small intestine, so there are various epithelia, connective tissues, and other structures in addition to the advertised smooth muscle layers.

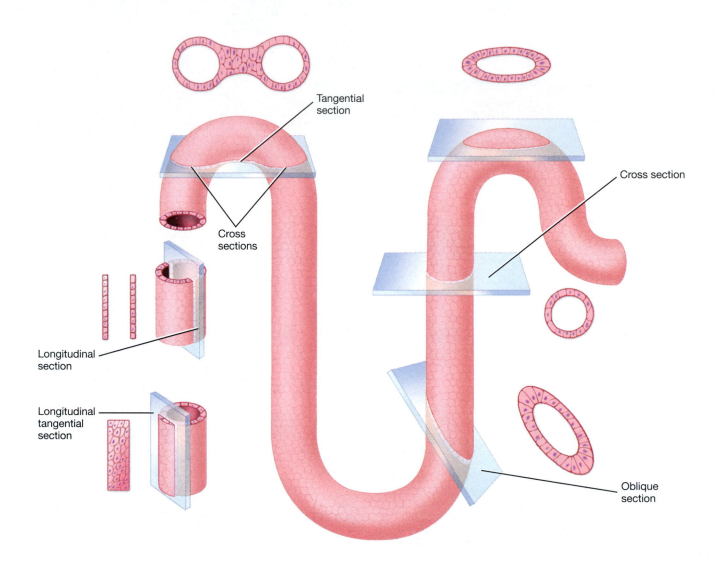

Tangential section

Cross sections

Cross section

Longitudinal section

Longitudinal tangential section

Oblique section

1-9 **Sections of a Tube** ■ Study this diagram to gain an understanding of how the cut sections relate to the three-dimensional whole. This is one of the toughest skills to learn as a histologist. Check the label of a microscope slide before you examine it. Usually it will tell you how the specimen was sectioned (or if not sectioned, how it was prepared).

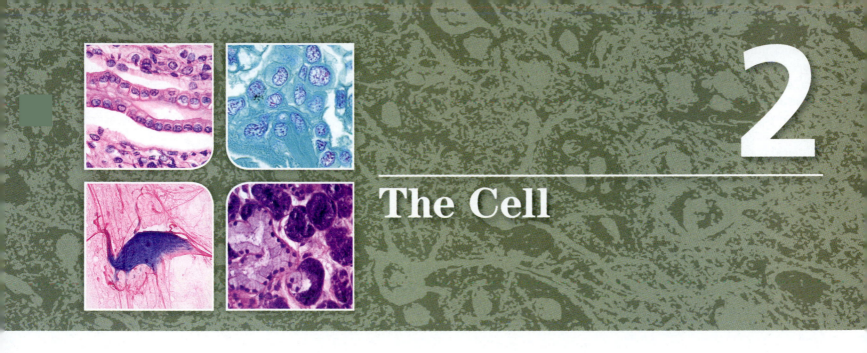

The Cell

2

Tissues are made of cells, so it is appropriate to study cell structure and ultrastructure before embarking on a study of the tissues that comprise organs.

Cells were first discovered and studied using the light microscope. For centuries, our understanding of cell structure was based on the view provided by the light microscope. However, due to the physical limitations posed by using light to create the specimen's image, a point was reached where cell biologists had basically "seen it all." Figure 2-1 illustrates two light micrographs of cells stained with different dyes. Notice that the cells appear to be little more than granular cytoplasm surrounded by a membrane with a nucleus inside.

With the development of the electron microscope in the middle 20th century, and its ability to produce much higher magnification with greater resolution, cells could be visualized with a new degree of clarity. Structural detail (cell ultrastructure) that was inaccessible before was now revealed and opened the door to further study of cell structure and function. An artist's rendition of a generalized animal cell based on electron microscopy is shown in Figure 2-2.

Although the electron microscope is used for most research applications, it is still the light microscope that is employed in introductory histology courses and routine examination of tissues in clinical settings. In this chapter, we briefly review cell ultrastructure as understood from electron micrographs, but the main emphasis is on what can be seen with the light microscope. For complete structural and functional details, the reader is referred to a standard reference text on general biology, histology, or cytology.

Plasma (Cell, Cytoplasmic) Membrane

Although a line in the region of the **plasma membrane** is often visible with the light microscope (Figure 2-3), it wasn't until the electron microscope was used that membranes could be visualized in detail. The electron microscope also revealed the presence of numerous membrane-bound organelles in the cytoplasm (see below).

Membranes are a double layer of phospholipids oriented with their hydrophobic fatty acid tails toward the interior of the membrane and the hydrophilic phosphate heads on each surface (Figure 2-4). Various proteins are embedded in the phospholipid bilayer or are positioned on its surface, depending on their function. Membrane protein functions include catalyzing reactions as enzymes, transporting materials across the membrane as pumps or carriers, acting as receptors of chemical signals, forming transmembrane channels, and transporting electrons during cellular respiration. Other lipids and carbohydrates are also found in or on membranes. Functionally, the cytoplasmic membrane is the primary permeability barrier between the cell's interior and the external environment.

In high-power electron micrographs, membranes appear as two dark lines separated by a lighter band in the center, with a total thickness of approximately 7–10 nm (Figure 2-5). Although membranes throughout the cell have the same appearance, they differ in the particular phospholipids, proteins, and other components, depending on their functions.

Nucleus

The **nucleus** (Figure 2-1) is generally the most prominent cellular structure when viewed with the light microscope. It contains the cell's hereditary material—deoxyribonucleic acid (DNA). Each DNA molecule (of which there are 46–comprising 23 pairs–in a normal human cell) is composed of two long, thin polynucleotides wound in a double helix. Figure 2-6, which was prepared with a stain to show DNA, gives no indication of the polymeric nature of the molecule, but does illustrate that DNA is localized in the nucleus. The genes of DNA contain information for production of cellular structures (and as a result, tissues, organs, and organ systems) as well as the enzymes that catalyze metabolic reactions.

In a dividing cell, each DNA molecule (and its associated proteins) is tightly coiled and becomes visible as a **chromosome** (Figures 2-7 and 2-8). Chromosomes are extremely compact and efficient forms in which to distribute genetic material to the daughter cells produced by division (see the section on mitosis at the end of this chapter).

In a nondividing cell, the DNA is in a dispersed form called **chromatin**. Chromatin granules are often visible in light micrographs of the nucleus, especially at the periphery (Figure 2-9). In many preparations, it is possible to differentiate between denser **heterochromatin** and less dense **euchromatin** (Figure 2-10). The former is inactive, whereas the latter is actively being transcribed into ribonucleic acid (RNA). In females, one entire X chromosome is inactive and is sometimes visible in light micrographs as a "drumstick" at the periphery of the nucleus of certain white blood cells (Figure 2-11).

Also often visible in the nucleus are the **nucleolus** and **nucleoplasm** (Figure 2-12). The nucleolus appears as a dark region and is involved in rRNA synthesis. The nucleoplasm comprises the remaining contents of the nucleus.

Surrounding the nucleus is the **nuclear envelope**, often visible as a line in light micrographs (Figure 2-12), but shown to be a double layer of membrane in electron micrographs (Figure 2-13). The outer nuclear membrane is continuous with the rough endoplasmic reticulum. Regions in the nuclear envelope, called **nuclear pores**, are formed where the two membranes of the envelope join. Simple diffusion and ATP-dependent transport mechanisms move materials between the nuclear and cytoplasmic compartments of the cell through the pores.

A last word about nuclei: Most cells you will examine have a single nucleus. But some cells may have two, many, or even none when mature. Remember that structure is related to function!

Cytoskeleton: Thin Filaments, Intermediate Filaments, and Microtubules

The **cytoskeleton** is composed of protein filaments that are responsible for movement and maintaining cell shape. It is difficult to view them in routine preparations with the light microscope, but filaments can be demonstrated in cells where they are particularly abundant (Figure 2-14).

Thin filaments (microfilaments) are composed of the protein actin and are found in many cell types. Actin filaments, along with the thicker myosin filaments, are present in muscle cells, where they form the contractile apparatus.

Although the individual filaments are not visible in light micrographs, their highly organized arrangement is reflected in the banding pattern seen in skeletal muscle cells (Figures 2-15, 7-1, and 7-4) and cardiac muscle cells (Figure 7-14). Actin filaments are also involved in pinching the cytoplasm into two parts during cell division.

Electron micrographs show **microtubules** to be hollow protein cylinders. They form the interior of structures such as cilia and flagella (see page 11), comprise the **centrioles** of the **centrosome** (Figure 2-16), and are involved in movement of chromosomes during mitosis as the **spindle apparatus** (Figure 2-17).

Intermediate filaments are involved in maintaining cell shape and are intermediate in size between thin filaments and microtubules. In association with actin filaments and other proteins, intermediate filaments form the terminal web in the cytoplasm near the surface of epithelial cells. The cytoskeleton visible in the neuron shown in Figure 2-14 is made up primarily of intermediate filaments (neurofilaments).

Ribosomes

Ribosomes are small, electron-dense structures composed of four different types of ribosomal RNA (rRNA) and multiple proteins. In eukaryotes, the ribosome is made up of a large subunit and a small subunit, distinguishable by their sedimentation coefficients (60S and 40S, respectively). Some ribosomes are attached to endoplasmic reticulum (Figure 2-18), whereas others are free in the cytoplasm (Figure 2-19). The former produce secreted proteins, whereas the latter are involved in synthesis of proteins for cytoplasmic use. Ribosomes are not visible individually with the light microscope, but because of their RNA composition, they are basophilic. Many protein-secreting cells have a dark purple or blue cytoplasm because of the abundance of ribosomes (Figure 2-20).

Endoplasmic Reticulum

The cytoplasm of eukaryotic cells is traversed by a network of membranous tubules called **endoplasmic reticulum**. **Smooth endoplasmic reticulum (SER)** appears to be involved in steroid, cholesterol, and triglyceride synthesis. In some cells its functions are more specialized. For example, in muscle cells it stores calcium ions, and in liver cells it is involved in detoxification of chemicals. The membranes of **rough endoplasmic reticulum (RER)** have ribosomes (Figure 2-18) involved in synthesis of proteins for secretion. RER is also involved in producing membranes and their specific proteins for other organelles within the cell. The endoplasmic reticulum is continuous with the outer nuclear membrane. The dark-staining regions in the micrographs in Figure 2-20 actually show the regions of RER.

Golgi Apparatus

The **Golgi apparatus** (Figure 2-21) is made up of a stack of curved, membranous sacs, called **cisternae,** and associated vesicles. The Golgi apparatus is involved in carbohydrate synthesis and modifying, sorting, and packaging proteins. It is visible with an appropriate stain or occasionally as a pale-staining region adjacent to the nucleus in the cytoplasm of some cells (Figure 2-22).

Mitochondria

Mitochondria (Figure 2-23) are double-membrane organelles that are the primary site of ATP production in the cell. The space surrounded by the inner membrane is the **mitochondrial matrix** and possesses the enzymes of the Krebs cycle as well as some DNA, thought to be a remnant of their Bacterial ancestry. Embedded in the inner membrane are the components of the mitochondrial electron transport system. Mitochondria are barely visible with the light microscope and appropriate stain.

Surface Modifications: Cilia, Flagella, Microvilli, and Stereocilia

Cilia and **flagella** are easily viewed with the light microscope (Figures 2-25 and 2-26). Both are long, thin, cellular projections involved in motility by producing sweeping motions. Typically, cilia are more numerous and shorter than flagella (which are found singly in humans). When first viewed with the electron microscope, it became apparent that both have the same basic construction. Both are surrounded by cell membrane and contain nine pairs of microtubules (doublets) around two single microtubules (singlets) (Figures 2-24 and 2-27). This 9+2 arrangement of microtubules constitutes the **axoneme.** At the base of each flagellum and cilium is a **basal body** composed of nine microtubule triplets with no central microtubules (identical to centrioles) into which the axoneme inserts.

Microvilli (Figures 2-24, 2-27a, and 2-28) are tiny projections that increase the surface area of cells and are especially abundant in those involved in absorption. Although not individually visible with the light microscope, they do appear as a **striated border** on cells of the small intestine and colon, and as a **brush border** on kidney tubules (Figure 2-29). Actin filaments inside each microvillus are joined by proteins to form a bundle, which is anchored to the terminal web by the actin (Figure 2-30).

Stereocilia are long microvilli found on cells lining the epididymis (Figure 2-31) and on the hair cells of the inner ear, where they are involved in producing a signal in response to sound waves.

Cellular Junctions (Junctional Complexes)

Light micrographs of intestinal epithelium provided the first evidence that certain adjacent cells are connected by specialized attachments. These were named **terminal bars** (Figure 2-32). The electron microscope has since revealed a number of structurally different types of attachments found not only in epithelium but also in cardiac and smooth muscle. These include the following:

- **occluding (tight) junctions** that bind adjacent epithelial cells tightly and seal the intercellular space. These are also known as **zonulae occludentes** (singular: **zonula occludens**).

- **adhering (anchoring) junctions,** of which there are two main types: **zonulae adherentes** (singular: **zonula adherens**), which are continuous rings of attachment to intracellular actin filaments; and **desmosomes,** also known as **maculae adherentes** (singular: **macula adherens**), which are spot attachments to intracellular intermediate filaments and hold the cells tightly together. Other adhering junctions anchor cells to underlying connective tissues.

- **communicating (gap) junctions** are found between cells whose activities must be highly coordinated. They are made up of tiny pores through which adjacent cells can transfer materials or electrical signals.

In epithelia, zonulae occludentes, zonulae adherentes, and maculae adherentes (desmosomes) collectively form **junctional complexes. Intercalated disks** (Figure 2-33) of cardiac muscle have been shown to be made up of highly interdigitated cell membranes and junctions resembling zonulae adherentes, desmosomes, and gap junctions.

Cellular Inclusions

Some cells are specialized to store carbon and energy as either lipid or glycogen. These materials can be demonstrated with special stains. Figure 2-12a shows testicular interstitial cells containing lipid droplets, and Figure 2-34 shows liver cells storing lipid and glycogen.

The Cell Cycle and Mitosis

The **cell cycle** marks the events of a cell between the time that it comes into existence until it divides into two new cells. These events are divided into two major parts: **interphase** and **mitosis/cytokinesis.** Interphase (Figure 2-35a) comprises the majority of the cell cycle and is recognized histologically by a typically appearing nucleus. Many activities occur throughout interphase, but certain events allow its subdivision into three stages: G_1 (**first gap) phase, S phase,** and G_2 (**second gap) phase.** During G_1, the cell grows and begins synthesizing macromolecules necessary for DNA replication, the hallmark event of the S phase. The G_2 phase is devoted to synthesis of materials necessary for division.

Mitosis is the part of the cell cycle during which replicated nuclear material is distributed to opposite ends of the cell prior to division of the cytoplasm, **cytokinesis**. In this way, the two daughter cells receive complete and identical amounts of nuclear DNA. The five stages of animal cell mitosis and cytokinesis are described below.

- The first is **prophase** (Figures 2-35a and 2-35b), in which the chromatin condenses into visible chromosomes, nucleoli disappear, and the spindle apparatus (made of microtubules) begins to form. At this point, the chromosomes each possess two **sister chromatids** attached at a **centromere**.

- During **prometaphase** (Figure 2-35c), the nuclear envelope disintegrates and the spindle fibers attach to a specialized region within each chromatid's centromere called the **kinetochore**.

- During **metaphase** (Figure 2-35d), the chromosomes are positioned at the cell's equator to form the **metaphase plate**.

- In **anaphase** (Figures 2-35e and 2-35f), centromeres split and sister chromatids are moved to opposite poles of the cell.

- Mitosis ends with **telophase** (Figures 2-35g and 2-35h), in which the events of prophase are undone: chromosomes disperse as chromatin, the nucleoli reappear, the spindle apparatus disintegrates, and the nuclear envelope reforms.

During late anaphase and telophase, cytokinesis begins with the formation of a **cleavage furrow** (Figures 2-35g and 2-35h). The cleavage furrow eventually pinches the cytoplasm into two separate compartments—the daughter cells—and the division is complete.

The specimens used to illustrate the stages of the cell cycle in Figures 2-35a through 2-35j were prepared exclusively for that purpose, but mitotically dividing cells may be observed in various tissues (Figure 2-36). However, the cell cycle is not uniform for all body cells. Some cells, such as those comprising the skin's surface and lining the intestine, continually divide, entering G_1 of interphase immediately following completion of mitosis/cytokinesis. Others, such as liver cells, enter a G_0 **phase** and divide only when disease or damage make it necessary. **Terminally differentiated cells**, such as neurons, have become so specialized that they have lost their ability to divide.

Some cells in mitotically active tissue might not present chromosome arrangements that fit the defined categories. In some instances it may be difficult to differentiate between late anaphase and early telophase, for example. This is to be expected, because mitosis is a continuous process and we see the cells stopped in the middle of their activity. Further, the orientation of the division plane may complicate interpretation. Figure 2-35h shows a cell whose division plane is parallel with the page, so we are observing it from one end, not above. This makes placing it in a particular stage very difficult.

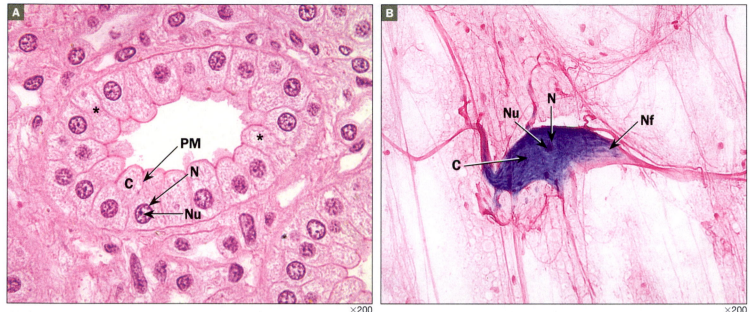

×200   ×200

2-1 **Cells as Viewed with the Light Microscope** ■ (**A**) Prominent purplish nuclei (N) and pinkish granular cytoplasm (C) characterize specimens stained with H&E. Darker purple nucleoli (Nu) are visible inside the nuclei, as are plasma membranes (PM) surrounding the cells. Realize that the single line of "membrane" is actually both membranes of adjacent cells. Notice the cells that apparently lack a nucleus (*). Their nuclei were not in the plane of the section, so they appear to be absent, a not uncommon occurrence when observing sectioned specimens. Compounding this is the fact that it was embedded in plastic, which allowed it to be sectioned to a thickness of approximately 2 μm—about one-fourth that of standard preparations. The trade-off is that the section's thinness produces the relative sharpness of its features. (**B**) The stain used in a preparation matters. This motor neuron from a spinal cord smear was stained with methylene blue and phloxine (pink). Notice that the nucleus (N) is not the most prominent feature of the cell, but rather is lightly stained with a darker nucleolus (Nu) within. Dark blue neurofilaments (Nf) are visible in the cytoplasm (C). Lastly, although the edges of this cell are obvious, there is no visible evidence of a membrane. (×200)

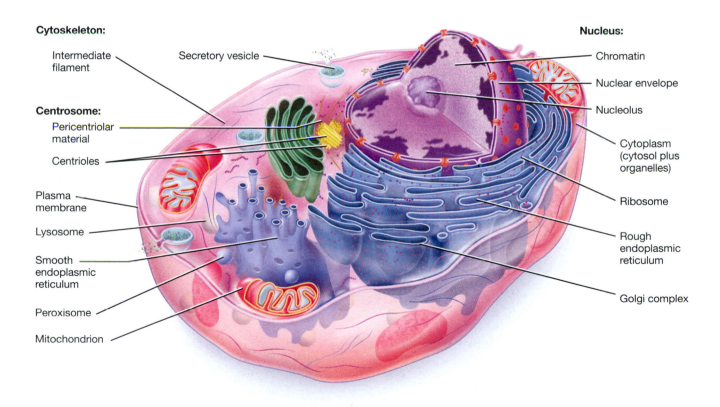

2-2 **An Artist's Rendering of Animal Cell Ultrastructure** ■ This illustrates the general features found in animal cells. Please see the text for brief explanations of their functions. (Specialized surface features are shown in Figure 2-24.)

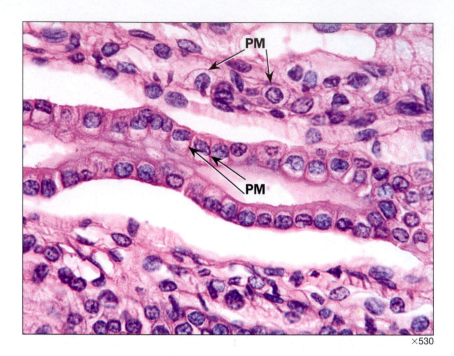

×530

2-3 **Plasma Membranes as Seen with the Light Microscope** ◾ Membranes (PM) are pretty obvious between the cells of the tubule running across the field, but they are less distinct on many of the other cells in the field. Remember that each line represents the membranes of adjacent cells. (×530)

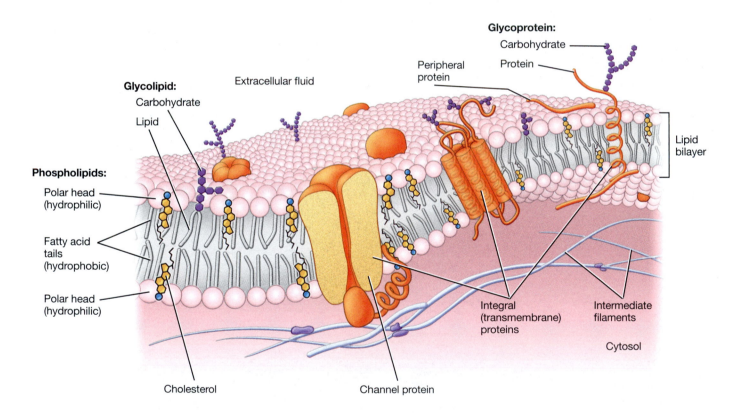

2-4 **An Artist's Rendering of a Typical Membrane** ◾ Membranes are composed of a phospholipid bilayer associated with various proteins and carbohydrates. The specific molecules and their locations are related to the membrane's function. Notice the orientation of the phospholipids, with their hydrophilic heads on each surface and their hydrophobic tails projecting to the membrane's interior.

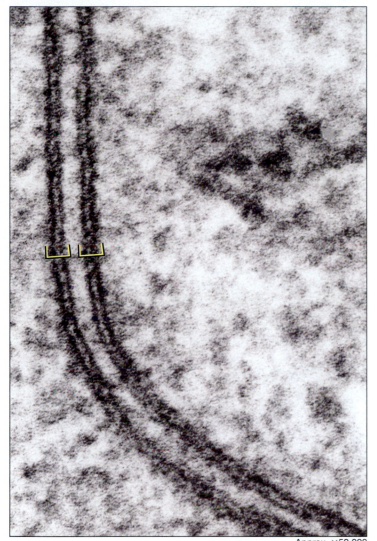

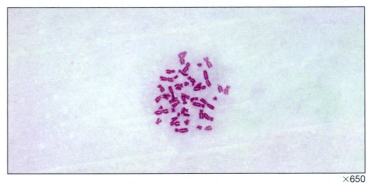

×650

2-7 **Chromosome Spread** ◼ Chromosomes are compact structures that are an efficient way of distributing the long DNA molecules to the two daughter cells during division. They are not visible during most of the cell cycle. These chromosomes are from a male cell grown in tissue culture. (×650)

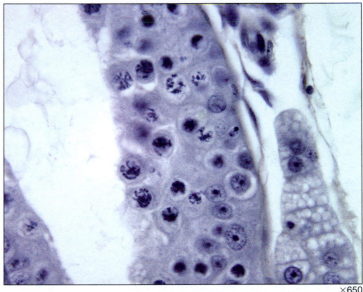

×650

2-8 **Chromosomes** ◼ Chromosomes are visible in tissues where the cells are actively dividing, as in these cells from the testis. (×650)

Approx. ×50,000

2-5 **Membrane Structure as Seen with the TEM** ◼ Each membrane (brackets) of these adjacent cells is approximately 8 nm thick. Note the "dark-light-dark" appearance of each and the comparatively large inter-cellular region between them. (Approx. ×50,000)

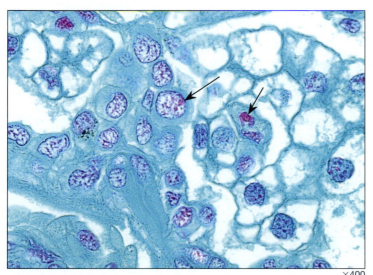

×400

2-6 **DNA Stain** ◼ DNA (arrows) appears reddish when treated with a Feulgen stain. Notice that the DNA is found in the nuclei. (×400)

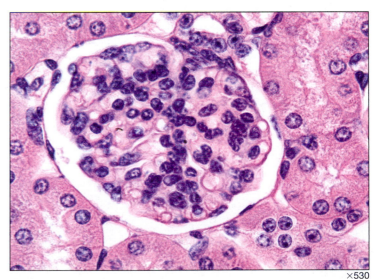

×530

2-9 **Chromatin Granules** ◼ Dense regions of chromatin in the nucleus are often visible in light micrographs and may be useful in cell identification. (×530)

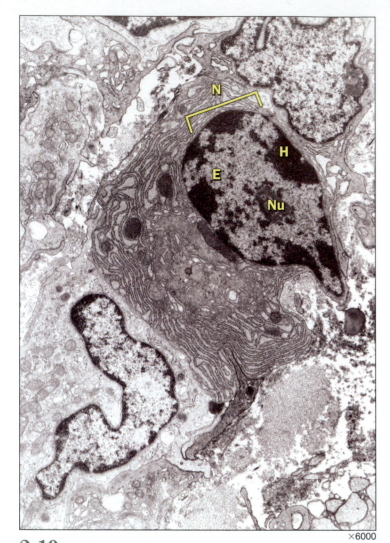

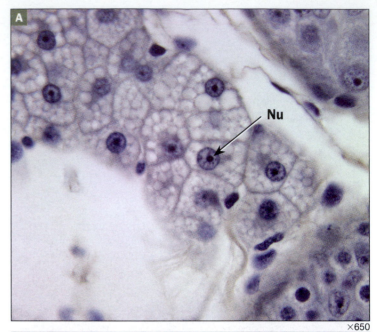

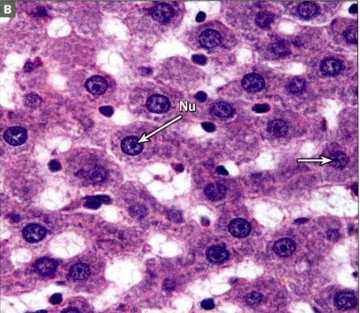

2-10 **Euchromatin and Heterochromatin** ◼ In this transmission electron micrograph, dense regions of inactive chromatin, called heterochromatin (H), are visible at the periphery of the nucleus (N). DNA that is being transcribed forms the lighter euchromatin (E). The medium gray region near the center is the nucleolus (Nu). Notice the irregularly shaped nucleus of the cell in the lower left. Not all nuclei are spherical! Also notice the different amounts of heterochromatin and euchromatin of the two cells. (×6000) (Courtesy of UCSD Medical Center)

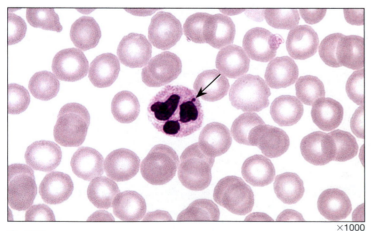

2-11 **A "Drumstick"** ◼ The inactive X chromosome in females is often visible as an appendage (arrow) of the nucleus in white blood cells called neutrophils. (×1000)

2-12 **Nucleolus and Nucleoplasm** ◼ The nucleolus (Nu) is a prominent dark region in light micrographs of the nucleus. It should not be confused with chromatin granules, which are usually toward the periphery. Nucleoli are the sites of rRNA synthesis and ribosome assembly. The nucleoplasm is the lighter, background material in the nucleus. The nuclear envelope is also visible as a dark line on the outside of the nucleus. **(A)** In addition to prominent nucleoli, these testicular interstitial cells display abundant lipid droplets characteristic of steroid-secreting cells. (×650) **(B)** Notice that some of these liver cells have more than one nucleolus (arrow). (×780)

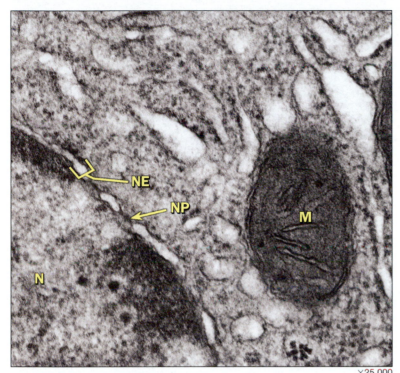

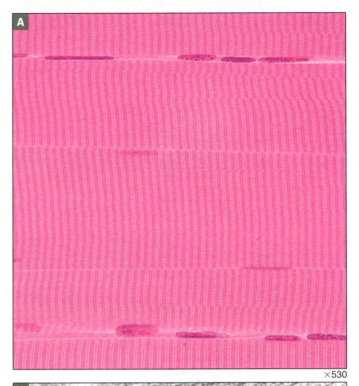

2-13 **Nuclear Envelope and Pores** ◾ In this transmission electron micrograph, the nucleus (N) is in the lower left (notice the euchromatin and heterochromatin) and the cytoplasm fills the remainder of the field. The double membrane of the nuclear envelope (NE) largely separates the two compartments, but nuclear pores (NP) allow movement of materials between them (ribosomes and mRNA out and nucleotides and hormones in, for examples). The outer membrane of the nuclear envelope is continuous with endoplasmic reticulum (ER), though no continuities are seen in this section. Several mitochondria (M) are also visible. (×25,000)

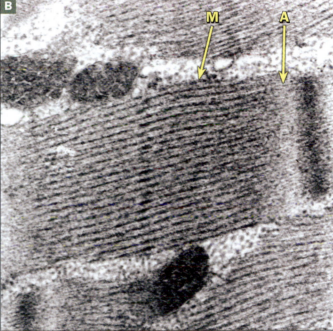

2-15 **Skeletal Muscle** ◾ (A) The banding seen in these skeletal muscle cells is due to the highly organized arrangement of the protein filaments actin and myosin. (×530) (B) This TEM of skeletal muscle shows the thick myosin (M) and thin actin (A) filaments that form the bulk of the muscle fiber's contractile apparatus. (×40,000) (Courtesy of UCSD Medical Center)

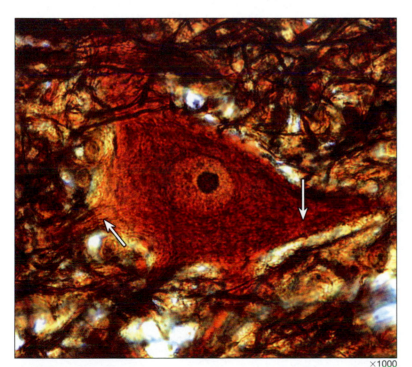

2-14 **Neurofilaments** ◾ The cytoskeleton is composed of many different kinds of protein filaments. The thin, brown lines (arrows) in the cytoplasm of this neuron are filaments. (×1000)

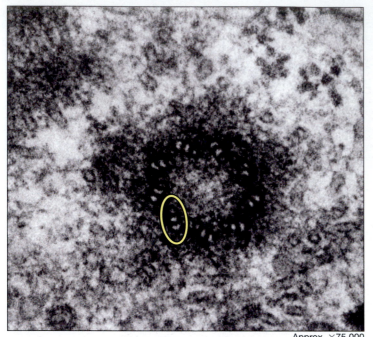

2-16 **Centrioles and the Centrosome** ◼ Centrioles are paired, cylindrical structures composed of nine triplets of microtubules. (One triplet is circled.) The centrioles are oriented at 90° to one another and together form the centrosome. In this specimen, the centriole in the upper left was sectioned longitudinally and the other was cut in cross section. (Approx. ×75,000)

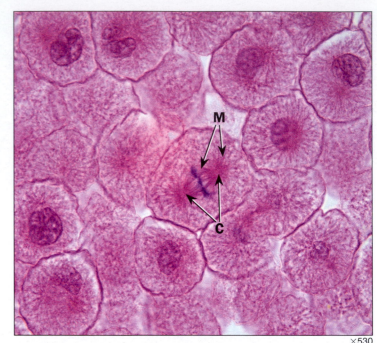

Approx. ×75,000

2-17 **Microtubules of the Spindle Apparatus** ◼ Microtubules (M) are barely visible with the light microscope. Here they are shown forming the spindle apparatus of mitosis. The spindle fibers radiate outward from the centrosome (C) regions, which are located at the apices of the spindle apparatus. (×530)

×530

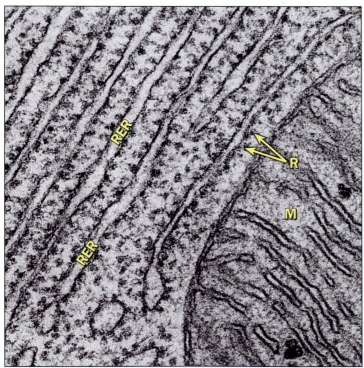

Approx. ×40,000

2-18 **TEM of Ribosomes on Rough Endoplasmic Reticulum** ◼ Ribosomes (R) are small, electron-dense particles that are the site of protein synthesis. Ribosomes responsible for producing proteins for secretion are bound to the endoplasmic reticulum to form rough endoplasmic reticulum (RER). Notice that the ribosomes are located on the same (cytoplasmic) side of the ER membrane. The proteins they transcribe pass into the ER lumen (cistern) for export. Also notice the large mitochondrion (M) in the field. (Approx. ×40,000)

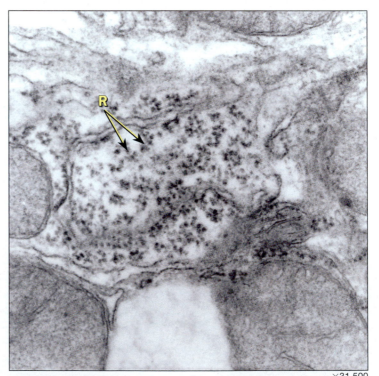

×31,500

2-19 **TEM of Free Ribosomes** ◼ These free ribosomes (R) are not bound to membrane and produce proteins for internal use. When found in chains, they are referred to as polyribosomes. (×31,500) (Courtesy of UCSD Medical Center)

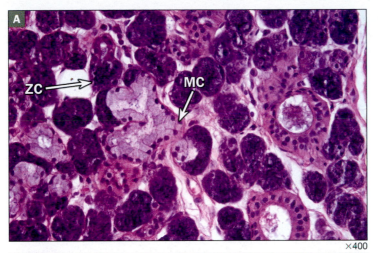

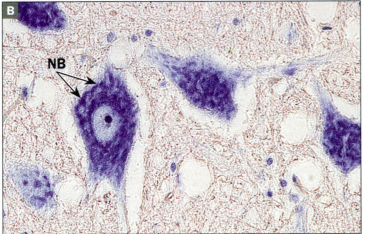

2-20 **RER Affects the Appearance of the Cytoplasm** 🔲 The light microscope cannot resolve the detail of RER. However, if it is abundant the cytoplasm appears granular and dark staining. (**A**) Zymogenic cells (ZC), such as these from a salivary gland, produce proteins (enzymes) for secretion. Contrast these with the pale-staining, mucus-secreting cells (MC) visible in the field. Although mucus contains glycoproteins, the RER is not as prominent in light micrographs of these cells. (**B**) Regions of RER in neurons appear as Nissl bodies (NB) with the light microscope. (Both ×400)

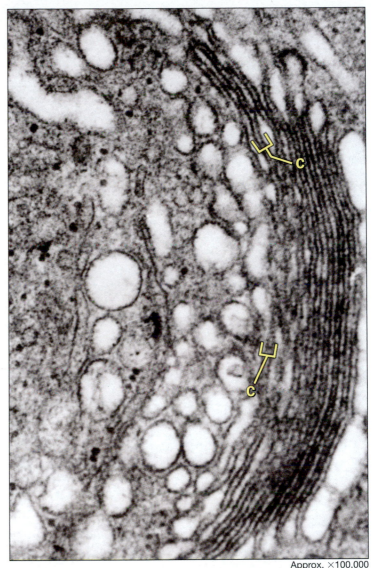

Approx. ×100,000

2-21 **Golgi Apparatus as Viewed with the TEM** 🔲 This organelle is formed by nesting membranous sacs called cisternae (C) and is responsible for processing and packaging materials for secretion. (Approx. ×100,000)

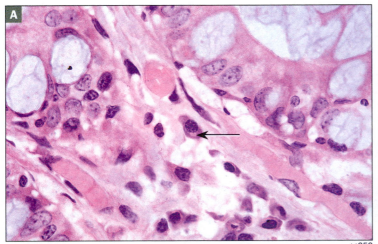

×650

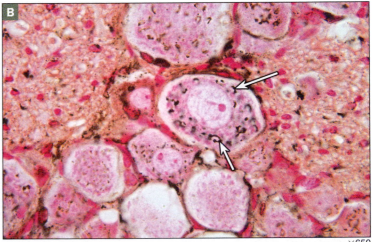

×650

2-22 **Golgi Apparatus as Viewed with the Light Microscope** 🔲 (**A**) The location of the Golgi apparatus is occasionally visible as a light-staining region near the nucleus of some cells. The cell indicated is an antibody-secreting plasma cell. (**B**) This specimen has been prepared using the Da Fano silver method, which darkens the Golgi bodies (arrows). (Both ×650)

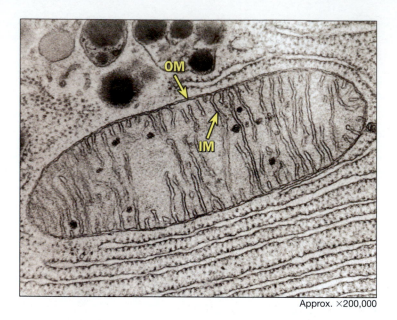

Approx. ×200,000

2-23 **Mitochondria** ■ Mitochondria are the organelles that house the enzymes and electron transport chain of aerobic respiration. The inner and outer membranes (IM and OM, respectively) are clearly visible in this TEM. (Approx. ×200,000)

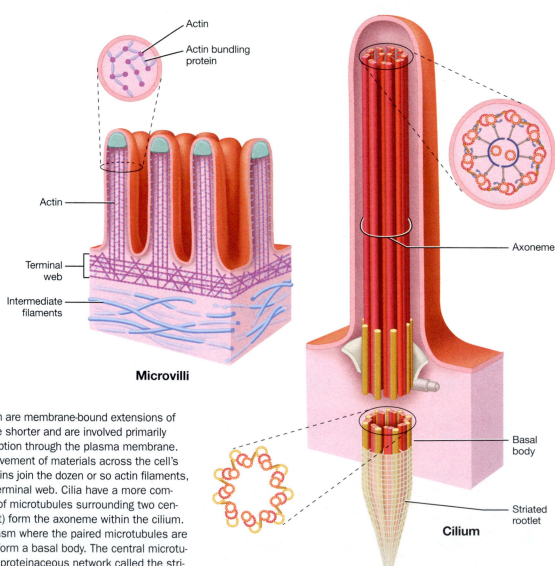

Actin

Actin bundling protein

Actin

Terminal web

Intermediate filaments

Microvilli

Axoneme

Basal body

Striated rootlet

Cilium

2-24 **Microvilli and Cilia** ■ Both are membrane-bound extensions of the cytoplasm, but microvilli tend to be shorter and are involved primarily with increasing surface area for absorption through the plasma membrane. Cilia are longer and are involved in movement of materials across the cell's surface. Internally, actin bundling proteins join the dozen or so actin filaments, which in turn bind the bundle to the terminal web. Cilia have a more complex internal organization. Nine pairs of microtubules surrounding two central microtubules (a 9+2 arrangement) form the axoneme within the cilium. The axoneme extends into the cytoplasm where the paired microtubules are each joined by a third microtubule to form a basal body. The central microtubules are absent in the basal body. A proteinaceous network called the striated rootlet anchors the basal body to the cytoplasm. Sliding of one microtubule in each pair across its partner provides the mechanism of ciliary movement. Cilia and flagella have the same internal structure, but cilia are more numerous and shorter than flagella.

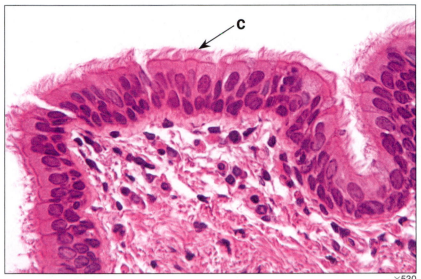

×530

2-25 **Cilia** ■ Cilia (C) are thin, motile projections responsible for moving materials across the cell's surface. They are more numerous and shorter than flagella (compare to Figure 2-26). These cilia are from the respiratory tract, where they sweep inhaled materials away from the lungs. Notice in this micrograph how the cilia resemble bent teeth on a comb. Do not confuse cilia with a brush border of microvilli (Figure 2-29). Cilia are longer than microvilli and can frequently be seen as individual hairs with the light microscope, which is not often the case with microvilli. (×530)

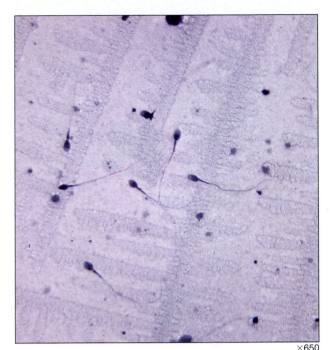

×650

2-26 **Flagella** ■ Sperm are the only human cells that have flagella. The tails of these sperm cells are the flagella. (×650)

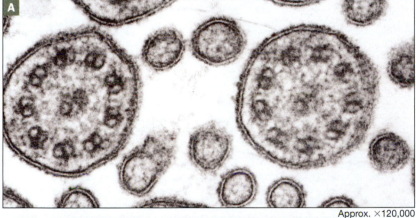

Approx. ×120,000

A

B

BB

×30,000

2-27 **TEMs of Cilia** ■ (A) The 9+2 microtubular arrangement is apparent in this TEM of cilia in cross section. Flagella have exactly the same arrangement. The smaller circular objects between the cilia are microvilli, which lack microtubules (see Figure 2-28). (Approx. 120,000) (B) The microtubules are visible in this longitudinal section of cilia, but their 9+2 arrangement is not. Located in the cytoplasm at the base of each cilium is a basal body (BB), which has the same construction as centrioles. (×30,000)

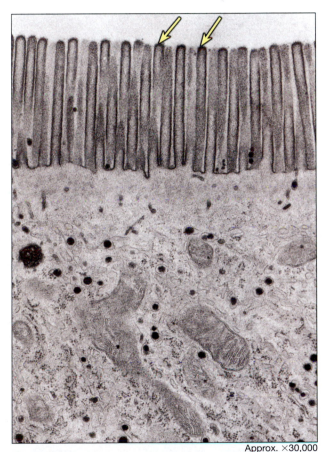

Approx. ×30,000

2-28 **Microvilli** ■ Microvilli (arrows) are folds of the surface membrane that increase surface area for absorption. Microvilli are shorter, narrower, and lack the microtubules of cilia. (Approx. ×30,000)

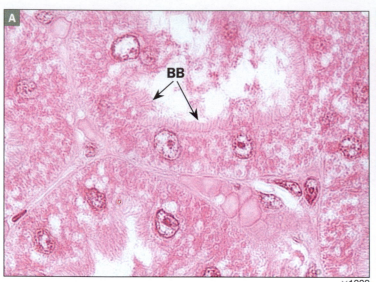

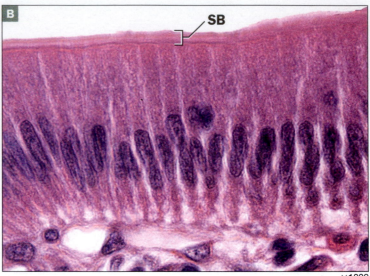

2-29 **Microvilli Viewed with the Light Microscope** ▣ **(A)** Microvilli are typically not individually visible with the light microscope, but in this thin section of the kidney they are barely discernible (arrows). More typically, they are seen as "fuzz" on the cell's surface and are called a brush border (BB). **(B)** These microvilli of the small intestine are not individually visible (even in this thin section), and form a striated border (SB). (Both ×1000)

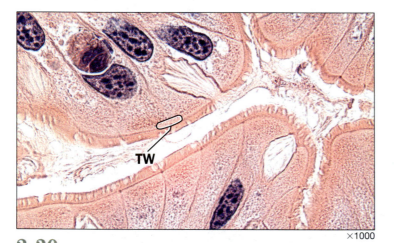

2-30 **Terminal Web as Seen with the Light Microscope** ▣ Although the individual actin, myosin, and other protein filaments of the terminal web (TW) are not visible, their presence is sometimes detectable by the cytoplasm staining more lightly just below the microvilli (circled region). The terminal web filaments can contract, thus pinching the cell's apex and spreading the microvilli. This increases the space between them and allows more fluid to contact their surface and improve efficiency of absorption. (×1000)

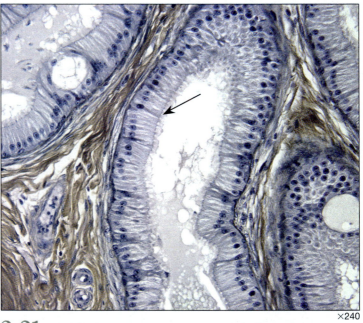

2-31 **Stereocilia** ▣ The misnamed stereocilia are actually long microvilli. These are from the epididymis. (×240)

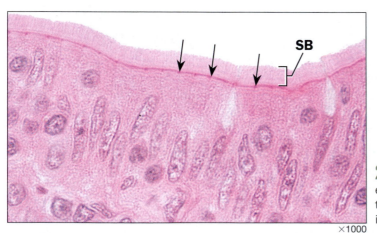

2-32 **Terminal Bars** ▣ The junctions between adjacent intestinal epithelial cells are sometimes seen as terminal bars (arrows). Use of the electron microscope has uncovered several different types of intercellular junctions. Also note the striated border (SB). (×1000)

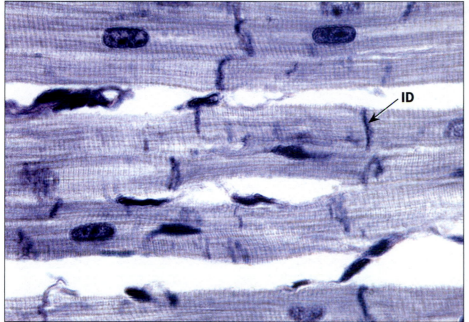

2-33 Intercalated Disks ▪ The junctions between adjacent cardiac muscle cells are complex and include highly interdigitated cell surfaces joined by several types of intercellular attachments. In the light microscope, these appear as the intercalated disks (ID). Do not confuse intercalated disks with the fainter striated pattern produced by the organized arrangement of actin and myosin filaments. (×1000)

×1000

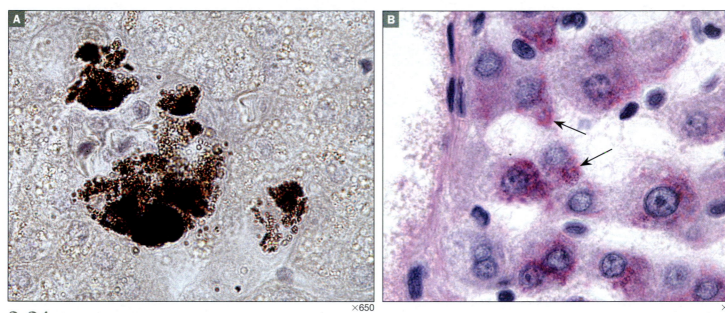

×650   ×1000

2-34 Cellular Inclusions ▪ Some storage products, such as glycogen and lipid, appear in the cytoplasm of cells. (**A**) This liver specimen has been stained for lipids with osmium tetroxide, which makes them appear brownish. (×650) (**B**) PAS positive glycogen in this liver specimen appears reddish (arrows). (×1000)

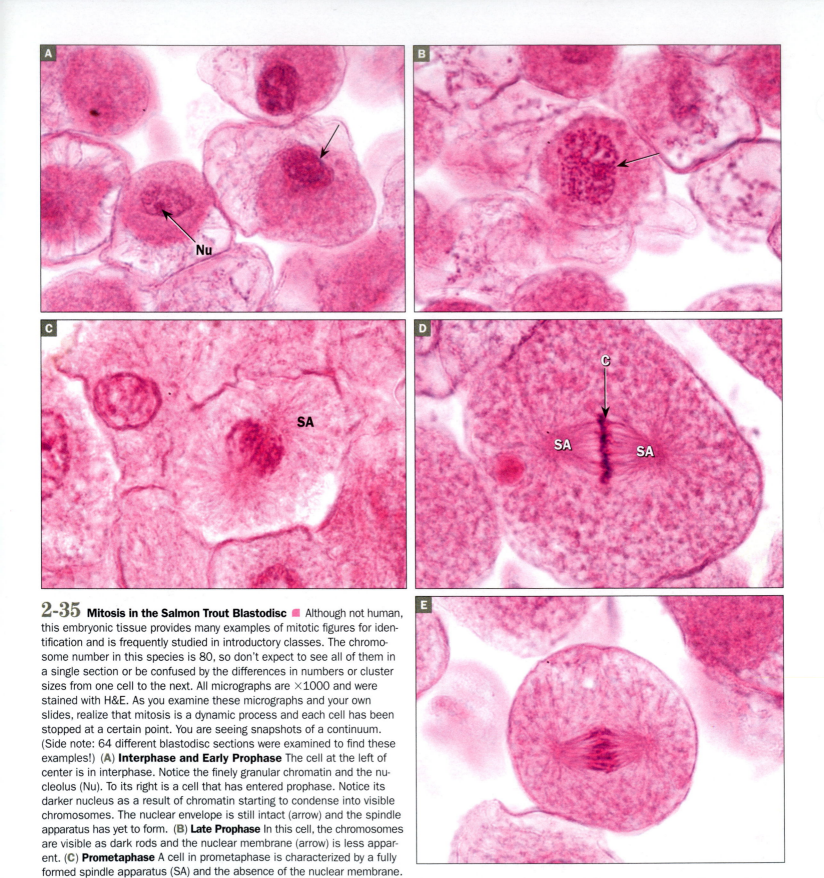

2-35 **Mitosis in the Salmon Trout Blastodisc** ◼ Although not human, this embryonic tissue provides many examples of mitotic figures for identification and is frequently studied in introductory classes. The chromosome number in this species is 80, so don't expect to see all of them in a single section or be confused by the differences in numbers or cluster sizes from one cell to the next. All micrographs are ×1000 and were stained with H&E. As you examine these micrographs and your own slides, realize that mitosis is a dynamic process and each cell has been stopped at a certain point. You are seeing snapshots of a continuum. (Side note: 64 different blastodisc sections were examined to find these examples!) (**A**) **Interphase and Early Prophase** The cell at the left of center is in interphase. Notice the finely granular chromatin and the nucleolus (Nu). To its right is a cell that has entered prophase. Notice its darker nucleus as a result of chromatin starting to condense into visible chromosomes. The nuclear envelope is still intact (arrow) and the spindle apparatus has yet to form. (**B**) **Late Prophase** In this cell, the chromosomes are visible as dark rods and the nuclear membrane (arrow) is less apparent. (**C**) **Prometaphase** A cell in prometaphase is characterized by a fully formed spindle apparatus (SA) and the absence of the nuclear membrane. The chromosomes continue to condense, although it is not apparent when comparing this cell with the cell in (**B**) because they are different cells from different specimens. (**D**) **Metaphase** The spindle fibers have moved the chromosomes (C) to the cell's equator. (**E**) **Early Anaphase** In anaphase each chromosome splits at its centromere with one chromatid (now called a chromosome) going to each pole. *(continues)*

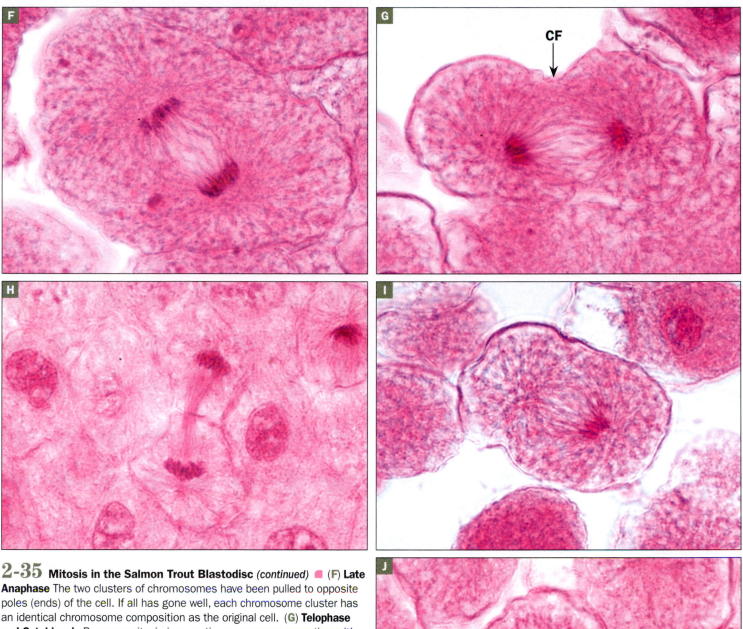

2-35 **Mitosis in the Salmon Trout Blastodisc** *(continued)* ◼ **(F) Late Anaphase** The two clusters of chromosomes have been pulled to opposite poles (ends) of the cell. If all has gone well, each chromosome cluster has an identical chromosome composition as the original cell. **(G) Telophase and Cytokinesis** Because mitosis is a continuous process, sometimes it's not possible to pinpoint exactly where a particular cell was when the slide was made. For example, an argument (though not a particularly fruitful one) could be made that the cell in **(F)** is in early telophase, not late anaphase. However, if you see a cleavage furrow (CF) the cell has more than likely reached telophase. In this cell you can even see that the chromosome clusters have "tightened up," that is, they are not as spread out as in **(F)**, which is another indication of telophase. **(H) Late Telophase** Cytokinesis is complete in these two cells. Notice the remnants of the spindle apparatus. **(I) Mitosis in Oblique Section** The cells of a blastodisc do not divide in a single plane–the developing fish is getting bigger in all dimensions. This means you will see chromosomes in cells from various views. Sometimes only one of the mitotic figures is in the plane of section, as in this specimen. Usually, these can be placed into one of the phases because the two sides are mirror images of one another. This cell is probably in early telophase, based on the fact that the chromosomes on the right seem to be as far as they can go. A hint of the spindle apparatus is visible in the other part of the cell; the plane of section missed the chromosomes. **(J) Mitosis in Polar View** The cell in this micrograph is clearly undergoing mitosis (because chromosomes are visible) and is at least to the point of prometaphase (because the nuclear membrane is gone). At first glance, you might be tempted to classify it as prometaphase (because the nuclear membrane is gone and the chromosomes are not particularly organized). But, notice there is no spindle apparatus (compare to **C**)—and that is a key recognition clue. You are seeing these chromosomes from one end (pole) of the cell–they were either moving toward you or away from you when the slide was made. You are seeing mitosis in polar view and without the spindle apparatus for orientation and perspective; it's not easy to identify the stage. This could be a vertical section through the chromosome cluster at metaphase, anaphase, or telophase.

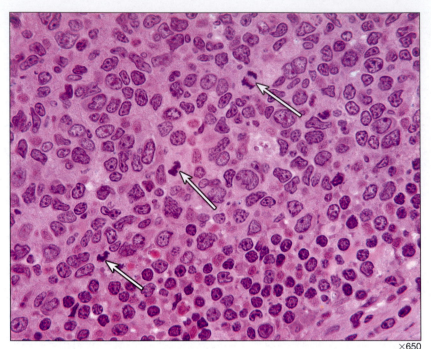

×650

2-36 **Mitosis in Lymphatic Tissue** ■ Careful observers may see mitotic figures in many different tissues. This is a plastic-embedded lymph node specimen. Several cells (indicated by arrows) are undergoing mitosis, but only the topmost is in an identifiable stage (anaphase). Most cells are in interphase, which is not unexpected because interphase is the longest stage of the cell cycle. Notice the chromatin granules and the nucleoli in these nondividing cells. (×650)

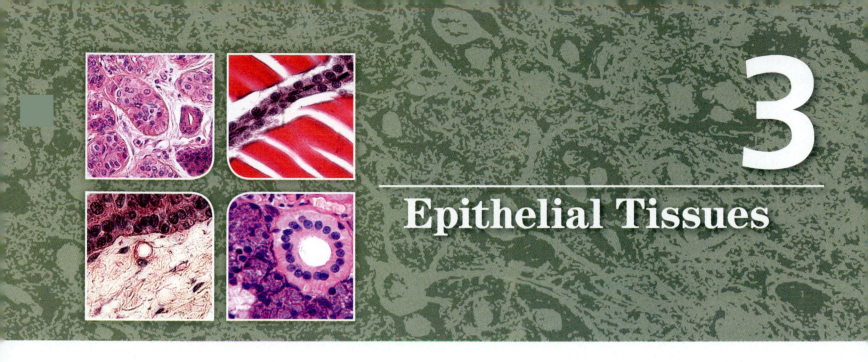

Epithelial Tissues

3

Basic Characteristics of Epithelial Tissues

Epithelial tissues, or **epithelia,** cover most surfaces in the body. By growing downward into deeper tissues, they also form glands. Typically, the cells are joined by junctional complexes (see Chapter 2) into sheets with little intercellular material (Figure 3-1). (For a graphic example, recall the last time you peeled after a sunburn!) Epithelia rest on a **basement membrane** that separates them from the underlying connective tissue (Figure 3-2). Electron micrographs reveal that the basement membrane is composed of a **basal lamina** (derived from the epithelial cells, Figure 3-3) and a **reticular lamina** (produced by fibroblast cells of the connective tissue, though some authors contend that this is an artifact of preparation). Blood vessels do not penetrate the basement membrane, making epithelia **avascular.**

Epithelial Membranes

Because epithelia are avascular, the majority rely on nourishment from capillaries of underlying connective tissues. The connective tissue also carries nerves, lymphatic vessels, and other structures that supply and support the epithelium in various ways. This results in a structural and functional association between an epithelium and its underlying connective tissue: an **epithelial membrane.** Epithelial membranes are of three types. **Mucous membranes** line surfaces open to the external environment and often secrete mucus* (Figure 3-4). Examples are the membranes lining the digestive, respiratory, urinary, and reproductive tracts. The connective tissue in these locations is frequently called **lamina propria.** The pericardial, pleural, and peritoneal cavities (ventral body cavities) are lined by **serous membranes.** These are named **pericardium, pleura,** and **peritoneum,** respectively.

The epithelial component of serous membranes is called **mesothelium. Cutaneous membrane** is the skin.

Functions of Epithelia

The structures of epithelia vary depending on their functions. Some functions of epithelia are:

- Mechanical protection from abrasive forces (e.g., epidermis of the skin).
- Absorption of substances from the **lumen** (inner portion) of a tubular organ (e.g., intestinal epithelium). The luminal surface is usually modified with **microvilli** to increase the surface area and improve efficiency of absorption.
- Secretion of materials (e.g., intestinal epithelium). This epithelium often contains single-celled, mucus-secreting **goblet cells** (see page 29).
- Lubrication of surfaces (e.g., mesothelium of serous membranes).
- Formation of a surface for diffusion (e.g., walls of lung alveoli and capillaries).

Epithelial Terminology

Some important terminology associated with epithelia is illustrated in Figure 3-5. If the cell is actually on the surface (and is not buried in the epithelium) the surface edge of the cell is called the **free, apical,** or **luminal surface.** The sides contacting other epithelial cells are called **lateral surfaces,** and the edge in contact with the basement membrane is called the **basal surface.** If the epithelium consists of more than one layer, the **basal cells** are closest to the basement

---

* "Mucus" is a noun; "mucous" is an adjective.

membrane. References may also be made to the **apical** and **basal poles** of epithelial cells.

Epithelia are named based on two main criteria: the number of cell layers and the shape of the cells at the surface. **Simple epithelia** have a single layer of cells, so all cells contact the basement membrane. **Stratified epithelia** are made of two or more cell layers and only the basal cells contact the basement membrane. **Squamous cells** are flat with flattened nuclei. (Note: The shape of the nucleus is important in identifying an epithelium, because nuclei tend to be the most obvious part of a cell.) **Cuboidal cells** are as tall as they are wide with spherical nuclei positioned in the cell's center. (Realize this is an approximation and doesn't imply geometric precision!) **Columnar cells** are taller than wide and frequently have an elongated, basal nucleus. To completely name an epithelium, both the number of cell layers and the shape of cells at the surface must be included.

Simple Epithelia

Simple squamous epithelium (Figure 3-6) is composed of a single layer of flat cells. It forms the alveoli of the lungs (Figure 3-7a), where it participates in forming the respiratory membrane through which gases diffuse, and glomerular capsules of the kidney where blood filtration occurs (Figure 3-7b). Two simple squamous epithelia have special names. The simple squamous lining of blood vessels and the heart is called **endothelium** (Figure 3-8a); **mesothelium** is the epithelial component of serous membranes and secretes a lubricating fluid (Figures 3-1 and 3-8b).

Simple cuboidal epithelium (Figure 3-9) is composed of a single layer of cube-shaped cells. It is found in glands (Figure 3-10a), where it is involved in secretion, and in kidney tubules where it is involved in secretion and absorption (Figure 3-10b), among other places.

Simple columnar epithelium (Figure 3-11) is made of a single layer of tall cells, frequently with basally positioned, elongated nuclei. It is typically involved in absorption and secretion, and often has microvilli and goblet cells (Figure 3-12).

Stratified Epithelia

Stratified squamous epithelium is composed of several to many layers of cells with the superficial layers being flattened. Because it is so thick, it is generally found in places subjected to abrasion. **Keratinized stratified squamous epithelium** (Figures 3-13 through 3-15) is found on dry surfaces (e.g., the skin). As basal cells divide their progeny get pushed to the surface and undergo changes, including accumulation of the protein keratin, and ultimately death. The dead cells so formed provide a waterproof, microbe-proof, abrasion barrier.

Nonkeratinized stratified squamous epithelium (Figures 3-13 and 3-16) is found in moist areas of the body not subjected to as much abrasion (e.g., oral cavity, esophagus, and vagina). Unlike the keratinized variety, the surface cells are living and have normal nuclei.

Stratified cuboidal (Figures 3-17 and 3-18) and **stratified columnar** (Figures 3-19 and 3-20) **epithelia** generally consist of only a couple of layers. They are fairly uncommon, but may be found in the ducts of some glands, with the cell height corresponding to the duct's size.

Other Epithelia

Some epithelia do not conform very well to the conventional naming criteria. These are considered in this section.

Transitional epithelium (Figures 3-21 and 3-22) is stratified and is found lining the renal calyces, urinary bladder, ureters, and male urethra. Also referred to as **urothelium**, it is specialized for stretching and forms a protective barrier against the hyperosmotic urine. When distended (stretched), only a few layers of flat cells are observed. In the relaxed state, the number of layers appears greater and the cells of the middle are columnar, while the surface cells are dome shaped and are called **umbrella cells**.

The surface umbrella cells are highly specialized and are often binucleate. Their apical membranes have thickened patches of the outer lipid layer. These **plaques** are separated by small regions of ordinary membrane that act as hinges and, along with underlying actin filaments, allow the cells to fold and unfold, depending on whether the epithelium is in the stretched or relaxed state. It is the plaques along with intercellular junctions that are responsible for providing protection against hyperosmotic urine.

Pseudostratified ciliated columnar epithelium (PSCC) is not a truly stratified epithelium, because all cells are in contact with the basement membrane (Figures 3-2, 3-23, and 3-24). However, not all cells reach the surface; some cells are short, some are tall, and others are intermediate in height. This variation in cell height results in nuclei being seen at different levels in the epithelium, giving the false impression of stratification—hence "*pseudo*stratified." And, because the cells that reach the surface are taller than wide, the epithelium is considered to be columnar. (Remember that epithelia are named based on the shape of the surface cells.) It is most associated with the respiratory tract, where it lines the nasal cavity, trachea, and bronchi. Goblet cells produce mucus that traps dust and other particles in inspired air, then the cilia sweep the mucus toward the pharynx, where it is swallowed. Pseudostratified epithelium is also found in parts of the male reproductive tract (epididymis– Figures 17-7b and 17-7c—and sometimes in the spongy urethra—17-9e).

Glandular Epithelia

Glandular epithelia are specialized for secreting materials. They develop from typical lining epithelium that grows down (*invaginates*) into deeper tissues during embryonic development and as such is not found on the surface. **Exocrine glands** remain connected to the surface and deliver their secretion to it by way of a duct. They are the subjects of this section. **Endocrine glands** (Chapter 10) lose the connection to the surface during development. Their secretion diffuses into the blood where it is distributed throughout the body.

Unicellular glands are represented by the abundant **goblet cells** of the respiratory and digestive tracts (Figure 3-25). Goblet cells secrete **mucinogen**, which converts to mucin when hydrated. Mucin is a major component of **mucus**.

Multicellular exocrine glands are more complex, with specialized duct cells and secretory cells (Figure 3-26). Photomicrographic examples are provided in Figures 3-27 through 3-34. Multicellular glands are classified according to their duct(s) and their secretory portions. If the duct is unbranched, the gland is **simple**; if it branches, the gland is **compound**. If the secretory portion is about the same size as the duct, the gland is **tubular**. If the secretory cells are larger than the duct, it is an **acinar** (or **alveolar**) **gland**. Some glands have both acinar and tubular secretory portions.

The secreting cells and the ducts comprise the **parenchyma** of the gland. In addition, there may be a connective tissue **stroma** in the gland that supports the parenchyma. In larger glands, the connective tissue **capsule** on the surface sends branches into the gland and divides it into **lobes** and **lobules**.

Myoepithelial cells (Figure 3-35) are associated with some acini. These are contractile epithelial cells that push the gland's secretion into the duct. They are found in salivary, mammary, and sweat glands.

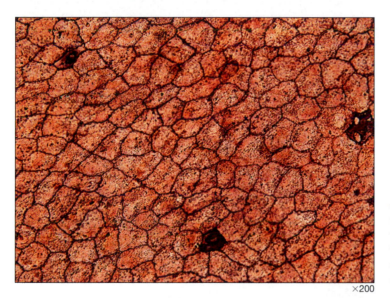

×200

3-1 **Epithelium Is a Cellular Tissue** ■ This is a whole mount of mesothelium, an epithelium composed of a single layer of flat cells, stained with silver nitrate to highlight cell membranes. Viewed from the surface, the very cellular and sheetlike nature of epithelial tissue is apparent. Most specimens you will encounter are viewed in section, so are seen from a lateral aspect or in cross or oblique section. (×200)

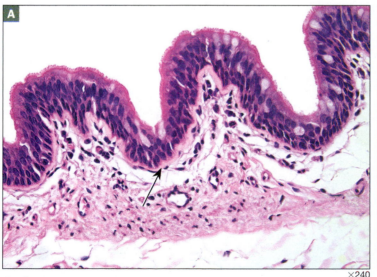

×240

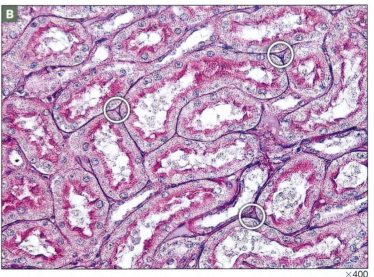

×400

3-2 **Light Micrographs of a Basement Membrane** ■ **(A)** Shown is an epithelium from the respiratory tract (PSCC) that has a prominent basement membrane (arrow) when stained with the standard H&E stain. In sections of most epithelia, the basement membrane is not as obvious because it is thin and stains the same as underlying connective tissue. In many cases, all that is visible is the junction between the epithelium and the underlying connective tissue. (×240) **(B)** PAS staining brings out the basement membrane. It can be seen as the dark (magenta) line outlining each of the kidney tubules. Although it appears to be a single layer where two tubules rest against one another, you can see at the junction of three cells (circled) that each tubule has its own. (×400)

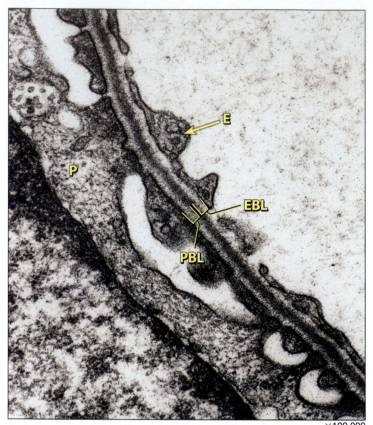

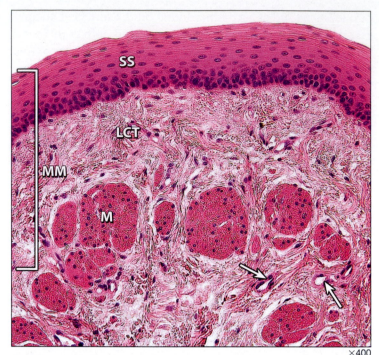

3-3 **TEM of Basal Laminae** ◼ This TEM is from the kidney, where two epithelial layers—capillary endothelium (E) and glomerular podocytes (P)—are back-to-back and their basal laminae are fused (PBL = podocyte basal lamina; EBL = endothelium basal lamina). There is evidence that the lighter layer of each basal lamina is an artifact of preparation. Where connective tissue is absent, no reticular lamina is seen. (×100,000)

×100,000

×400

3-4 **An Epithelial Membrane** ◼ All epithelial membranes (mucous, serous, and cutaneous membranes) are composed of an epithelium and its underlying connective tissue. In each, the avascular epithelium relies on the capillaries of the connective tissue for its oxygen and nutrients, and thus forms a functional as well as a structural unit. Shown here is the mucous membrane (MM) of the esophagus. The stratified squamous epithelium (SS) rests on a layer of loose connective tissue (LCT) that extends down to the pink, incomplete muscle layer (M). A couple of small blood vessels are indicated by the arrows. (×400)

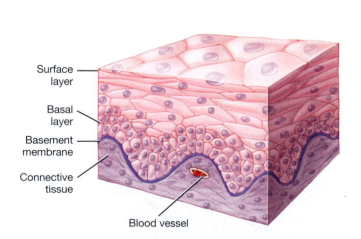

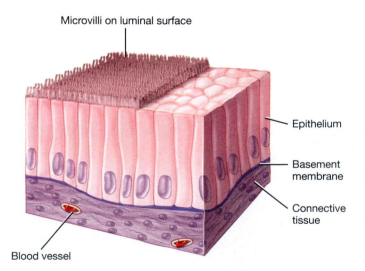

3-5 **Epithelial Terminology** ◼ Illustrated are standard descriptive terms associated with epithelia using nonkeratinized stratified squamous epithelium on the left and simple columnar epithelium with microvilli on the right as examples. Notice the importance of the basement membrane and surface as points of reference. Note also the presence of blood vessels in the underlying connective tissue and their absence in the epithelium.

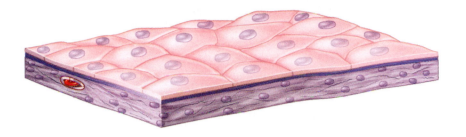

3-6 Illustration of Simple Squamous Epithelium ▪ Notice how thin the single layer of cells is and how the nuclei bulge from the cytoplasm. When cut, the plane of section won't pass through the nucleus of every cell (just like every bite of a chocolate chip cookie doesn't pass through a chocolate chip!). The result will be a layer of cells, some of which appear to be anucleate.

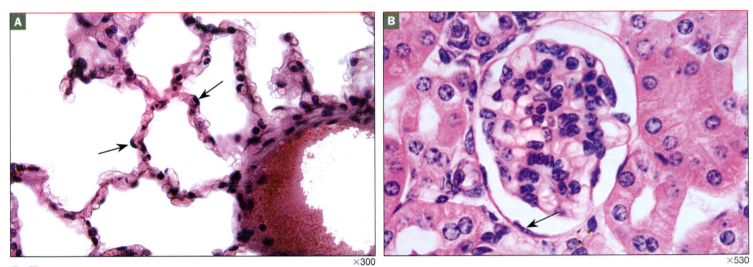

×300   ×530

3-7 Simple Squamous Epithelium ▪ (A) In this section of lung tissue, notice that the simple squamous cells lining the air sacs are so thin that only their nuclei are visible (arrows), making it difficult to believe that the epithelium is even there. In fact, partitions between air sacs are composed of a layer of simple squamous epithelium on both sides, with both simple squamous walls of a capillary between! (But it takes an electron microscope to see that kind of detail.) (×300) (B) Even though there is an obvious thin layer of cytoplasm surrounding the white space, the most prominent features of this simple squamous epithelium (arrow) are the flattened nuclei. Compare this micrograph with the illustration in Figure 3-6. Why are nuclei not seen in every cell? (×530)

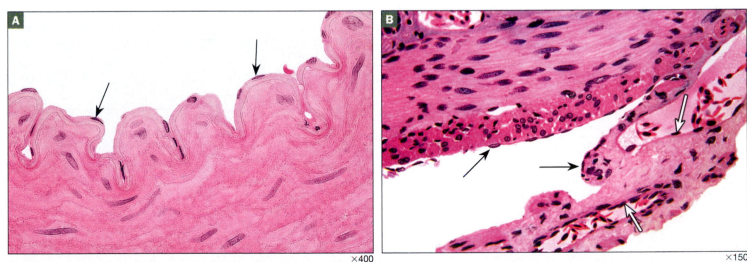

×400   ×150

3-8 Simple Squamous Epithelia with Special Names ▪ (A) Shown is a plastic-embedded section of an artery. The insides of all blood vessels and the heart are lined with a simple squamous endothelium (arrows). Note the different appearance of the epithelial cell nuclei from those nuclei in the deeper tissue. The red crescent is the sole remaining red blood cell after slide preparation. (×400) (B) The outer surface of organs in the ventral body cavity is lined with a serous membrane made of a connective tissue and a simple squamous mesothelium (black arrows). Also note the simple squamous endothelium (white arrows) lining the various blood vessels. This is a plastic-embedded section of a nonmammalian intestine (note the nucleated red blood cells). (×150)

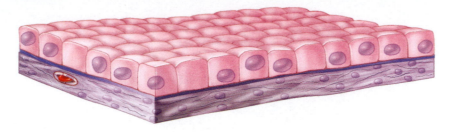

3-9 **Illustration of Simple Cuboidal Epithelium** ▪ Notice the single cell layer, the approximately uniform cell dimensions, and the central, spherical nuclei.

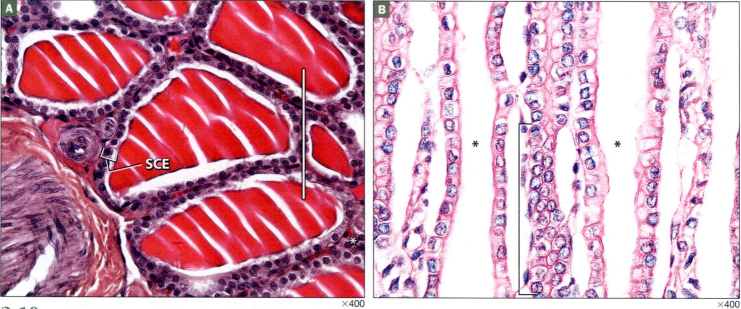

×400 ×400

3-10 **Simple Cuboidal Epithelium** ▪ **(A)** Shown is a section of the thyroid gland. It is composed of compartments (follicles) lined with a simple cuboidal epithelium (SCE). Notice that in most portions of the field the epithelium appears as a double layer. This is because the adjacent follicles are so close together that their simple cuboidal epithelia are almost back-to-back. The region indicated by the asterisk (*) in the lower right corner seems to be made up of the same cells as the follicles (same staining properties, same basic cellular shape) but they are not in a single layer. This is because those cells are part of follicles that have been cut through their edge. (Imagine the appearance of the cells sectioned along the line drawn on the follicle in the middle right of the field.) **(B)** Seen here are several kidney tubules (among other structures) lined with simple cuboidal epithelium that run parallel with one another. Asterisks (*) illustrate two lumina of the tubules through which urine passes during its formation. Notice the tubule that was sectioned longitudinally through its wall and is seen as a patch of cells (bracket). (Both ×400)

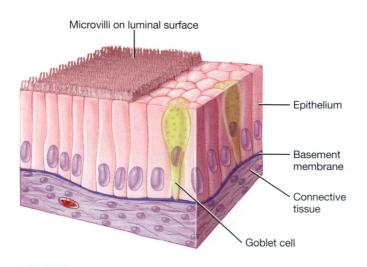

Microvilli on luminal surface

Epithelium

Basement membrane

Connective tissue

Goblet cell

3-11 **Illustration of Simple Columnar Epithelium with Goblet Cells** ▪ Columnar cells frequently have elongated and basally positioned nuclei. (But notice that the nuclei of all cells are not cut by the microtome blade, making some cells appear anucleate.) Simple columnar epithelial cells often have cilia or microvilli (as shown here) on their apical surfaces. In addition, single-celled mucus glands (goblet cells) may be present.

A Photographic Atlas of Histology

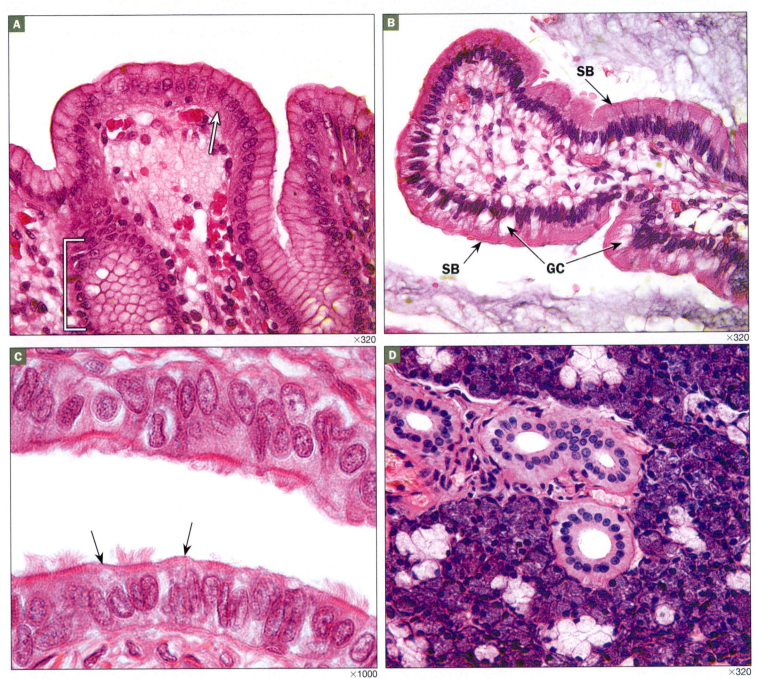

3-12 Simple Columnar Epithelium 🟥 (**A**) These simple columnar cells are characterized by a tall shape and a basal, elongated nucleus. The basement membrane is not apparent in this stomach specimen, but it is still clear where the epithelium ends and the connective tissue begins (arrow). The region indicated by the bracket is a curved surface lined by the same epithelium, but cut obliquely through the apical portions of the cells. A key to correctly interpreting this is, these cells have the same staining properties and texture as those clearly on the surface. (×320) (**B**) This simple columnar epithelium is from the small intestine. Microvilli, collectively referred to as a striated border (SB), are present on the apical surfaces of the columnar cells. Although not individually visible at this magnification, their presence is seen as the dark band. Imagine that you are seeing the lawn, but not the individual blades of grass. Microvilli increase surface area for absorption. The large, pale-staining cells are goblet cells (GC) that secrete mucus. (×320) (**C**) Shown is a section of uterine tube. What you see are two opposing surfaces lined with simple ciliated columnar epithelium. Nonciliated peg cells (arrows) are also visible. (×1000) (**D**) Our definitions of cuboidal and columnar cells are rigid, but nature is full of nuance! You may encounter epithelial cells that are difficult to pigeonhole because cell heights in the body represent a continuum rather than clearly defined groups. These pink cells are ducts in a salivary gland. They have spherical nuclei (a characteristic of cuboidal cells), but would be classified as columnar because they are two to three times taller than wide. Imagine that as the ducts get closer to their origin, they will be smaller in diameter and the epithelial cells will be shorter (more cuboidal). As the ducts get larger, farther away from their origin, the cells will be taller. The epithelial lining forms a continuum of cell heights. (×320)

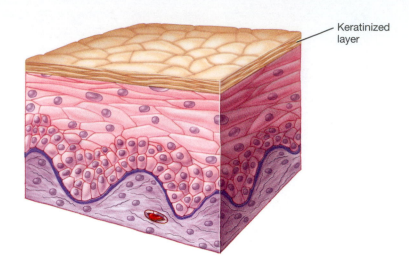

Keratinized layer

3-13 **Illustration of Stratified Squamous Epithelia** 🔲

Stratified squamous epithelium consists of a few to many cell layers, ranging in shape from cuboidal or irregular in most layers to flat at the surface. (Recall that epithelia are named after the shape of their surface cells.) The majority of cell division is in the basal layer (primarily because it is closest to the supply of oxygen and nutrients diffusing in from the underlying connective tissue). In all cases, the least healthy cells are on the surface and are regularly shed. In keratinized stratified squamous epithelia (left), the surface cells accumulate as they die and form the dry, keratinized layer. This epithelium is able to withstand mechanical abrasion and moisture loss and is found in the skin and a few other locations. Nonkeratinized stratified squamous epithelium lacks this layer of dead cells and is found in moist locations of the body not subject to severe abrasion, such as the oral cavity and esophagus.

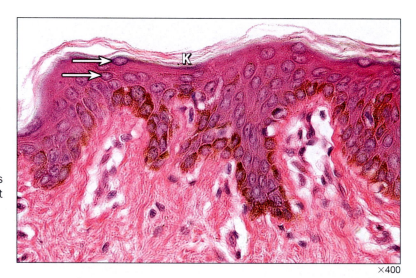

×400

3-14 **Thin Keratinized Stratified Squamous Epithelium** 🔲 This specimen is from abdominal skin and is only a few cells thick. The flat surface cells are dead and form the keratinized layer (K). Immediately beneath the keratin layer are one or two layers of flat, nucleated cells (arrows). Compare their shape to the cells near the basement membrane. Also note the pigment in the basal cells. (×400)

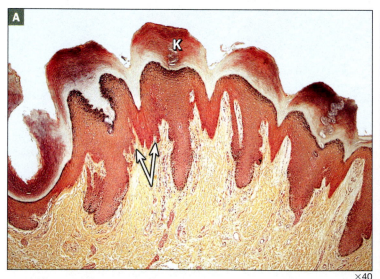

×40

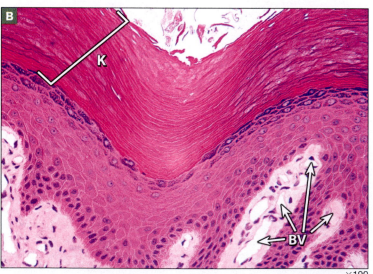

×190

3-15 **Thick Keratinized Stratified Squamous Epithelium** 🔲 (A) This specimen is from palmar skin. Notice the absence of nuclei in the thick, keratinized layer (K). Also, notice the typical, wavy interface (arrows) between the epithelium and the connective tissue—so typical, in fact, that it is often identifiable at low power without even seeing the individual cells. (×40) (B) In this higher magnification of a different specimen, some cell and nuclear outlines are still visible in the keratinized layer. Notice the wavy interface between the epithelium and the connective tissue, and the faint, prickly appearance in the light lines between living cells. These are due to intercellular attachments (desmosomes). Also notice the abundant blood vessels (BV) in the deeper connective tissue and their absence in the epithelium—remember that epithelia are avascular. The simple squamous endothelium of the blood vessels is also visible. (×190)

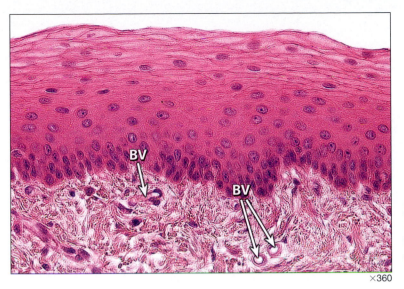

×360

3-16 **Nonkeratinized Stratified Squamous Epithelium** ◼
In this specimen from the esophagus, the cells are flat at the surface, but there is no keratin layer. Note the small blood vessels (BV) in the connective tissue. (×360)

3-17 **Illustration of Stratified Cuboidal Epithelium** ◼ This epithelium is most frequently seen in the larger ducts of glands.

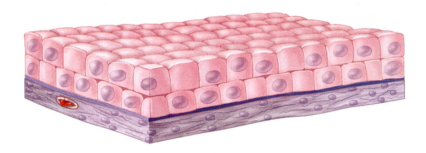

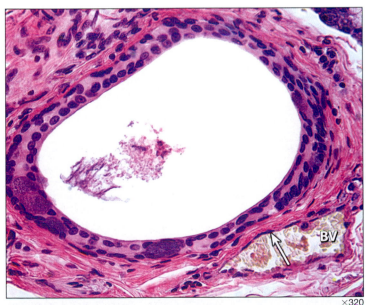

×320

3-18 **Stratified Cuboidal Epithelium** ◼ Ducts of glands may be lined with a stratified cuboidal epithelium. This stratified epithelium is only two cells thick. Notice the simple squamous endothelium (arrow) of the blood vessel (BV) in the lower right corner of the field. (×320)

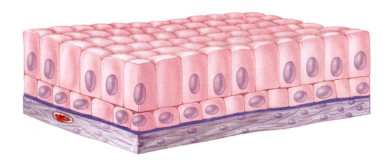

3-19 **Illustration of Stratified Columnar Epithelium** ◼ As with stratified cuboidal epithelium, stratified columnar epithelium is fairly uncommon. It is found in some larger ducts and parts of the male urethra. Notice that it is the surface cells that are columnar. Basal cells are usually shorter.

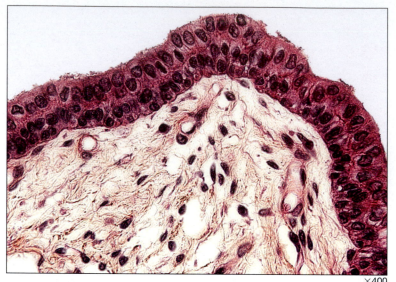

×400

3-20 **Stratified Columnar Epithelium** ■ This is a section of the male urethra. Notice that there are only two or three cell layers in this specimen (but there may be more in others) and only the surface cells are columnar. (×400)

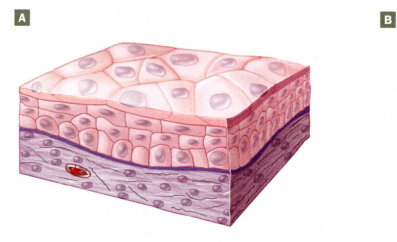

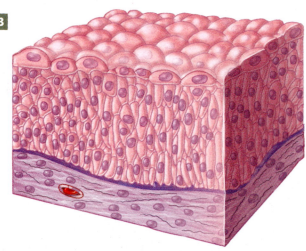

3-21 **Illustration of Transitional Epithelium (Urothelium)** ■ Transitional epithelium is specialized for stretching. In its stretched state (**A**) the surface cells are flat and there appear to be fewer layers than in the relaxed state. (**B**) The surface cells of relaxed transitional epithelium have a rounded appearance and are called umbrella cells.

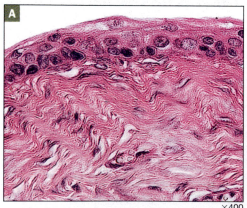

×400

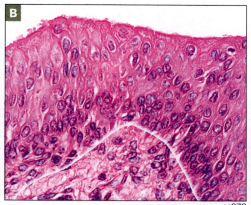

×270

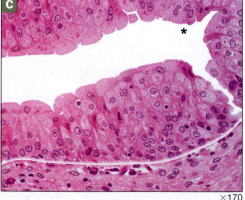

×170

3-22 **Transitional Epithelium (Urothelium)** ■ (**A**) Transitional epithelium is stratified and primarily is found in the urinary bladder and ureters. It is specialized for stretching. When stretched, the cells flatten, as in this micrograph. This might be confused with nonkeratinized stratified squamous epithelium, but notice the nuclei of the apical cells are rounded. (×400) (**B**) When the urinary bladder empties, the wall relaxes and the epithelium assumes the shape shown in this micrograph. Most of the cells are vertically elongated and the apical edge of the surface cells is rounded. (Please see the text for a description of the folding process.) The line indicates the level of the basement membrane. (×270) (**C**) The rounded apical surface of the umbrella cells is prominently displayed in this specimen of relaxed transitional epithelium. Umbrella cells are sometimes binucleate (or even multinucleate!). Two neighboring binucleate umbrella cells are above the asterisk (*). The line indicates the level of the basement membrane. (×170)

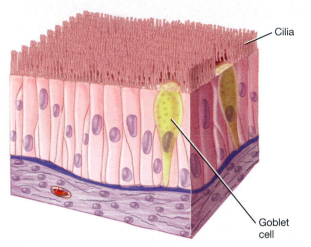
Cilia

Goblet
cell

3-23 **Illustration of Pseudostratified Ciliated Columnar Epithelium (PSCC) with Goblet Cells** ▪ PSCC is associated with the respiratory tract. Notice in the illustration that all the cells contact the basement membrane, so it really is a single cell layer. What gives it a stratified appearance is that not all cells reach the surface, resulting in nuclei being seen at different levels, which gives the appearance of stratification. Goblet cells and cilia on the tallest cells are also shown. Some organs, such as the ductus deferens, are lined with nonciliated pseudostratified columnar epithelium.

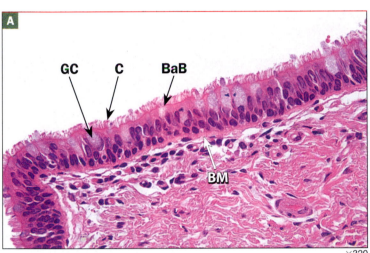

A
GC   C   BaB
BM
×320

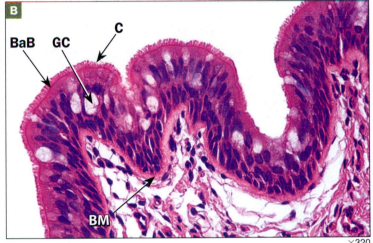

B
BaB   GC   C
BM
×320

3-24 **Pseudostratified Ciliated Columnar Epithelium (PSCC)** ▪ (**A**) This specimen is from the trachea. Short, intermediate, and tall cells, all of which touch the basement membrane, characterize it. It is the various heights of nuclei that give the impression of a stratified epithelium. Also present are cilia (C) on the tallest cells, mucus-secreting goblet cells (GC), and a prominent basement membrane (BM). (×320) (**B**) Because the actual cell boundaries are not very clear in this specimen of PSCC, one might confuse this with a stratified columnar epithelium. However, stratified columnar epithelium usually has only a couple of cell layers and the nuclear layers are fairly distinct, not jumbled as in this micrograph. Goblet cells (GC), cilia (C), and the basement membrane (BM) are clearly shown. At the apical poles of ciliated cells in both micrographs is a prominent magenta band. It is the location of the ciliary basal bodies (BaB). (×320)

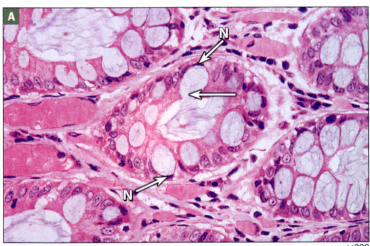

A
N
N
×320

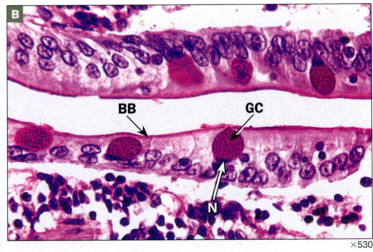

B
BB   GC
N
×530

3-25 **Goblet Cells** ▪ (**A**) Numerous goblet cells in the colon's simple columnar epithelium are visible. One cell, indicated by the arrow, has released its secretion, mucin, which when hydrated becomes mucus. Flat, dense-staining goblet cell nuclei (N) are visible below the mucin droplets in a couple of cells. (×320) (**B**) Due to their high polysaccharide content, the mucin granules of the goblet cells (GC) are PAS positive and appear red (see Table 1-1). Also notice the basal nuclei (N) of the goblet cells and the brush border (BB) on the simple columnar epithelium. In addition to PAS, this specimen from the small intestine was also stained with hematoxylin. (×530)

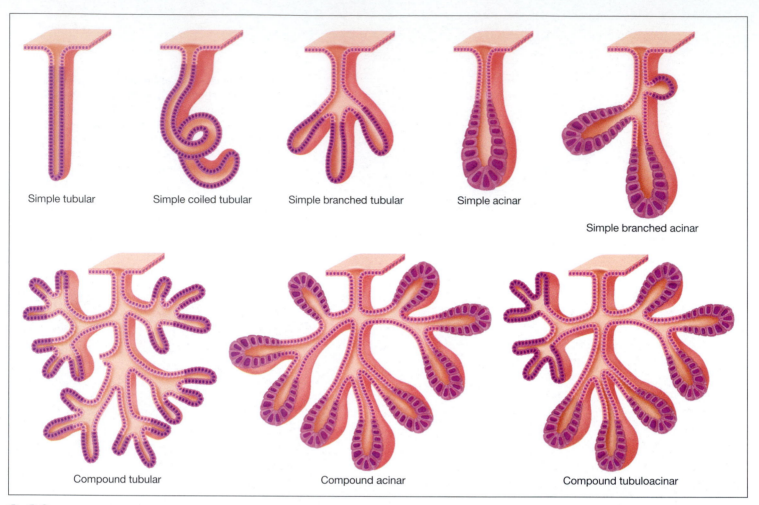

Simple tubular

Simple coiled tubular

Simple branched tubular

Simple acinar

Simple branched acinar

Compound tubular

Compound acinar

Compound tubuloacinar

3-26 **Multicellular Glands** ◖ Multicellular glands are composed of a duct (pink) and a secretory portion (darker purple). If the duct is unbranched, the gland is simple; if branched, the gland is compound. In tubular glands, the secretory cells are about the same size as the duct cells. If the secretory cells are larger than the duct cells, the gland is alveolar or acinar. All combinations of simple/compound and tubular/acinar glands are represented in the body. Be advised that your specimens are going to look more like the following micrographs. That is, they will be sectioned, not seen in three dimensions and in their entirety as illustrated here.

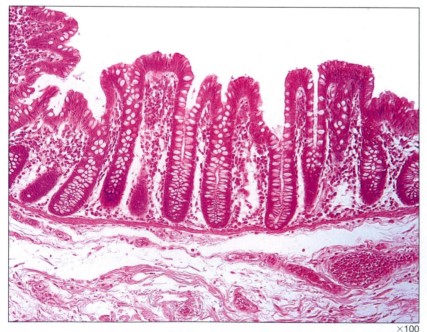

×100

3-27 **Simple Tubular Glands of the Colon** ◖ The straight depressions into the mucosa of the colon are called crypts of Lieberkühn. The crypts are simple tubular glands and are lined by simple columnar epithelium with abundant goblet cells. (×100)

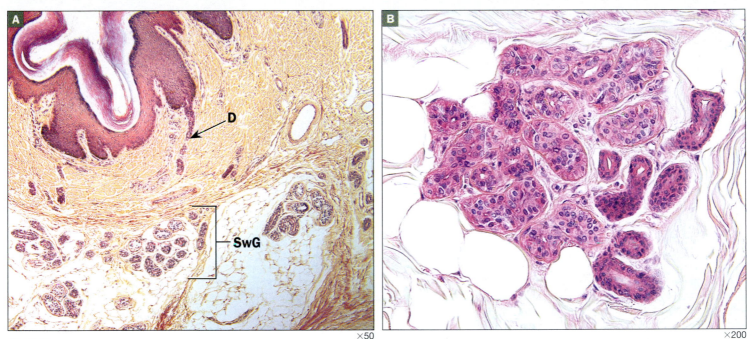

×50

×200

3-28 **Simple Coiled Tubular Gland** ■ (**A**) A relatively straight duct (D) connects the coiled secretory part of a sweat gland (SwG) to the skin's surface. Several sweat glands and their ducts are visible in this field. Also note the keratinized stratified squamous epithelium. (×50) (**B**) Shown is a higher magnification of the coiled gland from a different specimen. The pale-staining cells are secretory; the darker ones form the duct. (×200)

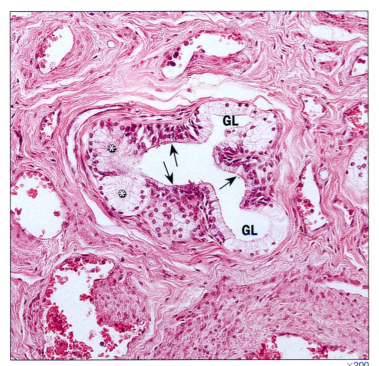

×200

3-29 **Simple Acinar Gland** ■ The glands of Littré (GL) are found in the connective tissue deep to the male penile urethra. They secrete mucus and are simple acinar glands. The pale cells forming pockets (acini) are the secretory cells. The regions between acini (arrows) are a pseudostratified columnar epithelium, the epithelium of the penile urethra. The acini, marked with asterisks (*), have been cut tangentially. (×200)

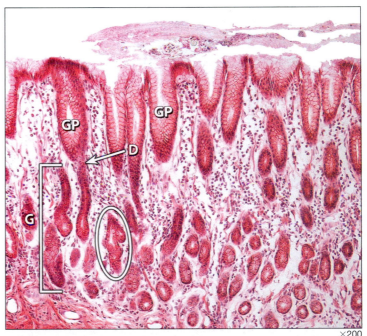

×200

3-30 **Simple Branched Tubular Glands** ■ The mucosal glands of the cardiac stomach are branched tubular glands (G) that open into mucosal depressions called gastric pits (GP) via a short duct (D). The straight, tubular nature of the glands is apparent, and a branching point is circled. Notice the difference in texture between the gland cells and the simple columnar epithelium lining the stomach surface and the pits. The latter cells are actually single-celled glands that secrete mucus. (×200)

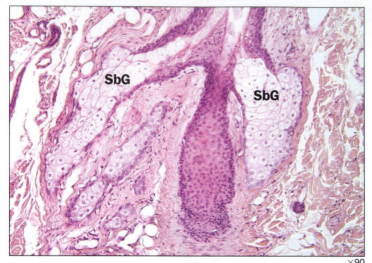

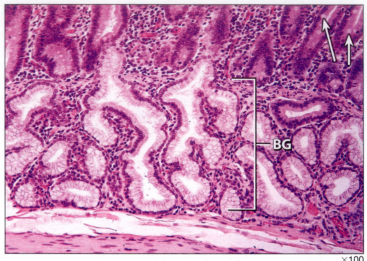

3-31 **Simple Branched Alveolar Gland** ◼ Sebaceous glands (SbG), associated with hair follicles, are branched alveolar glands with a very short duct. Two glands connected to the follicle are shown in this field. On the left are pieces of other branches that connect in a different plane. The secretory cells release their secretion by disintegrating, which is apparent in this specimen. (×90)

3-32 **Compound Branched Tubular Gland** ◼ Mucus-secreting Brünner's glands (BG) of the duodenum are compound branched tubular glands—that is, both the ducts and secretory parts are branched. The glands are composed of the lighter-staining cells in the middle third of the field. Their uniform diameter and branching are apparent in this specimen. Notice the goblet cells (arrows) in the simple columnar epithelium in the upper third of the field. (×100)

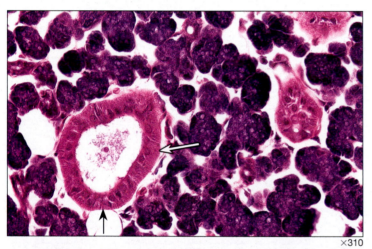

3-33 **Compound Acinar Gland** ◼ The dark cellular clusters are **serous acini** of the parotid salivary gland. Their secretion is rich in protein and has the purple (with H&E stain), granular appearance typical of many protein-secreting cells. The lighter pink, circular structures are parts of three ducts. Their different sizes are a fair indication that the ducts are branched and the gland is compound. The largest duct to the left of center is called a striated duct and is lined with a simple columnar epithelium. Notice the vertical lines in the basal portion of these cells (arrows). These are regions of membrane infoldings and numerous mitochondria. The former increase surface area for membrane pumps involved in final processing of saliva; the latter provide energy for the pumps. (×310)

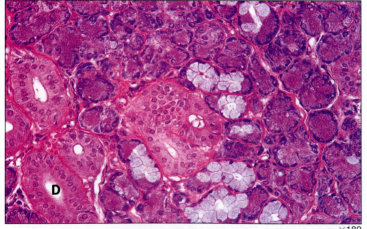

3-34 **Compound Tubuloacinar Gland** ◼ This submandibular salivary gland has tubular and acinar secretory portions, as well as numerous branched ducts. The gray secretory cells produce mucus, whereas the darker, more granular cells produce enzymes. The ducts (D) are lined with a simple columnar epithelium and have an obvious lumen (see Figure 3-12d for another example). (×180)

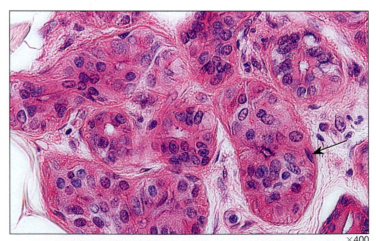

3-35 **Myoepithelial Cells** ◼ In sweat glands (as in this specimen) and salivary glands, myoepithelial cells (arrow) occupy the region between the secretory cells and the basement membrane. Their contraction assists movement of the secretion into the duct. (×400)

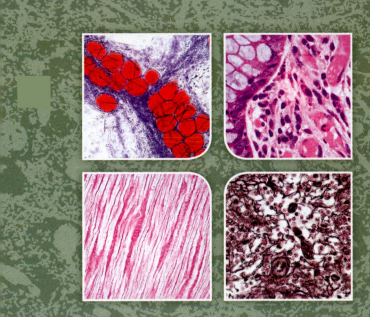

4

Fibrous Connective Tissue

Introduction to Connective Tissues

Chapters 4, 5, and 6 are devoted to connective tissues. The connective tissues make up a diverse grouping, both structurally and functionally, and there are several classification schemes used by different authors. The scheme used in this book is shown in Table 4-1.

Because the connective tissues are derived (primarily) from the same embryonic tissue, they have much in common, so there will be overlap between the chapters. Chapter 4 will introduce the basics of all connective tissues and describe those falling under the heading **connective tissue proper** as well as those that have been labeled **specialized connective tissues**. To keep chapters from becoming too cumbersome, other specialized connective tissues will be covered in their own chapters, with Chapter 5 devoted to **cartilage** and **bone**, and Chapter 6 covering **blood** and **bone marrow**.

Basic Characteristics of Connective Tissues

Connective (supporting) tissues anchor organs and join the other tissues of the body into a structurally integrated whole. In fact, most organs have a connective tissue covering that often penetrates it and binds the whole organ together. Unlike epithelia, connective tissues generally have abundant **extracellular (intercellular) matrix** and relatively few cells. The matrix consists of protein fibers, a ground substance, and other supporting biochemicals. Connective tissues may be vascular or avascular (cartilage, for example).

Functions of Connective Tissue Proper and Specialized Connective Tissues

The functions of connective tissues covered in this chapter are many and varied. Some examples are:

- Binding and support (e.g., ligaments)
- Defense (e.g., macrophages, lymphocytes, and mast cells of various tissues)
- Storage (e.g., adipose tissue)
- Protection (e.g., adipose tissue)
- Transport of materials between blood and other tissues (e.g., extracellular [interstitial, tissue] fluid in loose connective tissue and others)

Embryonic Connective Tissues— Mesenchyme and Mucous Tissue

Connective tissues of the adult are derived from an embryonic tissue called **mesenchyme** (Figure 4-1a), which is derived from embryonic **mesoderm** (Figure 4-2). Mesenchymal cells are angular or spindle-shaped and form a loose mesh that is functionally a rudimentary connective tissue with a viscous ground substance and few fibers. They are unspecialized and have the potential to differentiate into the cells typical of adult connective tissues (Table 4-1). In adults, mesenchymal cells play a role in tissue repair (along with **fibroblasts** and **pericytes**, which are found associated with capillaries).

Mucous tissue (Figure 4-1b) is found only in the umbilical cord and a few other locations in the embryo. It has fibroblasts and very few collagen fibers coursing through a jellylike ground substance in the umbilical cord, known as Wharton's jelly.

Extracellular Matrix of Adult Connective Tissues

The properties of a connective tissue are largely due to the properties of its **extracellular matrix (ECM)**. Comprising matrix are the ground substance, fibers, and structural glycoproteins.

Ground substance is an amorphous, gel-like material composed of charged glycosaminoglycans—GAGs—(mucopolysaccharides) and proteoglycans (mucoproteins) of various types. Both are polymers of disaccharide subunits, but the latter are also bonded to proteins. Their charges make them hydrophilic, resulting in tissue fluid mixing readily with the ground substance and helping create the gel-like state. Because of this association, the ground substance is an essential participant in the transport of nutrients and wastes between the blood and other tissues. Ground substance is not easily visualized in histological preparations.

Fibers are made of protein and come in two basic types: collagen and elastic. **Collagen fibers** (Figure 4-3) are made of the protein collagen and are the primary (most abundant) fibers of connective tissues. A collagen *molecule* consists of three polypeptide chains (α chains) wound in a triple helix. A collagen *fiber* is made of many (many!) collagen molecules packed together in a regular pattern. Each chain within a collagen molecule may have been produced by any of 42 different collagen genes! So far (as of 2011), 28 collagen types have been identified based on different chain combinations in the triple helix. Not surprisingly, these have different properties and serve different functions. The most abundant collagen is **Type I**, which has a high tensile strength and is flexible, but inelastic. **Type III collagen fibers** (Figure 4-4) are thin, branched, and formerly known as **reticular fibers**. These fibers form the framework of the liver, lymphatic tissue, and bone marrow. **Elastic fibers** (Figures 4-3 and 4-5) are made of the protein **elastin** and the glycoprotein **fibrillin**. The elasticity they confer is an important property of organs that can be deformed and then return to their original shape, such as larger arteries and the skin.

Structural glycoproteins are involved in anchoring and fastening cells to extracellular material, including basement membranes.

Cells of Adult Connective Tissues

There are many cell types in fibrous connective tissues. Fibroblasts, mast cells, macrophages, adipocytes, lymphocytes, and plasma cells are the most commonly encountered. Other cells characteristic of cartilage, bone, and blood will be discussed in their respective chapters.

Fibroblasts (Figures 4-3, 4-5, and 4-6) are derived from mesenchymal cells and are responsible for synthesis and maintenance of the matrix. Underscoring their relatively undifferentiated state, each fibroblast can produce all elements of the extracellular matrix. With H&E stain, only their granular, elongated nuclei and nucleoli are easily visible. The remainder of the cell with its elongated extensions can be better seen with other stains.

Macrophages (Figure 4-7) are derived from blood monocytes and are found in a variety of tissues. Their function is to phagocytose (engulf) foreign, dead and dying cells, and cellular debris. In their role as **antigen presenting cells (APCs)** they present antigens to lymphocytes as part of the immune response. **Resident (fixed) macrophages** (Figure 4-7a) are regular inhabitants of a particular tissue, whereas **elicited (wandering or free) macrophages** (Figure 4-7b) circulate in the blood and migrate to where they are needed. Connective tissue macrophages are difficult to identify with certainty using routine light microscope preparations. However, some characteristics to look for are an irregular shape; a basophilic, finely granular cytoplasm; and an oval- to kidney-shaped nucleus. Ingested particles would also be a useful clue.

Mast cells (Figure 4-8) originate in the bone marrow, but occupy various connective tissues. In many ways they resemble blood basophils, but are not developmentally related to them. They are large with prominent cytoplasmic, membrane-bound granules. The granules contain chemicals (such as heparin, histamine, chemotactic factors, and many others) that are involved in the inflammatory response. Release of the granules' contents is called **degranulation**.

Adipocytes are derived from mesenchymal cells and, perhaps, fibroblasts. They are specialized to store fat. **Unilocular fat cells** (Figure 4-9a) store the fat as a single, large droplet that pushes the nucleus and cytoplasm to the cell's periphery. Often, the fat is dissolved from the adipocytes during slide preparation, so all that is seen is empty cells (Figure 4-9b). **Multilocular fat cells** (Figure 4-10) are smaller, store fat in many droplets, and have a spherical nucleus.

Leukocytes (white blood cells) of various types may be seen in connective tissues, especially at the site of infection or inflammation. Most commonly seen in healthy tissue preparations are **lymphocytes** and **plasma cells** (Figures 4-11 and 4-12). Lymphocytes have a dark-staining nucleus surrounded by a thin layer of cytoplasm. Plasma cells are derived from lymphocytes and they secrete antibodies. They have a purplish cytoplasm (due to abundant RER necessary for antibody production) and an eccentric nucleus. A pale region next to the nucleus may also be visible. It is the site of the Golgi apparatus. **Neutrophils** (Figure 4-12) have a granular cytoplasm and a segmented (lobed) nucleus. They are phagocytic.

Types of Adult Connective Tissue

Fibrous connective tissues have traditionally been classified according to the arrangement and density of fibers. **Regular connective tissues** have the fibers oriented in the same direction; the fibers of **irregular connective tissues** are oriented in all directions. The fibers of **loose connective tissues** occur singly, whereas the fibers of **dense connective tissues** occur in bundles and are tightly packed together. Although these categories will be used here, it should be realized that they represent extremes and that intermediate connective tissue types exist. Further, some authors consider **adipose tissue** and **reticular tissue** as loose connective tissues, but they will be considered separately in this chapter.

Loose Areolar Tissue

Loose areolar tissue (Figures 4-3, 4-5, 4-6, 4-13, and 4-14) is the connective tissue component of serous and mucous membranes, acts as filler between muscles and between muscles and skin, and is found in various other locations in the body. Collagen and elastic fibers are present, as are fibroblasts, mast cells, macrophages, and most other connective tissue cells. Blood vessels, lymphatic vessels, and nerves are also present.

Dense Irregular Connective Tissue

Dense irregular connective tissue (Figure 4-15) is characterized by densely packed collagen bundles oriented in all directions. It is vascular and fibroblasts are the predominant cell type. It comprises the dermis and capsules of many organs.

Dense Regular Connective Tissue

Dense regular connective tissue is a poorly vascularized tissue that has fiber bundles arranged in parallel fashion. This fiber arrangement confers great tensile strength along their length. Fibroblasts are compressed and appear elongated between the compact fibers. Tendons provide an example of dense regular collagenous connective tissue (Figure 4-16).

Types of Specialized Connective Tissue

Elastic Connective Tissue

Elastic connective tissue has an abundance of elastic fibers. It can be found in the lungs (see Chapter 15) and some vertebral ligaments (4-17a). In elastic arteries (Figure 4-17b), the fibers form compact, concentric **laminae** (sheets). Elastic fibers in blood vessels are produced by smooth muscle cells instead of fibroblasts. Wherever it is found, elastic tissue is specialized for stretching and returning to its original shape.

Adipose Tissue

Adipose tissue is a vascular tissue and differs from other connective tissues in that it is very cellular with little intercellular material. **White adipose tissue** (Figures 4-9 and 4-18a) is composed of unilocular adipocytes and is commonly found in the subcutaneous regions as well as in serous membranes. Fixing slides by standard methods dissolves the fat, so "empty" adipocytes are typically seen. In some procedures, the fat is retained and can be stained, as with the oil-soluble dye Sudan red (Figure 4-9a).

Brown adipose tissue (Figure 4-18b) is primarily an embryonic tissue. By childhood, most has degenerated or been replaced by white adipose tissue. Some remnants may be found in the perirenal region and other locations in adults. It is composed of multilocular adipocytes and is much more vascular than white adipose tissue. It is involved in generation of body heat and is especially important in infants prior to developing the shivering response.

Reticular Connective Tissue

Reticular connective tissue (Figure 4-19) is a loose connective tissue with an abundance of reticular fibers (Type III collagen). The fibers are hard to distinguish with H&E, but can be visualized with silver stains. Reticular connective tissue forms the framework of bone marrow, lymphoid organs, and the liver sinusoids.

Table 4-1 Classification of Connective Tissues[1]
Connective Tissue Proper
Embryonic Connective Tissues
Mesenchyme
Mucous Connective Tissue
Adult Connective Tissues
Loose (Areolar) Connective Tissue
Dense Connective Tissue
Dense Regular Connective Tissue
Dense Irregular Connective Tissue
Specialized Connective Tissues
Adipose Tissue
White Adipose Tissue
Brown Adipose Tissue
Reticular Tissue
Elastic Tissue
Cartilage
Hyaline Cartilage
Elastic Cartilage
Fibrocartilage
Bone
Blood

[1] After Ovalle and Nahirney (2008).

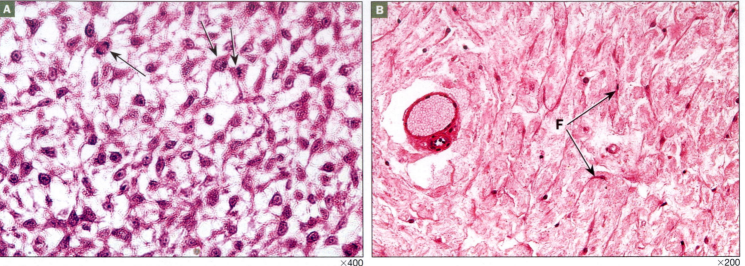

×400

×200

4-1 **Embryonic Connective Tissue** ◼ **(A)** Mesenchyme is a primitive connective tissue with few fibers. Its cells are angular and have the potential to develop into more specialized connective tissue cells. Note how the cellular processes join to form a three-dimensional lattice. Note also the mitotic figures in the field (arrows). (×400) **(B)** Mucous tissue is found only in the umbilical cord and a few other sites in the embryo. It contains fibroblasts (F) and a few fibers, so it is more specialized than mesenchyme. The ground substance is like jelly. (×200)

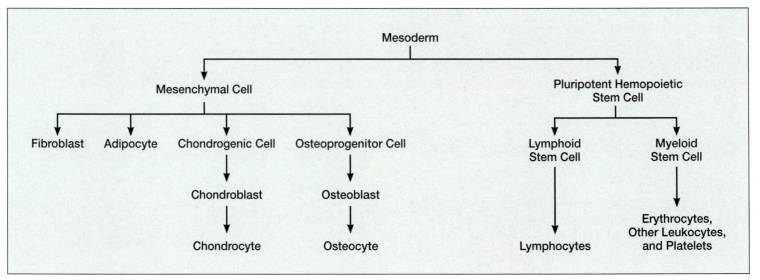

4-2 **Scheme of Connective Tissue Cell Development** ◼ Connective tissues develop from embryonic mesoderm, which gives rise to mesenchymal cells and pluripotent hemopoietic stem cells (HSC). Mesenchymal cells give rise to fibroblasts and adipocytes of connective tissue proper (covered in this chapter), and cartilage and bone cells (covered in Chapter 5). The HSC gives rise to all formed elements in blood (covered in Chapter 6).

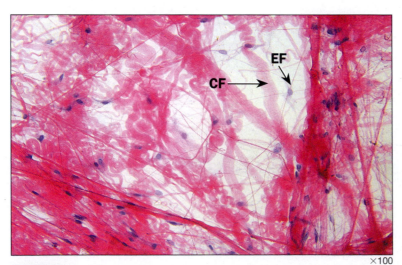

×100

4-3 **Collagen Fibers** ◼ Thick, strong, collagen fibers (CF) are seen in this specimen of loose areolar tissue. The thin fibers are elastic fibers (EF), and most of the cells are fibroblasts. (×100)

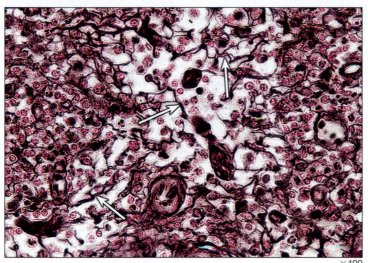

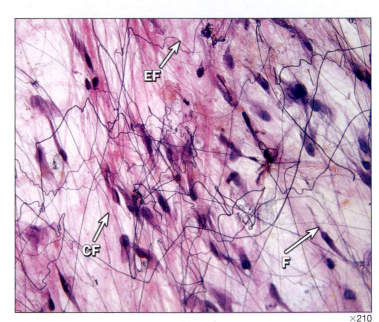

×400

4-4 **Reticular Fibers (Type III Collagen Fibers)** ■ Reticular fibers are thin and branched. This specimen is a lymph node, but they also form the structural framework of the spleen, bone marrow, and some other organs. These fibers are not easily seen when stained with H&E; a silver stain can be used to visualize them as black lines, some of which are indicated by arrows. (×400)

×210

4-5 **Elastic Fibers in Loose Areolar Tissue** ■ The thin, dark lines are elastic fibers (EF) in this loose areolar tissue stained for elastic fibers. Also visible are collagen fibers (CF) and fibroblasts (F). (×210)

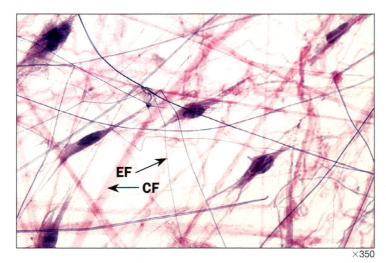

×350

4-6 **Fibroblasts** ■ Fibroblasts are very common cells of connective tissue proper. As seen in this spread of loose areolar tissue prepared with Verhoeff and eosin stains, they have an irregular shape. In H&E preparations, usually all that can easily be seen of them is their nuclei. Collagen (CF) and elastic (EF) fibers are also visible in this specimen. (×350)

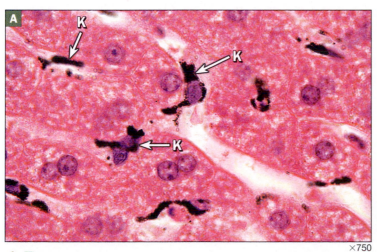

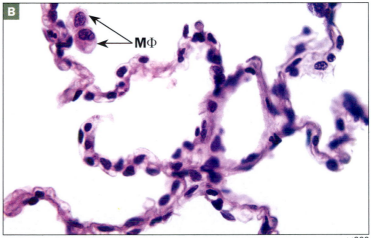

×750

×900

4-7 **Macrophages** ■ Macrophages may either be fixed or wandering, and both may be found in connective tissue proper, but they are difficult to identify without correct preparation. (**A**) Kupffer cells (K) are fixed macrophages that line the liver sinusoids and remove material from the blood. These macrophages have ingested carbon particles that make them stand out. Fixed macrophages may also be seen in the spleen and lymph nodes. (×750) (**B**) This micrograph of lung tissue shows a couple of wandering macrophages (MΦ). (×900)

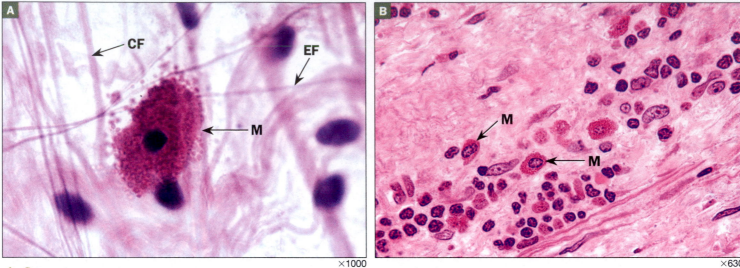

4-8 Mast Cells 🔲 Mast cells (M) are involved in the inflammatory response by degranulating and releasing histamine and other chemicals. (**A**) This is a loose areolar tissue spread stained to show a mast cell, fibroblasts, and elastic (EF) and collagen (CF) fibers. When stained properly, the mast cell with its granules is unmistakable. (×1000) (**B**) Several mast cells (arrows) are visible in this plastic-embedded tonsil specimen. (×630)

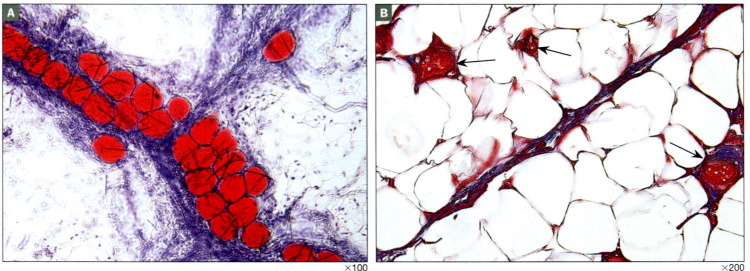

4-9 Unilocular Adipocytes 🔲 The cytoplasm and nucleus of unilocular adipocytes are pushed to the periphery and the single, large fat droplet occupies the majority of the cell. (**A**) These are unilocular adipocytes stained with Sudan red, a fat-soluble dye that stains the fat droplet red. (×100) (**B**) Standard slide preparation dissolves and removes the fat droplet and all that remains of the adipocytes is the membrane and some cytoplasm. Notice the blood vessels (arrows) in this vascularized tissue. (×200)

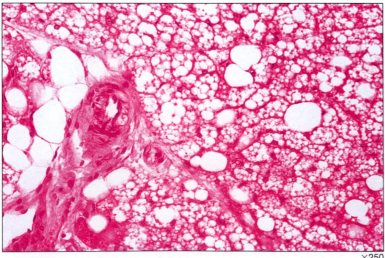

4-10 Multilocular Adipocytes 🔲 The obvious difference between unilocular and multilocular fat cells is that in the latter, fat is stored as several droplets rather than as one large droplet. (×250)

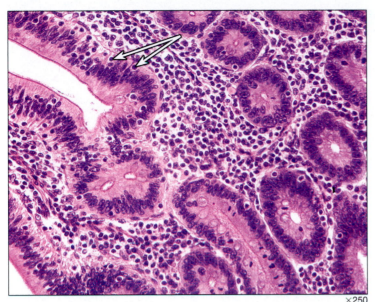

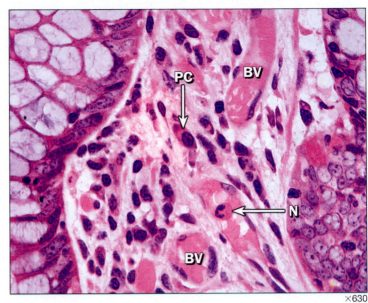

4-11 **Lymphocytes** 🔴 The lamina propria of mucous membranes is often infiltrated with lymphocytes, cells of the immune system that can differentiate into antibody-secreting plasma cells and perform other protective functions. They are small, round cells with dark-staining nuclei. In this specimen from the small intestine, the lymphocytes are quite dense. Some have even entered the simple columnar epithelium (arrows). (×250)

4-12 **Plasma Cell and Neutrophil** 🔴 Plasma cells (PC) are lymphocytes actively secreting antibodies. They are elongated cells with the nucleus toward one end. The nucleus may look like a clock face because of the chromatin distributed around its periphery. A pale region of cytoplasm near the nucleus is the site of a Golgi apparatus. A phagocytic neutrophil (N) is also visible in the field. Its granular cytoplasm is not very apparent, but the segmented nucleus is. Notice the blood vessels (BV) in the field. (×630)

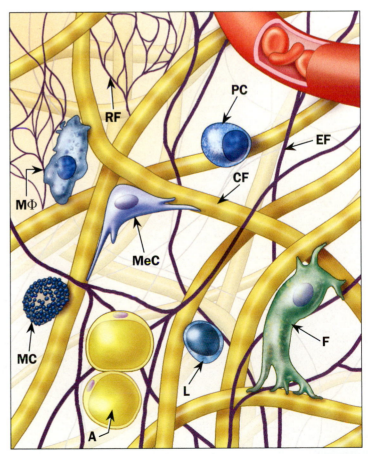

4-13 **Illustration of Loose Areolar Tissue** 🔴 A loose weave of collagen (CF), reticular fibers (RF), and elastic fibers (EF) characterizes loose areolar tissue. As seen in this illustration, LAT contains a variety of connective tissue cells, but the most abundant are the fibroblasts (F). Other cells include mast cells (MC), macrophages (MΦ), adipocytes (A), lymphocytes (L), plasma cells (PC), and mesenchymal cells (MeC). In routine spreads of LAT, not all cells will be easily identified. Note the blood vessel. LAT is found as a supporting tissue and as filler between organs (fascia).

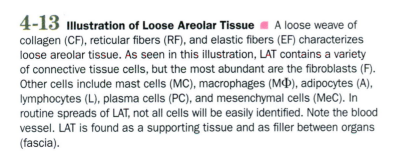

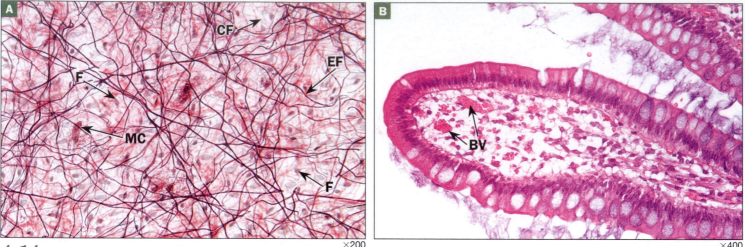

4-14 **Loose Areolar Tissue (LAT)** 🔲 **(A)** This specimen is from mesentery. The darker gray nuclei mostly belong to fibroblasts (F). Degranulated mast cells (MC) are also visible, as are elastic (EF) and collagen (CF) fibers. Also see Figures 4-3, 4-5, 4-6, and 4-9. (×200) **(B)** Loose fibrous connective tissue comprises the lamina propria of many epithelial membranes. This specimen is from the small intestine. Notice the blood vessels (BV). (×400)

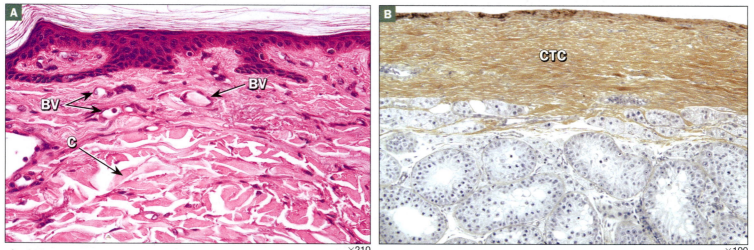

4-15 **Dense Irregular Connective Tissue** 🔲 **(A)** The dermis of the skin is composed of an irregular weave of tightly packed fiber bundles. Although all fiber types are present, collagen bundles (C) are the most obvious. Notice that the bundles are sectioned longitudinally, obliquely, and in cross section, indicating their irregular arrangement. Most of the cells are fibroblasts with only their nuclei seen clearly. Blood vessels (BV) indicate this tissue is vascular. (×210) **(B)** Many organs, including the testis shown here, are covered by a dense fibrous connective tissue capsule (CTC) composed mostly of collagen bundles. (×100)

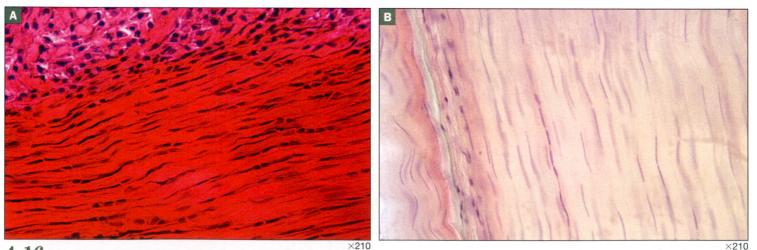

4-16 **Dense Regular Connective Tissue** 🔲 **(A and B)** Tendons, shown here, and ligaments are made of closely packed collagen bundles all oriented in the same direction. Dense regular connective tissue is poorly vascularized. The cells, seen only as nuclei, are fibroblasts, and they are typically in rows. (Both ×210)

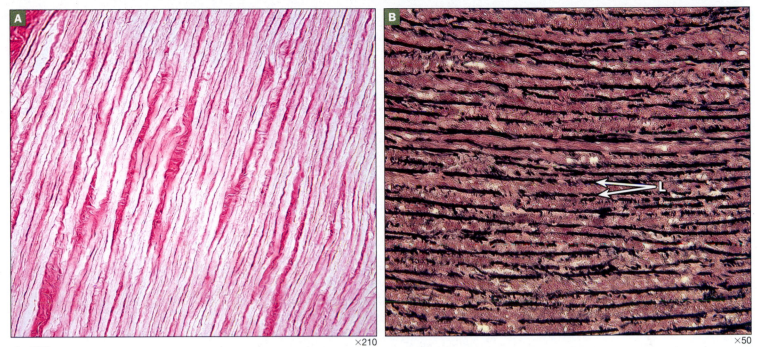

×210   ×50

4-17 **Elastic Tissue** ◾ (**A**) This specimen is an elastic ligament from the cervical spine. The waviness of the fibers is an indication of their elasticity. (×210) (**B**) This specimen is from the aorta. The dark lines are sheets of elastic fibers called laminae (L). Their elasticity allows the aorta to stretch when blood is pumped into it, then recoil and push the blood farther when the heart relaxes. Unlike most fibers, these are produced by smooth muscle cells, not fibroblasts. (×50)

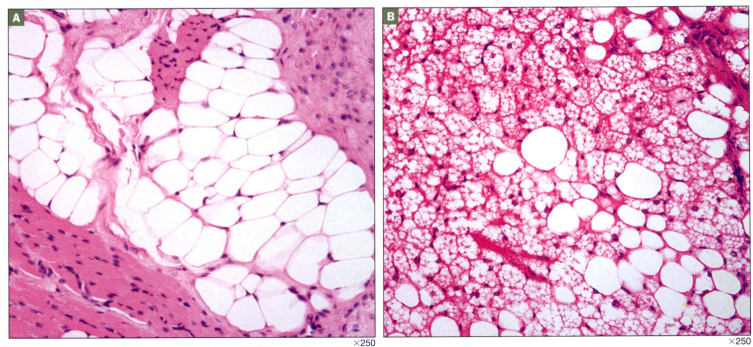

×250   ×250

4-18 **Fat Tissue** ◾ (**A**) White fat is made of unilocular adipocytes and may be found most anywhere loose connective tissue is found. This specimen is from a skeletal muscle. You can see fat filling the space between the muscle fiber bundles. (×250) (**B**) Brown fat is made of multilocular adipocytes, and in humans is primarily found in the embryo. (×250)

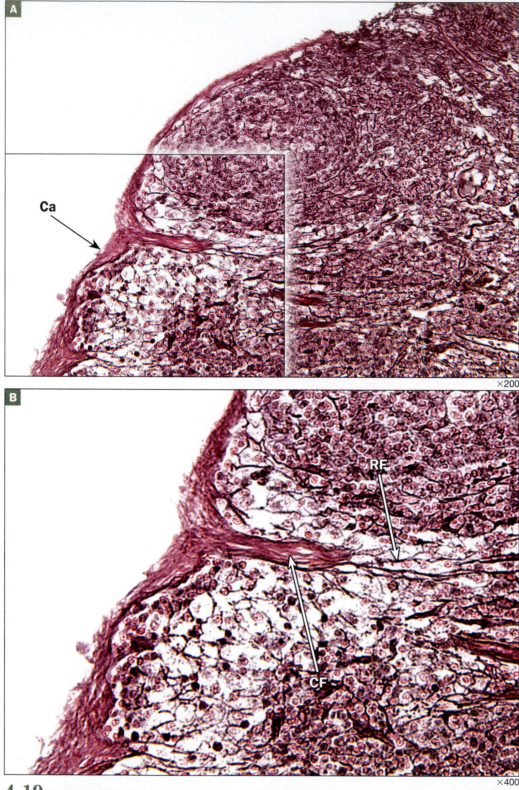

A

Ca

×200

B

RF

CF

×400

4-19 **Reticular Connective Tissue** 🔴 **(A)** Lymphoid organs and bone marrow have a reticular connective tissue framework. This lymph node specimen was prepared with a silver stain so the reticular fibers (dark lines) can be seen. Contrast the thin, black, branching, reticular fibers (Type III collagen) with the light brown, thicker, collagenous fibers of the capsule (Ca). (×200) **(B)** This is an enlargement of the boxed region in **A**. Branched reticular fibers (RF) and collagen bundles (CF) are visible. Most of the cells are lymphocytes. (×400)

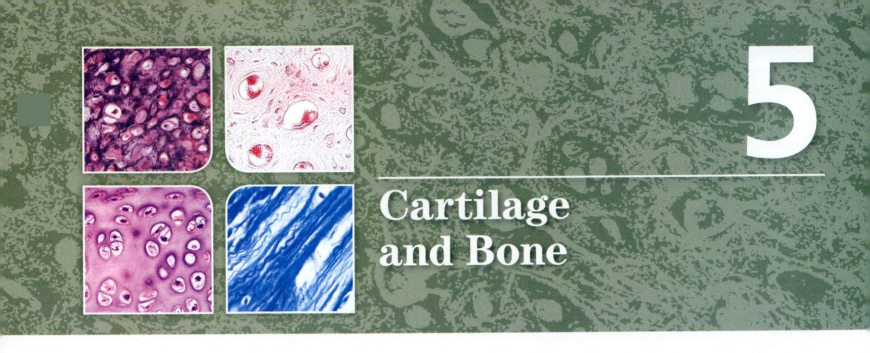

5

Cartilage and Bone

Introduction to Skeletal Tissues

Cartilage and bone are specialized connective tissues with a firm to rigid **matrix,** suiting them for their supportive and protective functions (Figure 5-1).

Basic Characteristics of Cartilage— Matrix, Cells, and Perichondrium

Cartilage is on joint surfaces; forms the framework of the nose, ears, respiratory tree, and part of the rib cage; and is located between vertebrae. It also comprises a majority of

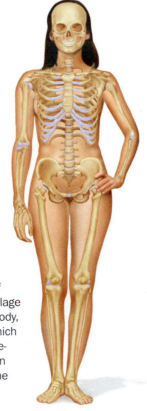

5-1 Skeletal System ◾
The skeleton is composed of bone tissue (beige) and cartilage (light blue). It supports the body, acts as a lever system on which muscles act to produce movement, and provides protection for vital organs, such as in the rib cage and skull.

the embryonic skeletal system before it is replaced by bone. The semirigid matrix makes cartilage well suited for these supporting functions.

Embryonically, cartilage begins developing from mesenchyme in chondrification centers. The mesenchymal cells differentiate into **chondroblasts,** which begin secreting cartilage matrix. When they become surrounded by matrix, they are called **chondrocytes** and the space each chondrocyte occupies is called a **lacuna** (Figures 5-2 and 5-3). When a chondrocyte grows and divides, it forms an **isogenous group** of cells in the lacuna. These cells continue producing matrix and become separated into different lacunae. The result is cartilage growth from the interior of the matrix, a process known as **interstitial growth.**

The characteristic consistency of the matrix is due to the grouped arrangement of proteoglycans and its degree of hydration. The matrix immediately around each lacuna is basophilic and is called **territorial matrix; interterritorial matrix** is found between lacunae (Figure 5-3). **Collagen** and **elastic fibers** (only in elastic cartilage) are present in the matrix and confer strength and flexibility, respectively. Most of the time collagen fibers are not easily seen in cartilage, even though they are abundant. A silver stain (or other specialized elastin stain) must be used to visualize elastic fibers because H&E does not differentiate them.

Cartilage is **avascular** (and also lacks lymphatics and nerves), but receives nourishment from blood vessels in the **perichondrium,** the fibrous membrane that surrounds most cartilage (Figure 5-4). It is composed of a superficial **fibrous layer** and a deeper **chondrogenic cell layer.** In **appositional growth,** the chondrogenic cells differentiate into chondroblasts that secrete new matrix on the cartilage's surface.

Types of Cartilage

There are three types of cartilage: hyaline cartilage, elastic cartilage, and fibrocartilage. Of the three, **hyaline cartilage** (Figures 5-3 through 5-5) is the most abundant. It is found in the nose and respiratory tree, on the sternal ends of the ribs, and on articular surfaces. It also forms the cartilage model for most of the skeleton during development. The matrix of hyaline cartilage is glassy in appearance (hence, "hyaline") and has Type II collagen fibers in it, though they are not easily seen with the light microscope. The pliancy of hyaline cartilage is attributable to the high degree of matrix hydration (between 60% and 80% of its weight). Water also provides a medium through which oxygen and nutrients can diffuse from the blood vessels in the perichondrium to the chondrocytes.

Articular cartilage (Figure 5-6) is a remnant of the embryonic hyaline cartilage bone[1] prior to **ossification** (bone formation). It differs slightly in chemical composition from adult hyaline cartilage, but the most obvious difference is its lack of perichondrium on the articular surface. In its stead, chondrocytes are nourished by the **synovial (joint) fluid.**

Elastic cartilage (Figure 5-7) is found in the ears and epiglottis. It is very similar to hyaline cartilage, except that its matrix has numerous elastic fibers in addition to the Type II collagen fibers. The chondrocytes also tend to be larger (at the expense of the matrix) and more numerous than in hyaline cartilage. A perichondrium is present.

Fibrocartilage (Figure 5-8) can be found joining bones (e.g., pubic symphysis and intervertebral disks) and within joint cavities (e.g., menisci of the knees). The abundance of Types I and II collagen fibers in the matrix make fibrocartilage resistant to compressive and shearing forces. Chondrocytes (identifiable by their rounded nuclei) tend to be seen in rows parallel to the fiber bundles, whereas fibroblasts (identifiable by flattened nuclei) may be seen among the fibers. There is no perichondrium.

Basic Characteristics of Bone— Matrix and Cells

Bone matrix is composed of about 25% organic (mostly Type I collagen) and 65% inorganic (calcium hydroxyapatite crystals) materials, with most of the remainder being water. The collagen provides some flexibility and tensile strength to the bone, whereas the inorganic materials confer hardness. There are four major cells of bone tissue. These are osteoprogenitor cells, osteoblasts, osteocytes, and osteoclasts.

Osteoprogenitor cells (Figure 5-9) are derived from mesenchymal cells and have the ability to differentiate into osteoblasts, and under some circumstances, into chondrogenic cells. They are elongated cells and are found associated with periosteum and endosteum of adult bones (see "Membranes of Bone").

Osteoblasts (Figure 5-9) develop from osteoprogenitor cells and therefore are also found lining external and internal bone surfaces, but they have more of a cuboidal shape. Osteoblasts are actively involved in secreting collagen-rich **osteoid,** the precursor to true bone matrix, during bone growth, repair, and remodeling. Osteoblasts subsequently calcify osteoid to make the bony matrix hard.

Osteocytes (Figure 5-9) are osteoblasts that have become surrounded and trapped by matrix. They occupy **lacunae** in the matrix and are responsible for maintaining and modifying matrix composition. They are connected to each other by long, thin cytoplasmic extensions (processes) and are discussed in "Types of Bone Tissue."

Osteoclasts (Figures 5-9 and 5-10) are large, multinucleate cells responsible for bone resorption; that is, they destroy bony matrix. They are often found associated with a pit in the bone called a **Howship's lacuna,** or **resorption bay.** Osteoclasts are active during the growth, repair, and remodeling processes. Their activities are balanced with those of osteoblasts so that (normally) bone mass remains constant.

Membranes of Bone

Bone surfaces are lined with one of two fibrous membranes: periosteum or endosteum. **Periosteum** (Figure 5-11) is the fibrous membrane that surrounds bone. Like its counterpart in cartilage, periosteum has a superficial **fibrous layer** and a deeper **cellular layer**. The cellular layer has osteoprogenitor cells that have the ability to become bone-forming cells. Periosteum is attached to bone by **Sharpey's fibers,** collagen bundles that penetrate the bone matrix (Figure 5-12). All internal surfaces are lined with a reticular connective tissue called **endosteum,** which is also associated with osteoprogenitor cells (Figure 5-13).

Types of Bone Tissue

Bone tissue is of two types: **spongy (cancellous) bone** and **compact bone** (Figure 5-14). Both types are in all bones, but their relative amounts differ depending on the particular bone and the specific part of the bone.

Compact bone is found on the bone's surface (deep to periosteum or articular cartilage) and has a dense bony matrix composed of lamellae (plates). **Circumferential lamellae** encircle the diaphysis of long bones on both inner and outer surfaces. Other lamellae will be described below.

Because diffusion is poor through calcified tissue, osteocytes embedded in the dense matrix are supplied by local blood vessels, which travel through canals in the matrix. Nerves are also found in these canals. **Volkmann's (perforating) canals** penetrate from the surface and **Haversian canals** run more or less parallel to the surface (Figures 5-15 and 5-16). The structural and functional unit of compact bone is the **Haversian system** or **osteon** (Figure 5-17). Each Haversian system consists of a central Haversian canal with its

---

[1] Notice that in this context, "bone" refers to an organ, not a tissue.

neurovascular bundle. The bony matrix is arranged in rings of **concentric lamellae** around the canal with osteocytes occupying lacunae at their junctions. Osteocytes maintain contact with other osteocytes by way of cellular processes that pass through tiny **canaliculi**. (These connections were first made when the cells were osteoblasts.) In this fashion, nutrients and oxygen from the blood vessel can diffuse from cell to cell outward toward the periphery of the Haversian system. A calcified cement line encircles the outer margin of the Haversian system. **Interstitial lamellae** can be seen as remnants of old Haversian systems as a consequence of bone remodeling.

Spongy bone (Figure 5-18) is found in the interior of bones. It is made of a delicate network of bony **trabeculae** that are arranged to strengthen the bone according to the mechanical loads placed on it. Irregular arrangements of lamellae are present, but Haversian systems are not.

:: Bone Growth

There are two basic mechanisms of bone growth. In **intramembranous ossification**, bone forms within a mesenchymal membrane. In **endochondral ossification**, bone tissue replaces a hyaline cartilage model. In both mechanisms, bone is initially formed as woven (nonlamellar or bundle) bone, which differs from mature bone in its less organized arrangement of collagen fibers and cells, higher cell density, and lower mineral content.

Intramembranous ossification (Figure 5-19) is responsible for producing the flat bones of the skull. The process is relatively straightforward.

1. Mesenchymal cells differentiate into osteoblasts at the **primary center of ossification** and begin depositing bony matrix to form **trabeculae** (strips) of bone.

2. Ossification continues radially from the ossification center, like ripples spreading from dropping something in water.

3. Bone marrow develops in the spaces between trabeculae.

4. Periosteum and endosteum develop from the unossified mesenchyme membrane.

5. The surfaces are remodeled to form compact bone. In the skull, these layers are called **inner** and **outer tables**. The spongy bone between them is the **diploë**.

Endochondral ossification produces most bones of the skeleton, and is most easily understood by studying appendicular long bones. While studying this process, it is important to remember that the cartilagenous model grows in length and diameter, even as parts of it are being replaced by bone. (After all, the skeleton must be functional and an appropriate size at all times during embryonic and postnatal growth.) Endochondral ossification is outlined in Figure 5-20 and can be summarized by the following steps:

1. Hyaline cartilage occupies the **zone of reserve cartilage** and acts as a source of cartilage to undergo the process described below.

2. Normal chondrocytes multiply in the **zone of proliferation (multiplication)**.

3. The chondrocytes enlarge (hypertrophy) in the **zone of hypertrophy**.

4. The cartilage matrix calcifies in the **zone of calcification**.

5. Chondrocytes deteriorate and die, and bone is deposited on the remaining fragments of calcified matrix in the **zone of ossification**.

6. Osteoclasts remove the newly formed bone to make the marrow cavity in the **zone of erosion**.

Examine the photomicrographs in Figures 5-21 through 5-27 as you read the details of this process. (Remember, this description is for long bones. The same events occur in other bones, but the zones are not as clearly defined, making the process more difficult to understand.)

1. Endochondral ossification begins with a bone made of hyaline cartilage. A **primary center of ossification** (Figure 5-21a) appears at the center of the shaft (diaphysis). There, osteoblasts develop deep to the perichondrium and deposit a ring of periosteal bone called a **bony collar** (Figure 5-21a). The bony collar acts as a splint to support the bone as the internal cartilage is eroded away. The perichondrium develops into a periosteum.

2. Chondrocytes internal to the bony collar begin multiplying and enlarging at the expense of the matrix. What matrix is left becomes calcified and appears more basophilic. Because the calcified matrix retards diffusion of oxygen and nutrients, chondrocytes begin to deteriorate and eventually die within the enlarged lacunae. This process accomplishes two things: It reduces the amount of cartilage matrix remaining in the bone and it provides space for bone tissue to be deposited.

3. Blood vessels (**periosteal buds**) grow into the enlarged lacunae (which form primary marrow spaces, Figures 5-21b and 5-21c). They bring mesenchymal cells that differentiate into osteoprogenitor cells in the marrow spaces. The latter differentiate into osteoblasts that deposit osteoid and then bone on the remaining cartilagenous fragments. **Hemopoietic stem cells** also enter and begin producing marrow.

4. After a region has ossified, osteoclasts move in and resorb the bone to form the marrow cavity (Figure 5-21d). This will not occur during endochondral ossification of short or irregular bones that lack a marrow cavity (although osteoclasts are present and active during remodeling of all bones).

5. The process of bone replacing cartilage spreads toward the ends of the bones (**epiphyses**), following the same sequence of events as occurred in the primary center: enlargement and multiplication of chondrocytes, calcification of matrix, death of chondrocytes, and deposition of bone (Figures 5-22 and 5-23).

6. Growth in diameter occurs as **periosteal bone** is deposited on the surface while osteoclast activity removes bone from the marrow cavity side of the diaphysis (Figure 5-24).

7. All bone tissue initially forms as woven bone, so it must be remodeled on the surface to become compact bone. The process involves deposition of the lamellae from outermost to innermost around the neurovascular bundle, which ends up in the remaining space, the Haversian canal (Figure 5-25).

8. At about the time of birth, **secondary centers of ossification** appear in one or both ends (epiphyses) of the long bone (Figure 5-26). These ossify the epiphyses, leaving cartilage in two places: on the surface of the epiphysis as **articular cartilage**, and in the **epiphyseal plate** that joins the epiphysis with the diaphysis (Figure 5-27). The epiphyseal plate continues to produce new cartilage on its epiphyseal side at the same rate it is being replaced by bone on the diaphyseal side. In this fashion, the plate remains the same thickness, but appears to grow away from the center of the bone. This results in longitudinal growth of the bone. At some time during development (typical for each bone), the epiphyseal plate ossifies and longitudinal growth is completed. Frequently, an **epiphyseal line** is visible in the spongy bone where the epiphyseal plate ossified.

■■ Synovial Articulations

Synovial joints (Figure 5-28) are characterized by having a **synovial (joint) cavity**. This makes them freely movable. Lining the bones' surfaces is articular cartilage. It is made of modified hyaline cartilage (from the original cartilage model that remained unossified) without a perichondrium. Lining the cavity is a vascular and fibrous **synovial membrane** that secretes a lubricating **synovial fluid** (Figure 5-29). The membrane's surface is lined with cells called **synoviocytes**. Strengthening the joint from the outside is a fibrous **joint capsule** that is continuous with the periosteum of the articulating bones. The capsule may contain thickenings that act as **ligaments**, or the ligaments may be separate from the capsule. Other cartilages (generally fibrocartilage) may be associated with the interior of the joint. The **menisci** of the knee joint are an example.

■■ Muscular Attachments to Bone

Skeletal muscles either attach to bone directly or by way of a **tendon**. In the first instance, the muscle fibers extend to the periosteum and the connective tissue components of the muscle blend in with the connective tissue fibers of the periosteum (Figure 5-30). The periosteum itself is attached to the bone by Sharpey's fibers, which are especially substantial at the point of muscular attachment. If the muscle attaches by way of a tendon, then it is the tendon fibers that mix with the periosteal fibers.

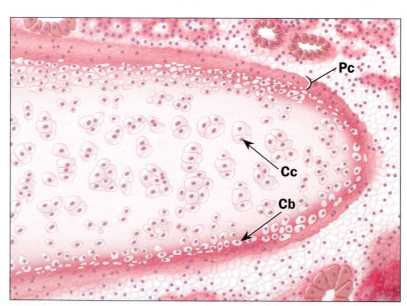

5-2 **Illustration of Cartilage Structure** ■ Cartilage is composed of chondrocytes (Cc) embedded in a firm, gel-like matrix containing collagen fibers. Surrounding hyaline and elastic cartilage is the fibrous and vascular perichondrium (Pc); fibrocartilage has no perichondrium. Growth of the cartilage is due to activity of chondroblasts (Cb) located at the junction of the perichondrium and cartilage. The main difference between the three types of cartilage is the abundance and type of fibers reinforcing the matrix.

A Photographic Atlas of Histology

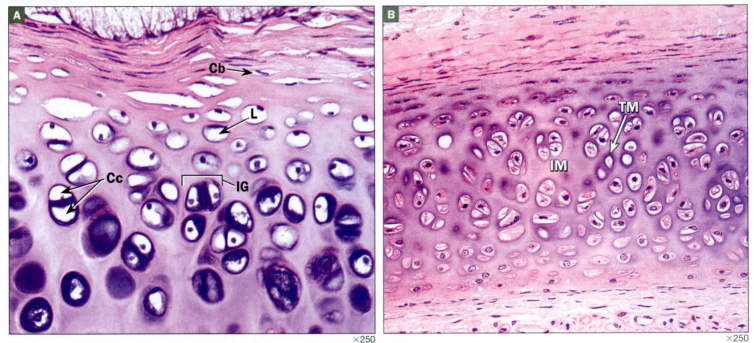

×250

×250

5-3 Cartilage Components ■ Two specimens of hyaline cartilage are shown; each with different components labeled (though all are visible in both micrographs). (**A**) Cells include chondroblasts (Cb) near the surface and chondrocytes (Cc) toward the interior. Where a chondrocyte has divided, the cluster is called an isogenous group (IG). Chondrocytes occupy lacunae (cavities) in the matrix (L). These are only seen as artifacts of preparation—either the chondrocyte fell out or shrinkage exposed the space. (×250) (**B**) The matrix is not of uniform molecular composition and this is manifested in different staining properties. Territorial matrix (TM) around the chondrocytes has less collagen, more sulfur-containing molecules, and stains darker than the interterritorial matrix (IM) between lacunae. (×250)

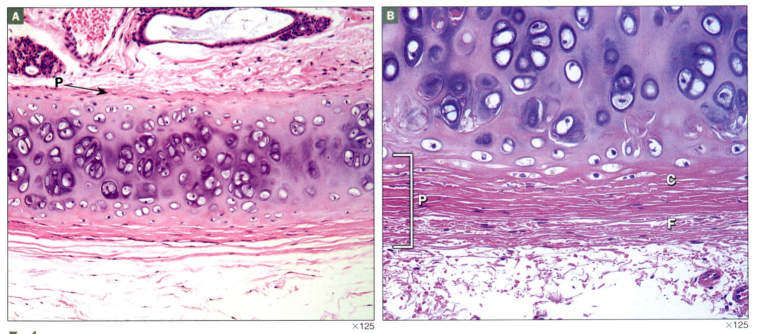

×125

×125

5-4 Perichondrium ■ The vascular fibrous membrane around cartilage is called perichondrium (P). (**A**) The pink layer is the perichondrium surrounding hyaline cartilage. The distinction between the outer fibrous layer and inner chondrogenic layer is not sharp. (×125) (**B**) This hyaline cartilage specimen has a thicker perichondrium. The outer fibrous (F) and inner chondrogenic (C) layers are visible, but still are not sharply separated. (×125)

5-5 **Hyaline Cartilage** ■ This section of the nasal septum illustrates hyaline cartilage, the most common cartilage in the body. Note the chondrocytes (Cc), the perichondrium (P), and the smooth matrix (M) lacking obvious fibers (though they are present). Figures 5-3 and 5-4 are also hyaline cartilage. (×250)

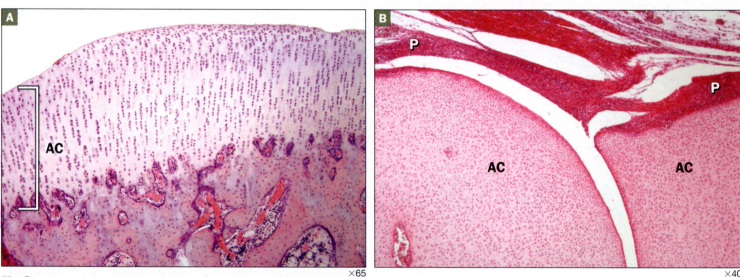

5-6 **Articular Cartilage** ■ The modified hyaline cartilage covering joint surfaces, called articular cartilage, lacks a perichondrium. (**A**) This bone has been removed from its joint during preparation, but the articular cartilage (AC) on its joint surface is apparent—as is the absence of perichondrium. (×65) (**B**) This micrograph shows two bones in an embryonic pig foot. They have not undergone ossification and remain as cartilage models of the bones they will become. Notice the perichondrium (P) connects these bones without extending over their articular surfaces. (×40)

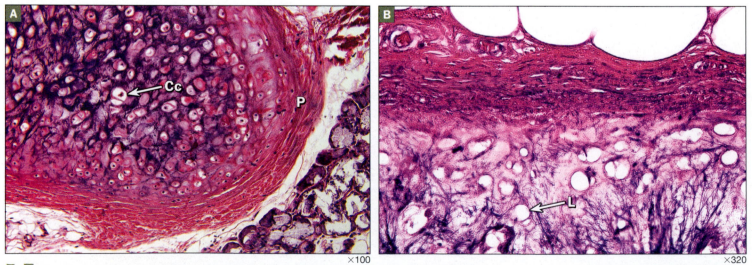

5-7 **Elastic Cartilage** ■ The framework of the ear and epiglottis is made up of elastic cartilage. A silver stain was used to highlight the elastic fibers in these two epiglottis specimens. They are the black lines. (**A**) Notice the perichondrium (P) and relatively large chondrocytes (Cc). (×100) (**B**) This higher magnification clearly shows the individual elastic fibers. Most chondrocytes have been lost during preparation, so mostly you see lacunae (L). (×320)

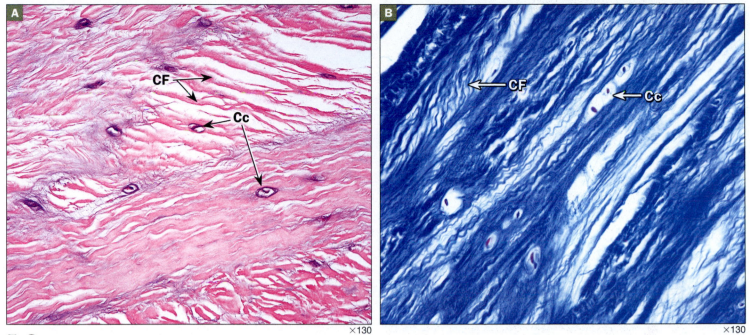

5-8 Fibrocartilage ◼ Intervertebral disks and the pubic symphysis are made up of fibrocartilage. It is characterized by dense bundles of collagen fibers (CF) in its matrix and the absence of a perichondrium. Often the chondrocytes (Cc) occur in lines, as in (**B**). Both specimens are from intervertebral disks. (Both ×130)

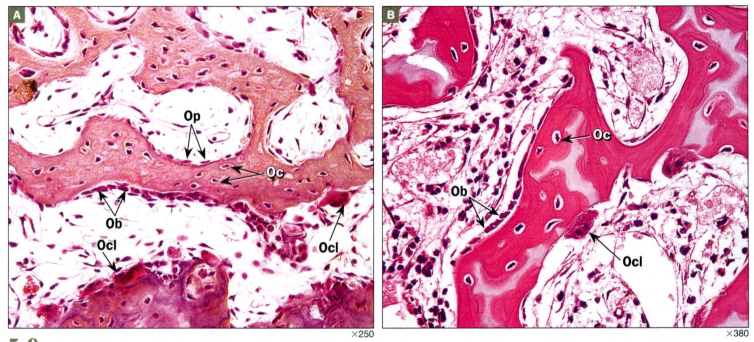

5-9 Bone Cells ◼ These two micrographs show the four types of bone cells. Osteoprogenitor cells (Op) and osteoblasts (Ob) are found in rows on the surface of bone, associated either with endosteum or periosteum. Osteoprogenitor cells are flatter than osteoblasts. Osteocytes (Oc) are cells of mature bone and are encased by the bony matrix. Osteoclasts (Ocl) are large, multinucleate cells found on the surface of bone. Micrograph (**A**) was magnified ×250. Micrograph (**B**) was magnified ×380.

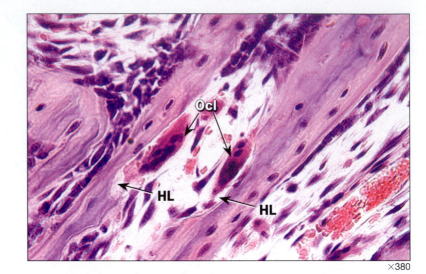
×380

5-10 Osteoclasts ■ Bone is resorbed by multinucleate osteo-clasts (Ocl). They often erode a pit in the surface of the bone called a Howship's lacuna (HL). (×380)

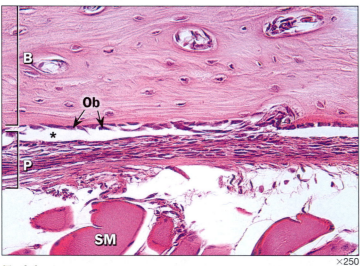
×250

5-11 Periosteum ■ Periosteum (P) is the fibrous membrane around bone (B). It has an outer fibrous layer and an inner osteogenic layer with osteoprogenitor or osteoblast (Ob) cells. In this specimen, the space (*) is an artifact of preparation. The pink tissue at the bottom of the field is skeletal muscle (SM). (×250)

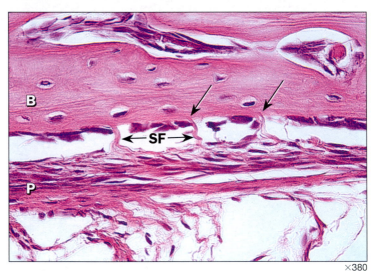
×380

5-12 Sharpey's Fibers ■ Periosteum (P) is anchored to the bone (B) by collagen bundles called Sharpey's fibers (SF), which penetrate the bony matrix (arrows). (×380)

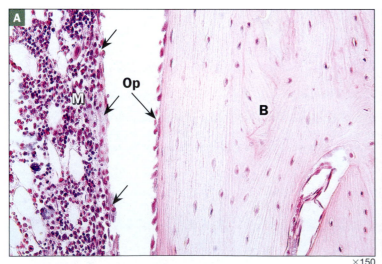
×150

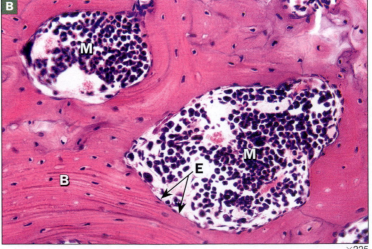
×225

5-13 Endosteum ■ All inner surfaces of bone (B) are lined with a delicate connective tissue, called endosteum (E), associated with a layer of osteopro-genitor cells (Op). (**A**) The endosteal cells form a clearly defined layer in this image, because the marrow (M) and much of the fibrous endosteum (arrows) shrunk during slide preparation. (×150) (**B**) The two cavities are filled with red bone marrow, but the endosteal cell layer is still recognizable (arrows). (×225)

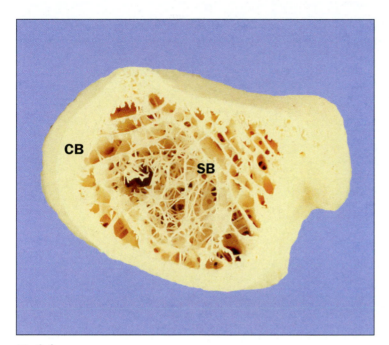

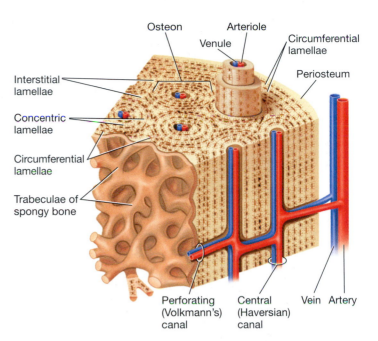

Osteon   Arteriole
Venule   Circumferential
                    lamellae
Interstitial   Periosteum
lamellae
Concentric
lamellae
Circumferential
lamellae
Trabeculae of
spongy bone
                Perforating   Central   Vein Artery
                (Volkmann's)   (Haversian)
                canal   canal

5-14 **Types of Adult Bone Tissue** ◼ Dense, compact bone (CB) covers outer surfaces, whereas the interior of a bone is composed of more delicate spongy bone (SB) tissue. Both types are found in all bones, but in different proportions. (Photograph by Gary D. Wisehart)

5-15 **Lamellae and Canal System of Compact Bone** ◼ Compact bone is deposited in lamellae (plates). Shown are circumferential lamellae around both surfaces, concentric lamellae of the Haversian systems (osteons), and interstitial lamellae between Haversian systems. Volkmann's (perforating) canals allow passage of blood vessels and nerves into the bone from both surfaces, whereas Haversian canals run parallel to the surface and form the center of Haversian systems.

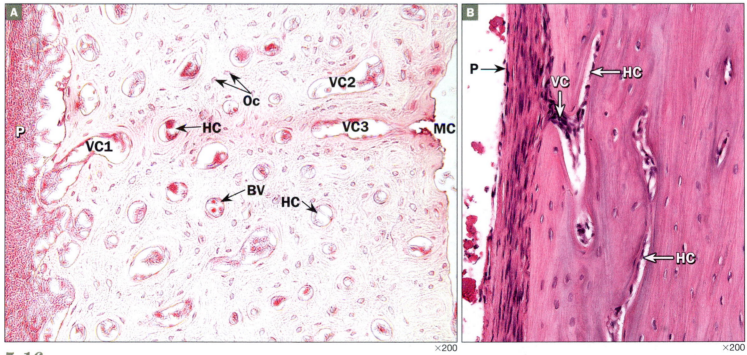

×200   ×200

5-16 **The Canals of Compact Bone** ◼ Shown are two decalcified bone specimens. Using this preparation method (as opposed to a ground bone preparation; see Figure 5-17) preserves the osteocytes (Oc) in their lacunae and blood vessels (BV) in the canal system. The periosteum (P) is also visible. (**A**) In this cross section, Volkmann's canals are cut longitudinally (VC1 and VC3) or obliquely (VC2). Notice that VC1 shows continuity with the outer bone surface, whereas VC3 appears to open to the marrow cavity (MC) but in a different plane. Haversian canals (HC) are cut in cross section. In this specimen, the Haversian system is better defined by the osteocytes' circular arrangement around the canal than by the faintly visible concentric lamellae. (×200) (**B**) In this longitudinal section, Haversian canals are cut longitudinally and run along the length of the bone. The single Volkmann's canal is cut longitudinally over its short length and shows continuity with the surface. (Note: it is possible for Volkmann's canals in a longitudinal section of the bone to be cut in cross section if the plane of section were 90° to this one.) Note the absence of circular lamellae and the random osteocyte arrangement in the vicinity of the Volkmann's canal. (×200)

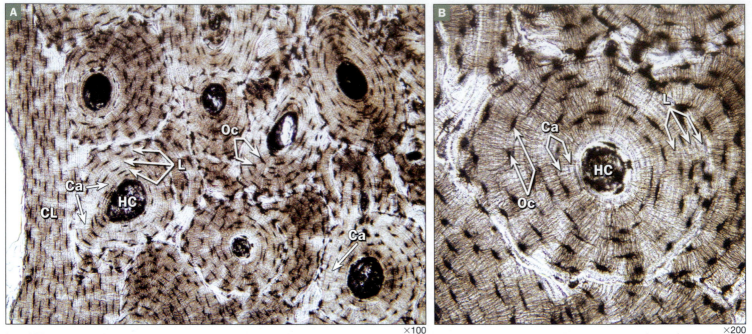

×100

×200

5-17 **Compact Bone in Cross Section (Ground Bone Preparation)** ▪ Due to the hardness of compact bone matrix, these specimens were not sectioned with a microtome, but instead were ground down to their final thickness. The osteocytes and blood vessels often are absent from preparations such as these; what you see in the canals and lacunae is debris left from grinding. The central Haversian canals (HC), concentric lamellae (L), osteocytes (or at least their lacunae) (Oc), and canaliculi (Ca), are visible in both specimens. Circumferential lamellae (CL) are visible in (**A**) at the left. (**A**) (×100) (**B**) (×200)

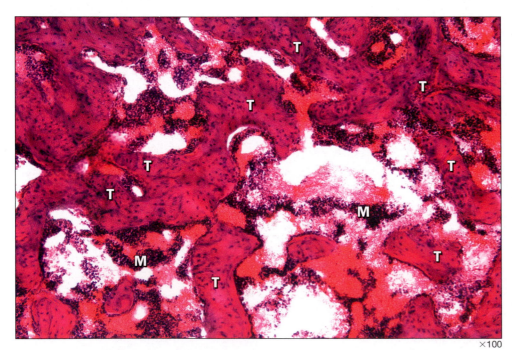

×100

5-18 **Spongy Bone** ▪ Trabeculae (T) of spongy bone contain osteocytes and lamellae of bone, but these are not organized into Haversian systems. Red bone marrow (M) fills the spaces. This specimen is from the skull where spongy bone is called diploë. (×100)

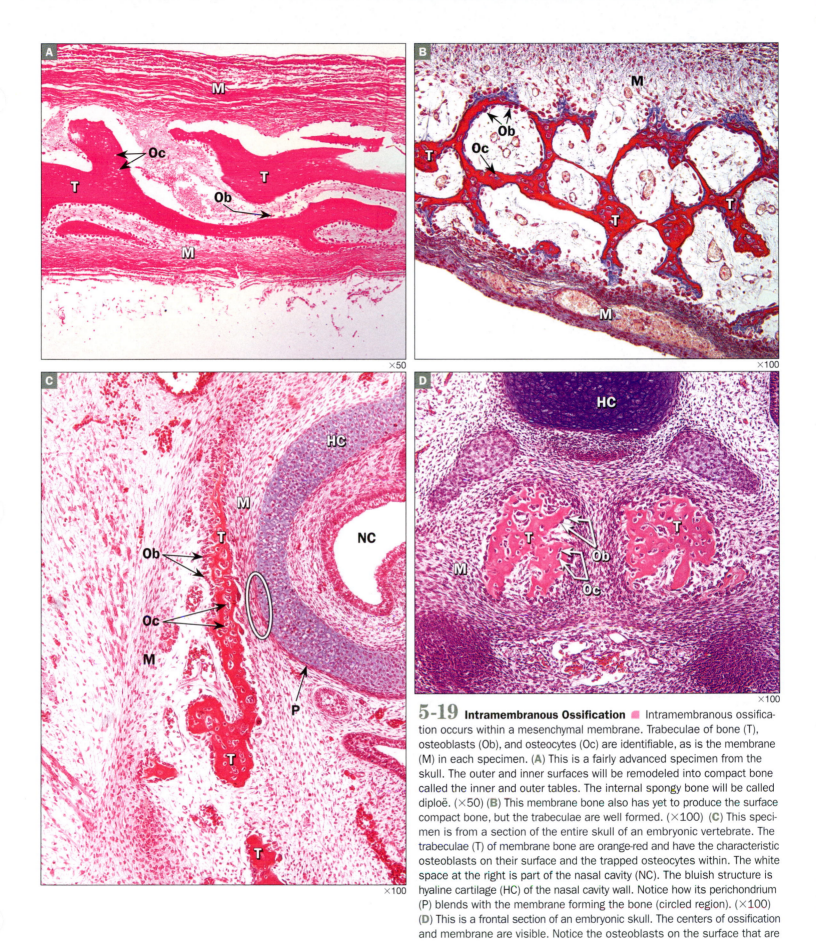

5-19 **Intramembranous Ossification** ■ Intramembranous ossification occurs within a mesenchymal membrane. Trabeculae of bone (T), osteoblasts (Ob), and osteocytes (Oc) are identifiable, as is the membrane (M) in each specimen. (**A**) This is a fairly advanced specimen from the skull. The outer and inner surfaces will be remodeled into compact bone called the inner and outer tables. The internal spongy bone will be called diploë. (×50) (**B**) This membrane bone also has yet to produce the surface compact bone, but the trabeculae are well formed. (×100) (**C**) This specimen is from a section of the entire skull of an embryonic vertebrate. The trabeculae (T) of membrane bone are orange-red and have the characteristic osteoblasts on their surface and the trapped osteocytes within. The white space at the right is part of the nasal cavity (NC). The bluish structure is hyaline cartilage (HC) of the nasal cavity wall. Notice how its perichondrium (P) blends with the membrane forming the bone (circled region). (×100) (**D**) This is a frontal section of an embryonic skull. The centers of ossification and membrane are visible. Notice the osteoblasts on the surface that are partially surrounded by bone. The hyaline cartilage (HC) of the nasal septum is the purple object at the center top. (×100)

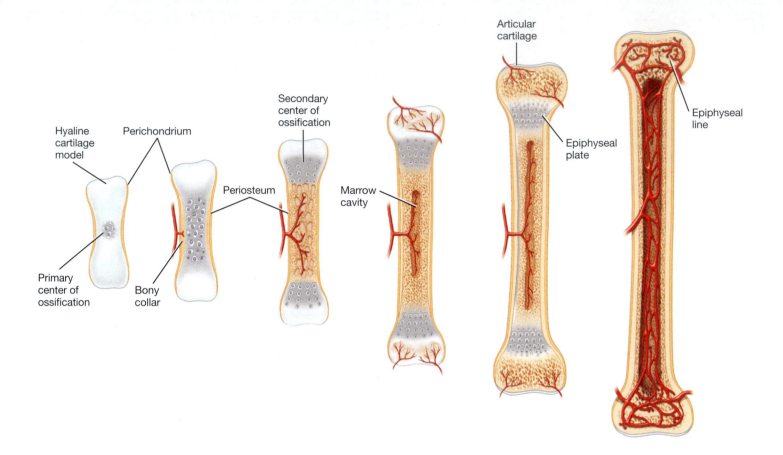

5-20 Endochondral Ossification in a Long Bone 🔲 This complex process starts with a hyaline cartilage model of the bone. The cartilage is replaced by bone tissue as the bone grows in size. See page 52 for details.

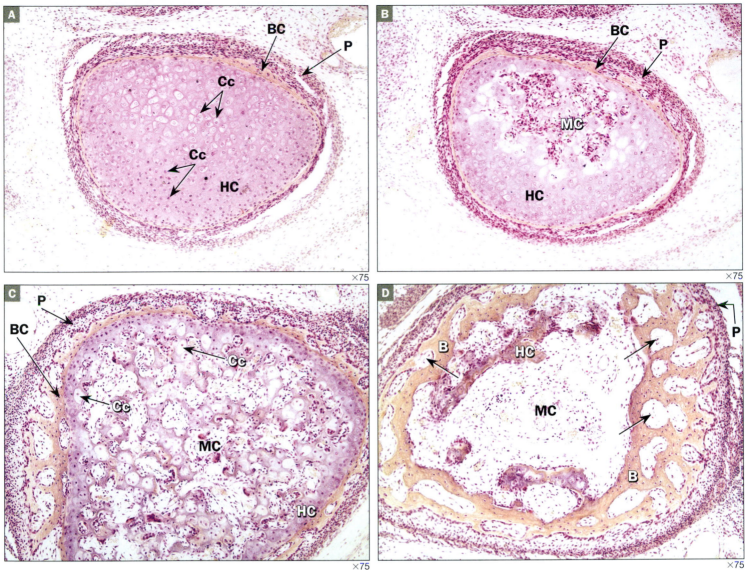

5-21 Endochondral Ossification at the Primary Center Shown in Cross Section ■ Although they are from different bones, this collection of images should allow the reader to piece together the dynamic process of endochondral ossification as it occurs in the diaphysis to produce circumferential growth. All images were magnified (×75). (**A**) The primary center of ossification has become active, as evidenced by the enlarged chondrocytes (Cc) at the center and the orangish bony collar (BC) produced by subperiosteal osteoblasts. The periosteum (P) is also visible and has partially separated from the bone during preparation. Notice that the hyaline cartilage (HC) at the periphery still looks like typical hyaline cartilage. (**B**) The chondrocytes and matrix in the bone's center have enlarged and some have died from lack of oxygen due to the calcified matrix. Osteoblasts and other marrow cells are visible in the primitive marrow cavity (MC). (**C**) The marrow cavity has gotten larger, the bony collar has gotten more complex, and the chondrocytes at the periphery have enlarged. That is, those that remain have reached the stage the interior chondrocytes were at in micrograph (**A**), but very little cartilage remains in the bone's center, having been removed as the chondrocytes enlarged. (**D**) Very little cartilage remains and the marrow cavity has been formed through osteoclast activity on the bone recently produced. The surface bone (B) has begun remodeling into compact bone (note the circular regions that will become Haversian systems—see arrows).

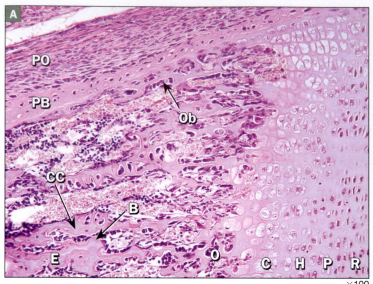

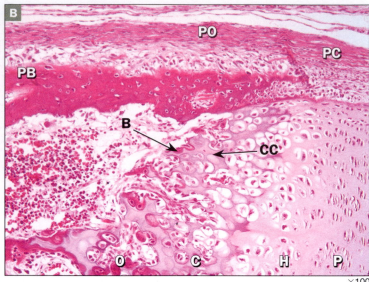

×100 (A)

×100 (B)

5-22 Endochondral Ossification in Longitudinal Section ▪ The zones of endochondral ossification are visible in both specimens, which are oriented so that the process is further along toward the left. Zones of reserve cartilage (R), proliferation (P), hypertrophy (H), calcification (C), ossification (O), and erosion (E) are visible, as are the periosteum (PO), perichondrium (PC), and periosteal bone (PB). (A) Bone tissue is pink in this specimen (see periosteal bone for the shade) as is calcified cartilage (which is somewhat paler). Notice how the spaces produced by deteriorated chondrocytes allow entry of osteoblasts (Ob) that deposit new bone (B) on the remaining slivers of calcified cartilage (CC). (×100) (B) The calcified cartilage (CC) is noticeably darker in this specimen than the normal matrix, but this is not always the case. Bone (B) is a deep pink. (×100)

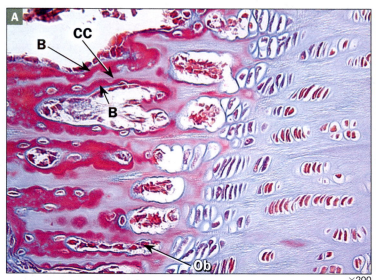

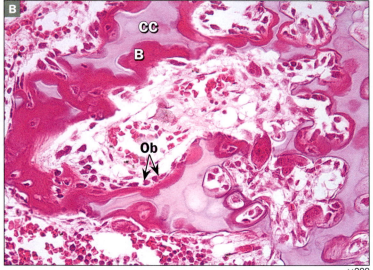

×200 (A)

×200 (B)

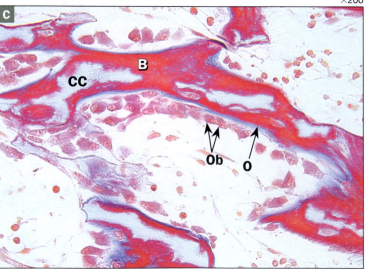

×320 (C)

5-23 Details of Endochondral Ossification ▪ (A) Chondrocytes enlarge and multiply at the expense of matrix. When they die from lack of oxygen in the calcified matrix (CC), there is little of the original cartilage that remains. Bone (B) is deposited on the slivers of calcified cartilage. Osteoblasts (Ob) have aligned themselves in rows on the surface of the growing bone, a very distinctive feature of them. (×200) (B) This image is of the zone of ossification. Bone tissue (B) is deep pink and calcified cartilage (CC) is lavender. Osteoblasts are visible in their characteristic rows on the bone's surface. (×200) (C) In this specimen, bone is orange-red and calcified cartilage is light blue. The blue just deep to the osteoblasts is osteoid (O), the precursor to true bone matrix. (×320)

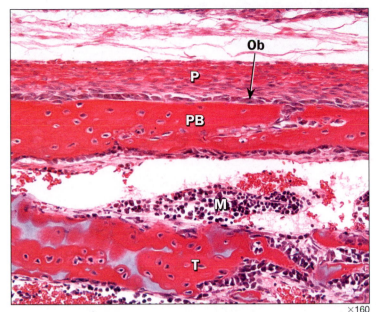

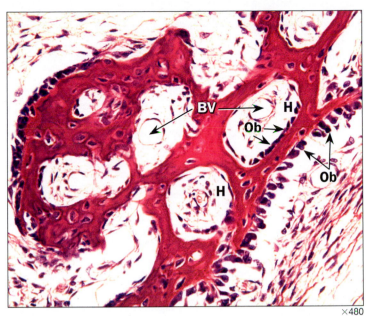

5-24 **Periosteal Bone** ▪ The bony collar is produced by subperioste-al osteoblasts (Ob) located deep in the periosteum (P) and is considered periosteal bone (PB). Growth of the bone in girth (circumferential growth) occurs through the continued pre- and postnatal activity of subperiosteal osteoblasts adding bone tissue to the outside. Meanwhile, osteoclasts resorb bone from the interior to keep the thickness of compact bone appropriate to the bone's size. If this occurs in the diaphysis, the osteoclasts hollow out the interior of most of its bone tissue and form the marrow cavity filled with bone marrow (M). Otherwise, the interior remains spongy bone with marrow filling in the spaces between trabeculae (T). (×160)

5-25 **Surface Remodeling** ▪ Bone tissue is produced as woven bone. The compact bone on bone surfaces is the result of remodeling this bone. Developing Haversian systems (H) are visible in this specimen, as are blood vessels (BV). Osteoblasts (Ob) deposit concentric lamellae in the open region until all that remains is the Haversian canal with its neurovascular bundle. (×480)

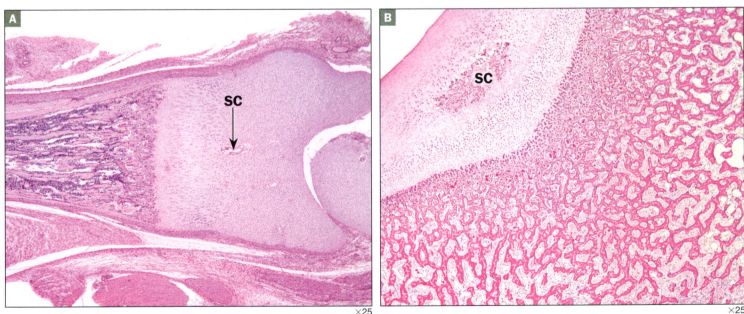

5-26 **Secondary Center of Ossification** ▪ In long bones and some other bones, a secondary center (SC) of ossification opens in the epiphysis sometime after birth. The secondary center completely ossifies the epiphysis except for two regions that remain hyaline cartilage: the epiphyseal plate that connects the epiphysis and diaphysis, and the articular cartilage. Both micrographs are ×25 and show early activity in the secondary center.

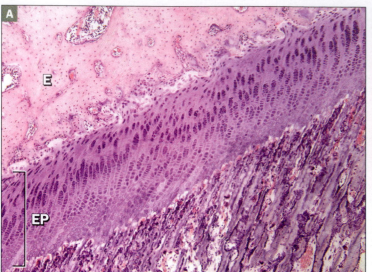

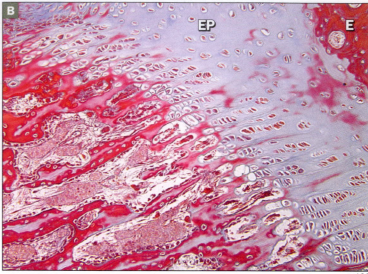

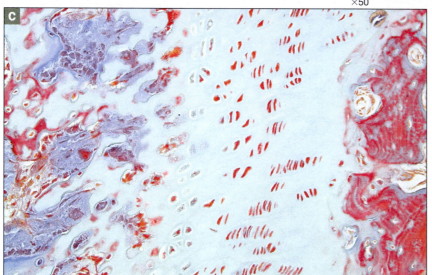

5-27 Epiphyseal Plate ▪ After birth, longitudinal growth in long bones is due to the activity of the epiphyseal plate (EP) of hyaline cartilage that joins the epiphysis with the diaphysis. All the zones of cartilage being replaced by bone are compressed into the epiphyseal plate; all are there, but there may be some overlap. New cartilage is formed on the epiphyseal side at the same rate as cartilage is replaced by bone on the diaphyseal side of the plate. (**A**) New bone is forming on the lower side of this epiphyseal plate, so the epiphysis (E) is being pushed upward in this micrograph. (×50) (**B**) The epiphysis is toward the upper right in this micrograph. Bone is red, reserve cartilage is light blue, and calcified cartilage is lavender. (×100) (**C**) The epiphysis is toward the right in this specimen prepared with Mallory triple stain. Chondrocyte nuclei are red, as is bone tissue. Hyaline cartilage is light blue and calcified cartilage is darker blue. (×200)

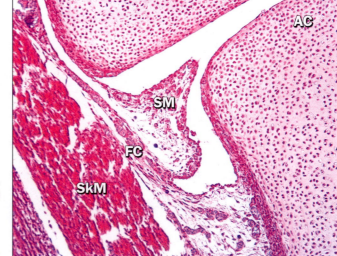

5-28 Embryonic Synovial Joint ▪ Synovial joints are freely movable. The bones involved (which have yet to ossify in this embryonic specimen) are held together with a fibrous articular capsule (FC). The joint cavity is lined with a vascular synovial membrane (SM) that secretes a lubricating synovial fluid. Also notice the articular cartilage (AC) lacking a perichondrium. Developing skeletal muscle (SkM) is visible in the lower left of the field. (×100)

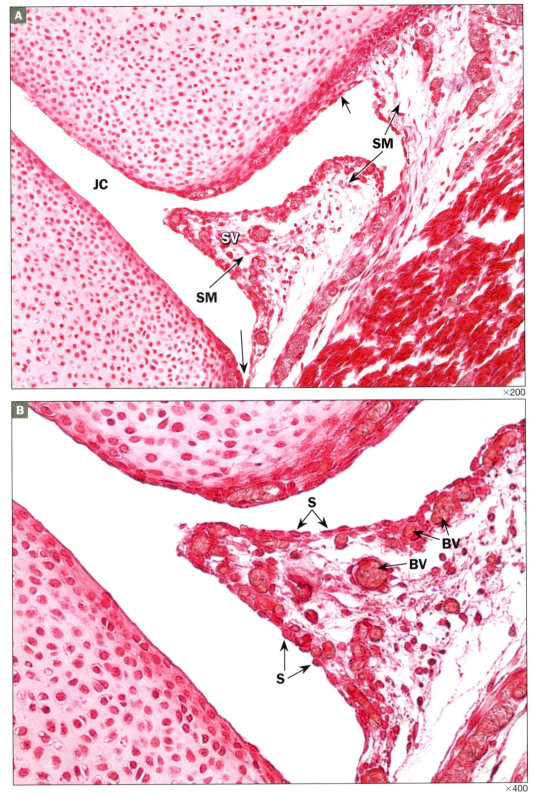

5-29 **Embryonic Synovial Membrane** ■ The source of synovial fluid is the vascular synovial membrane (SM). (**A**) In this view of a developing synovial joint, notice the continuity of the synovial membrane from one bone to the other (arrow to arrow). The synovial sac formed from this membrane encloses the joint cavity (JC) (think in three dimensions) and is filled with synovial fluid. The projection is a synovial villus (SV). (×200) (**B**) This is a higher magnification of the same villus. In it notice the synoviocytes (S) lining the membrane and the abundant blood vessels (BV) in the loose connective tissue in its interior. (×400)

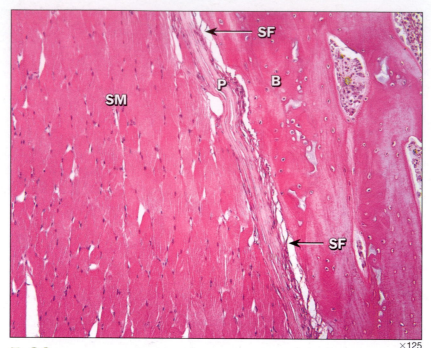

×125

5-30 **Muscular Attachment to Bone** ■ In this specimen the connective tissue of the skeletal muscle (SM) blends with the periosteum (P), which in turn is attached to the bone (B) with Sharpey's fibers (SF). If the muscle had a prominent tendon, it would do the same (see Figure 7-9). Notice that in this specimen all tissues are pink, so identification relies on differing textures and distribution of nuclei. (×125)

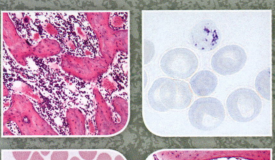

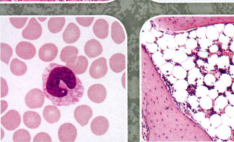

6

Blood and Bone Marrow

:: Introduction to Blood

Blood functions as a transport medium between organs specialized for contacting and exchanging materials with the environment and the remainder of cells buried in the body. It transports oxygen from the lungs to other body cells and carbon dioxide from these same cells back to the lungs. It distributes nutrients absorbed by the intestines and stored in the liver throughout the body, and it picks up wastes and transports them to the kidneys for excretion. In addition, it is involved in transporting cells of the body's defenses to sites where they are needed and distributing heat and hormones throughout the body.

Blood is a specialized connective tissue, with cells dispersed in a fluid intercellular material called **plasma**. Because some blood cells are not actually cells when functional, the "cellular" portion is said to be made of **formed elements** (Figure 6.1).

:: Formed Elements of Blood

When blood is spun in a centrifuge tube, the plasma separates from it and is found on top of the formed elements (Figure 6-2). Comprising the majority of the formed elements is a red layer made up of **erythrocytes (red blood cells, RBCs)**. On top of the erythrocytes is the narrow **buffy coat layer** made up of leukocytes (white blood cells, WBCs) and **platelets (thrombocytes)**. The formed elements constitute 45% of the blood volume, of which the erythrocytes and buffy coat layers account for 44% and 1%, respectively. Plasma comprises the remaining 55%. The following are typical cell densities for each (Figure 6-3):

■ Red blood cells: 4.2 to 5.4 million and 4.7 to 6.1 million RBCs per cubic millimeter (or microliter–μL) of blood in females and males, respectively

■ White blood cells: between 4,800 and 10,800 (average 8,000) per cubic millimeter (or μL) of blood

■ Platelets: between 150,000 and 350,000—it is difficult to get an accurate count—per cubic millimeter (or μL) of blood.

Erythrocytes (Figure 6-4) are biconcave disc-shaped cells with an average diameter of 7 to 8 μm

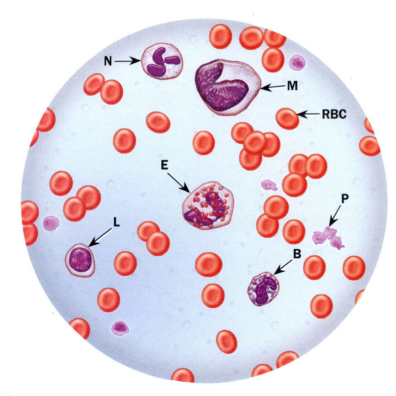

6-1 Blood Cells ■ The formed elements of blood include erythrocytes (red blood cells, RBC), leukocytes (white blood cells), and thrombocytes (platelets, P). White blood cells include neutrophils (N), monocytes (M), eosinophils (E), lymphocytes (L), and basophils (B).

and a thickness of 1.5 to 2.5 μm. They develop from cells in bone marrow, lose most organelles (including their nucleus) during maturation, and are little more than bags of the red oxygen-carrying pigment **hemoglobin** (plus a few soluble enzymes) when functional in the blood. Their shape increases surface area for oxygen exchange and makes them pliable enough to fit through the smallest blood vessels (3 to 4 μm in diameter).

Leukocytes differ from erythrocytes in a number of ways: they are larger, nucleated, and although found in the blood during transport, they usually function outside of it in the tissues. They are divided into two major groups: **granulocytes** and **agranulocytes**. Granulocytes have prominent cytoplasmic granules whose staining properties are a primary basis for differentiating the three major types (**neutrophils, eosinophils,** and **basophils**—see below). They are produced in the bone marrow and have **azurophilic** cytoplasmic granules in addition to the specific granules of each cell type. These are modified lysosomes and stain light purple. In addition, they have multi-lobed, or segmented, nuclei, which leads to the other name for this group: **polymorphonuclear leukocytes (PMNs)**. The characteristics of each granulocyte follows.

Neutrophils (Figure 6-5) are the most abundant leuko-cytes, accounting for between 60% and 70% of all leukocytes in blood. They are slightly larger than RBCs (9 to 12 μm in diameter) and have a multilobed nucleus with the lobes often joined by thin nuclear strands. Their cytoplasmic granules are unstained or are slightly lavender in standard blood smear preparations (Wright's or Giemsa stains). Functionally, they are short-lived (days) phagocytic cells.

Eosinophils (Figure 6-6) comprise less than 5% of all leukocytes in the blood. They are somewhat larger than neutrophils (10 to 14 μm in diameter), have a two-lobed nucleus, and their cytoplasmic granules stain red in stan-dard blood smears. They are active in combating parasitic infections, phagocytose antigen-antibody complexes, and temper allergic reactions.

Basophils (Figure 6-7) are rare in the blood, comprising less than 1% of all leukocytes. They are slightly larger than RBCs (8 to10 μm in diameter) and have prominent, dark-purple cytoplasmic granules that make seeing the S-shaped nucleus difficult. They are involved in the inflammatory re-sponse and like mast cells, are involved in hypersensitivity reactions.

Agranulocytes have unlobed nuclei and azurophilic granules, but lack the prominent specific granules of granu-locytes. Lymphocytes and monocytes are the two types of agranulocytes and they are produced in the bone marrow.

Lymphocytes (Figure 6-8) account for between 20% and 25% of all leukocytes in blood. They are slightly larger than RBCs (8 to 10 μm in diameter) and have a round nucleus that fills most of the cell, leaving only a thin ring of cytoplasm at the cell's periphery. There are three functionally distinct, but morphologically indistinguishable, types of lymphocytes.

These are **B cells, T cells,** and **null cells**. B cells differentiate into antibody-secreting **plasma cells** when exposed to the proper antigen (Figure 6-9). They are responsible for the **humoral immune response**. T cells do not secrete antibodies in response to antigen, but they do have antigen receptors in their membranes. Depending on the type of T cell, it may execute a **cell-mediated immune response** as a **cytotoxic T cell**, or it may regulate activity of other cells either as a **T-helper** or **T-suppressor cell**. **Null cells** are so named because they lack the membrane markers that identify T and B cells. **Natural killer (NK) cells** are null cells that kill foreign or infected cells without antigen-antibody interaction.

Monocytes (Figure 6-10) comprise between 3% and 8% of all blood leukocytes. They are about twice the size of RBCs (12 to 15 μm in diameter). The cytoplasm is bluish-gray in standard blood smears and the nucleus is often indented (but irregular shapes are also seen). Monocytes are the blood form of tissue **macrophages**, which, unlike neutrophils, are long-lived in tissues (weeks to months). In addition to phagocytic activity, some macrophages act as **antigen-presenting cells (APCs)** that phagocytose and digest foreign material, then carry the antigen on their own surface to "show" cells of the immune system and stimulate a response.

Platelets (Figure 6-11) are cell fragments derived from **megakaryocytes** in bone marrow (see page 71). They are involved in the clotting process.

Composition of Bone Marrow

Marrow is found in the marrow cavity of long bones and fills spaces between trabeculae in spongy bone of all bones (Figure 6-12). It is a highly vascular tissue that contains numerous and connected blood sinusoids, a framework of reticular fibers, and cells of various types. **Red bone marrow** is found in all fetal bones, but as the individual ages, its distribution is limited to ribs, sternum, vertebrae, and flat bones of the skull. Its primary function is hemopoiesis (formation of blood cells—see below). **Yellow bone marrow** (Figure 6-13) replaces red bone marrow during aging, although it maintains the ability to revert to red marrow if the need for more blood cells arises. It contains abundant fat cells.

Postnatal Blood Cell Development

Hemopoiesis is the production of blood cells, which is a complex process that occurs in the bone marrow. While some details remain sketchy (and others have been omitted by the author) here is the big picture. **Pluripotent stem cells**[1] in the bone marrow produce two kinds of stem cells: **myeloid stem cells** and **lymphoid stem cells**, each of which can produce different **progenitor cells** (that are more limited in the kinds of cells they produce). Myeloid stem cells produce **erythrocyte**

---

[1] "Pluripotent" means the cell has the potential to produce daughter cells that can develop into a variety of specialized cells.

progenitors that produce erythrocytes during **erythropoiesis**, **megakaryocyte progenitors** that produce megakaryocytes during **thrombopoiesis**, and **granulocyte/monocyte progenitors** that produce granulocytes and monocytes during **granulopoiesis** and **monopoiesis**, respectively. Lymphoid stem cells produce **common lymphoid progenitors** that give rise to lymphocytes during **lymphopoiesis**.

Granulopoiesis, illustrated in Figure 6-14, is the production of granulocytes. Each granulocyte type goes through similar developmental stages, and all begin with undifferentiated **myeloblasts** followed by **promyelocytes**, which contain primary (nonspecific, azurophilic) cytoplasmic granules. When a promyelocyte develops specific granules characteristic of each granulocyte it becomes a **myelocyte**. **Metamyelocytes** are smaller and have an indented nucleus. **Stab (band) cells** follow and are the last stage prior to a mature granulocyte. Stab cells are characterized by a U-shaped to slightly segmented nucleus. (By convention, if the nuclear indentation is less than half the nuclear diameter, the cell is a metamyelocyte. If more than half of the nuclear diameter, it is a stab cell.) Mature granulocytes have the segmented or lobed nucleus and appear as they do in blood. Examples of developmental stages are shown in Figure 6-15.

Monopoiesis is the production of monocytes (Figure 6-16). Monocytes develop from the same stem cell as granulocytes and pass through **monoblast** and **promonocyte** (Figure 6-17) stages before the mature monocyte is formed. During development, the cells become smaller and the nuclear indentation becomes more prominent. Both of these cells are rare in bone marrow smears.[2]

Lymphopoiesis is the production of lymphocytes (Figure 6-18). **Lymphoblasts** and **prolymphocytes** are the developmental stages a lymphocyte passes through prior to maturity. These are differentiated primarily by size, with the cells becoming smaller with maturity, but they are rarely seen in normal bone marrow. A mature lymphocyte is shown in Figure 6-17.

Erythropoiesis is the process of RBC formation and the sequence is shown in Figure 6-19. Examples of these cells are shown in Figure 6-20. **Proerythroblast**s are large cells with a prominent nucleus, little basophilic cytoplasm, and no hemoglobin. These develop into a series of **erythroblasts (normoblasts)** that show a progressive decrease in size, a loss of organelles (along with a loss of basophilic staining), and an increase in hemoglobin (along with increasing eosinophilia). The stages are **basophilic erythroblast, polychromatophilic erythroblast,** and **orthochromatophilic erythroblast**. The orthochromatophilic erythroblast has a pinkish cytoplasm and a small, densely staining nucleus. The final developmental stage before the cell is a mature RBC is the **reticulocyte**. It is anucleate and appears very similar to RBCs except its cytoplasm contains a bluish network when stained with

brilliant cresyl blue. It is estimated that erythropoiesis produces 250 billion RBCs each day!

Thrombopoiesis (Figure 6-21) is the production of platelets. **Megakaryocytes** are derived from a unipotent stem cell, that undergoes several rounds of DNA replication as a **megakaryoblast** without cytokinesis or nuclear division. The resulting megakaryocyte is a large (up to 100 μm in diameter), polyploid cell (averaging 16N) with a lobed nucleus—each of which contains the diploid amount of DNA. It has been estimated that collectively they produce 150 billion platelets by cytoplasmic fragmentation each day. These cells are shown in Figures 6-22 and 6-23.

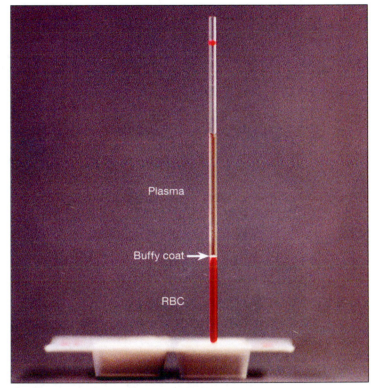

6-2 **Hematocrit** ■ This capillary tube contains blood that has been centrifuged to separate the plasma (above) from the formed elements (below). A thin buffy coat (composed of white blood cells and platelets) is visible at the RBC and plasma junction.

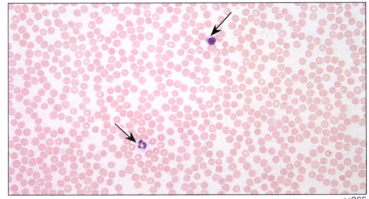

×265

6-3 **Blood Smear** ■ Blood is usually examined as a smear on a slide stained with either Giemsa (as in this preparation) or Wright's stain. RBCs outnumber leukocytes about 1,000 to 1. Two leukocytes (lymphocyte above, neutrophil below) are visible in this field (arrows). (×265)

---

[2] The cells in many lineages are difficult to find in bone marrow smears. Much has been learned from in vitro cell culture and experimental introduction of cultured cells into spleens and seeing what they produce.

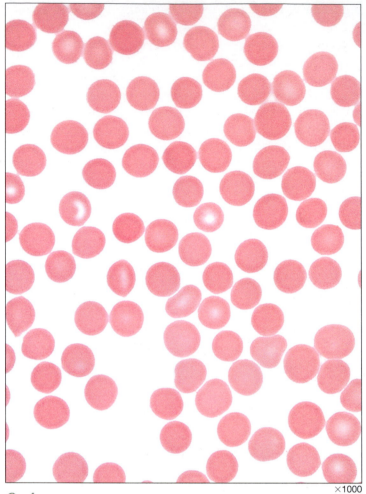

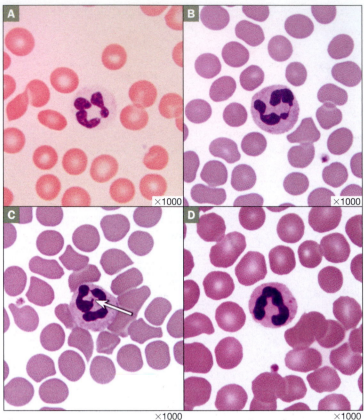

6-4 Erythrocytes ◼ The biconcave disc shape of the RBCs (as evidenced by their thin, lighter-staining centers) is seen in some cells of this Giemsa preparation. RBCs are very sensitive to osmotic conditions and their shape may change if the staining conditions are not isosmotic. They are also pliable. (×1000)

6-5 Neutrophils ◼ Neutrophils are granulocytes with a pinkish to gray cytoplasm. They are the most abundant leukocyte and are slightly larger than RBCs. Mature neutrophils have a segmented nucleus (as in micrographs **A**, **B**, and **C**) with lobes joined by a thin strand of nuclear material. Immature neutrophils have an unsegmented nucleus and are called band cells (as in micrograph **D**). About 30% of neutrophils in blood samples from females demonstrate a "drumstick" protruding from the nucleus, indicated by the arrow in micrograph (**C**). This is the region of the inactive X chromosome. Micrograph (**A**) was stained with Giemsa stain; the others were prepared with Wright's stain. (All micrographs are ×1000)

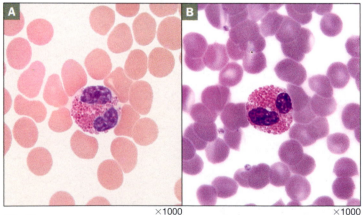

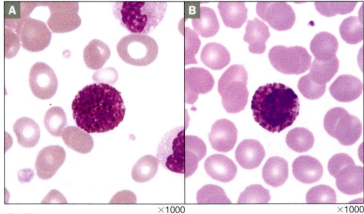

6-6 Eosinophils ◼ These granulocytes are relatively rare and are about twice the size of RBCs. Their cytoplasmic granules stain red, and their nucleus usually has two lobes. Micrograph (**A**) was prepared with Giemsa stain; (**B**) was prepared with Wright's stain. Both were magnified ×1000.

6-7 Basophils ◼ Basophils comprise only about 1% of all leukocytes. They are slightly larger than RBCs and have dark-purple cytoplasmic granules that obscure the nucleus. Micrograph (**A**) was prepared with Giemsa stain and (**B**) was prepared with Wright's stain. Both were magnified ×1000.

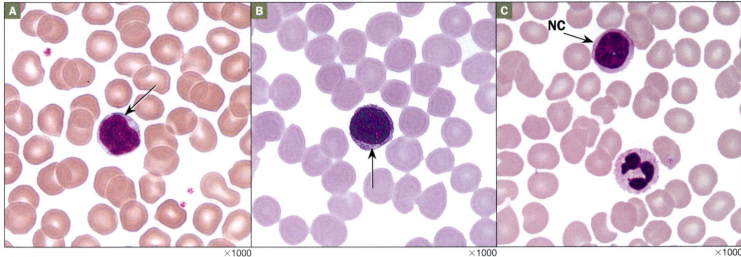

×1000   ×1000   ×1000

6-8 Lymphocytes ◻ Lymphocytes are common in the blood, comprising up to 25% of all leukocytes. Most are about the size of RBCs and have only a thin halo of cytoplasm (arrow) encircling their round nucleus. (If you don't see that halo, you will probably misidentify the cell as a basophil.) They belong to functional groups called B cells and T cells, which are morphologically indistinguishable. Micrographs (A) and (B) are small lymphocytes and were prepared with Giemsa and Wright's stains, respectively. Some lymphocytes are larger, as in micrograph (C). These are natural killer cells or some other type of "null" cell (NC). A neutrophil is also seen in (C). All micrographs are ×1000.

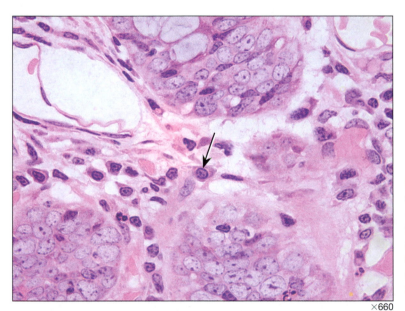

×660

6-9 Plasma Cells ◻ B lymphocytes develop into plasma cells when stimulated by the appropriate antigen. Plasma cells secrete protective antibodies against a specific antigen–conveniently the one that stimulated their conversion from a B lymphocyte. This plasma cell (arrow) is recognizable because of its elongated shape, eccentric nucleus with "clock face" chromatin, and a pale region near the nucleus (the site of the Golgi apparatus). This specimen is from the colon. Also see Figure 2-10. (×660)

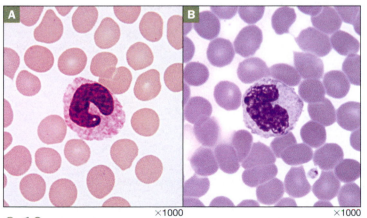

×1000   ×1000

6-10 Monocytes ◻ Monocytes are the blood form of macrophages. They are about twice the size of RBCs and have a round or indented nucleus (horseshoe shaped on the left, kidney shaped on the right). Both micrographs are ×1000. (A) Giemsa stain. (B) Wright's stain.

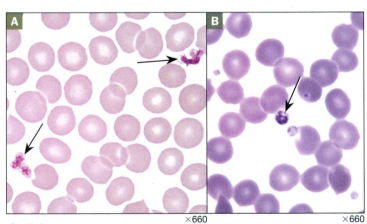

×660   ×660

6-11 Platelets ◻ Platelets (arrows) are cell fragments involved in clotting. (A) Giemsa stain. (B) Wright's stain. Platelets may also be seen in Figures 6-5b, 6-5c, and 6-7b. Both micrographs are ×660.

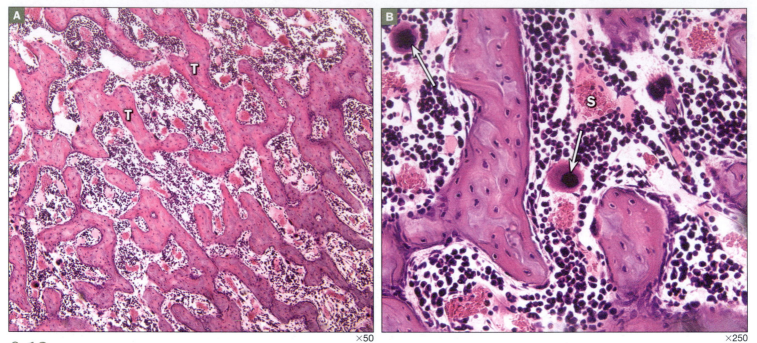

6-12 Red Marrow 🔲 (A) The spaces between trabeculae of spongy bone (T) are often filled with red marrow. It consists of various developmental stages of blood cells. (×50) (B) Blood sinusoids (S), marrow cells, and two megakaryocytes (arrows) are visible. (×250)

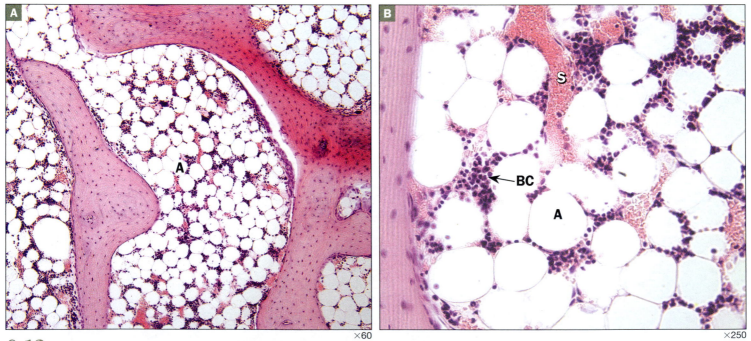

6-13 Yellow Marrow 🔲 (A) In most bones, red marrow is replaced by yellow marrow in adults. The majority of cells are adipocytes (A). (×60) (B) Adipocytes, sinusoids (S), and some remaining developing blood cells (BC) are seen more clearly in this higher magnification. (×250)

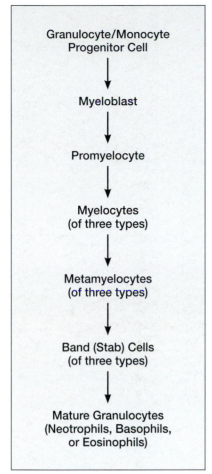

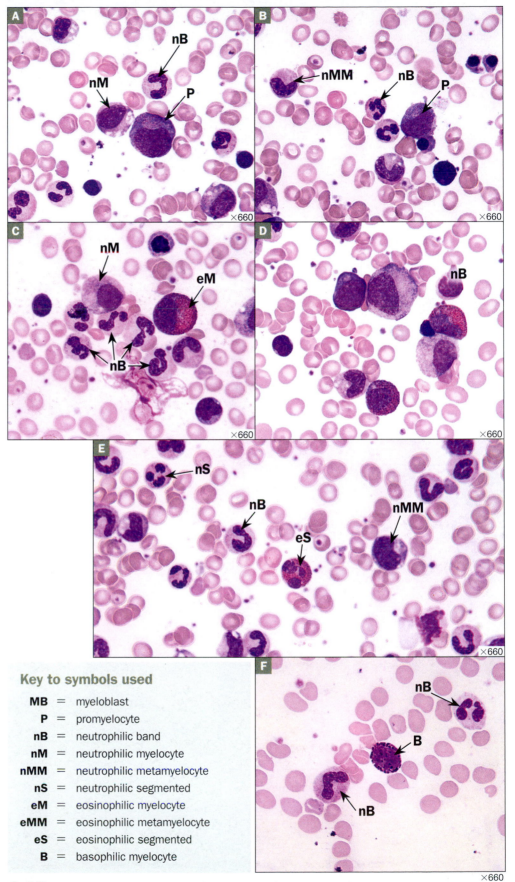

6-14 Granulocyte Development (Granulopoiesis) ◾ Through the promyelocyte stage, the precursors of neutrophils, basophils, and eosinophils are indistinguishable. Once myelocytes begin accumulating granules specific to each granulocyte, each developmental series can be traced separately. The overall pattern involves accumulation of cytoplasmic granules and progressive indentation and segmentation of the nucleus.

Key to symbols used

MB	=	myeloblast
P	=	promyelocyte
nB	=	neutrophilic band
nM	=	neutrophilic myelocyte
nMM	=	neutrophilic metamyelocyte
nS	=	neutrophilic segmented
eM	=	eosinophilic myelocyte
eMM	=	eosinophilic metamyelocyte
eS	=	eosinophilic segmented
B	=	basophilic myelocyte

6-15 Bone Marrow Smears Illustrating Granulocyte Development ◾ These marrow smears illustrate most of the cells in the granulocytic developmental series. Some cells will be encountered frequently (e.g., neutrophilic cells) whereas others are much less common (e.g., basophils). (**A** through **F**, ×660)

6-16 Monocyte Development (Monopoiesis)

Granulocyte/Monocyte Progenitor Cell

↓

Monoblast

↓

Promonocyte

↓

Monocyte

Note that the progenitor is the same cell that gives rise to the granulocytic cells. Cells of monocyte development are difficult to find in marrow smears.

6-17 Bone Marrow Smear Illustrating Monocyte and Lymphocyte Development

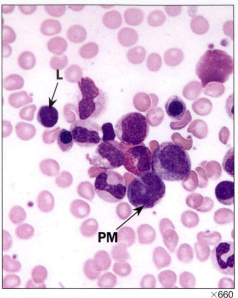

×660

The precursors of lymphocytes and monocytes are relatively rare in marrow smears. Shown here are a promonocyte (PM) and lymphocyte (L). Early stages of lymphocyte development are often difficult to tell apart. If there is doubt as to a cell's identity, by convention it is just called a lymphocyte. (×660)

6-18 Lymphocyte Development (Lymphopoiesis)

Lymphoid Stem Cell

↓

Lymphoblast

↓

Prolymphocyte

↓

Lymphocyte

Lymphocytes go through only two stages in development in marrow. Unlike other blood cells, they continue their development outside the marrow in lymphoid tissue throughout the body.

6-19 Erythrocyte Development (Erythropoiesis)

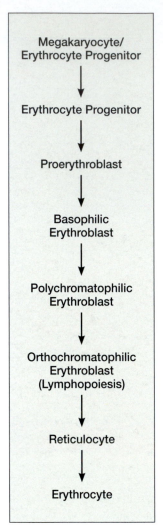

Megakaryocyte/Erythrocyte Progenitor

↓

Erythrocyte Progenitor

↓

Proerythroblast

↓

Basophilic Erythroblast

↓

Polychromatophilic Erythroblast

↓

Orthochromatophilic Erythroblast (Lymphopoiesis)

↓

Reticulocyte

↓

Erythrocyte

The major changes in erythrocyte development are a decrease in size, loss of organelles (most notably, the nucleus), and an increase in cytoplasmic hemoglobin.

6-20 Bone Marrow and Blood Smears Illustrating Erythrocyte Development

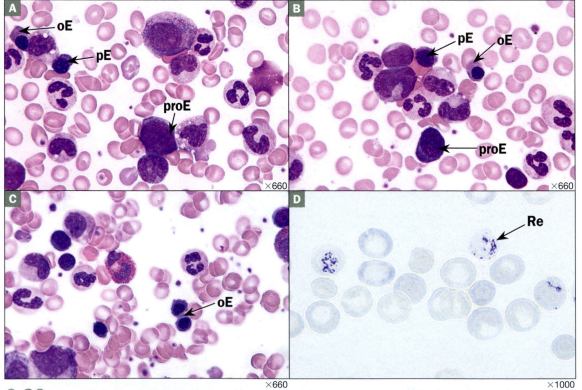

(A) through (C) are bone marrow smears. All are ×660. Key to symbols used: proE = proerythroblast, pE = polychromatophilic erythroblast, oE = orthochromatophilic erythroblast. Note the oE extruding its nucleus in (B) and the dividing oE in (C). Both are indicated with arrows. (D) This blood smear stained with new methylene blue shows reticulocytes (Re). These cells comprise 0.5% to 2% of RBCs in circulation. An elevated number (as in this specimen) may be indicative of anemia, with bone marrow delivering immature cells to circulation to compensate. The dark blue material is RNA. (×1000)

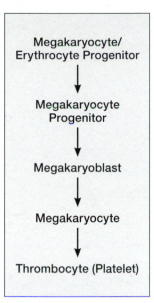

Megakaryocyte/
Erythrocyte Progenitor

↓

Megakaryocyte
Progenitor

↓

Megakaryoblast

↓

Megakaryocyte

↓

Thrombocyte (Platelet)

6-21 Thrombocyte (Platelet) Development (Thrombopoiesis) ◼

Megakaryoblasts develop into megakaryocytes by repeated DNA replications without cytokinesis or mitosis. Once formed, a megakaryocyte undergoes fragmentation to produce hundreds to thousands of thrombocytes.

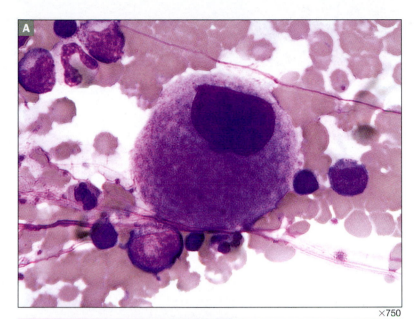

×750

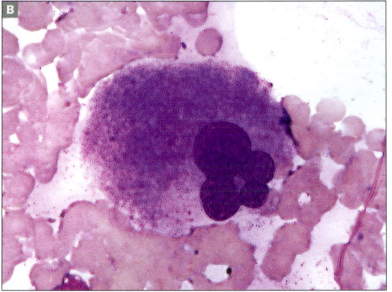

×750

6-22 Bone Marrow Smears Illustrating Thrombocyte Development

◼ (A) Megakaryoblast with a single, unlobed nucleus. Compare its size to the RBCs and leukocyte precursors in the field. (×750) (B) The characteristic lobed nucleus in this megakaryocyte is visible. Again, note its size. (×750)

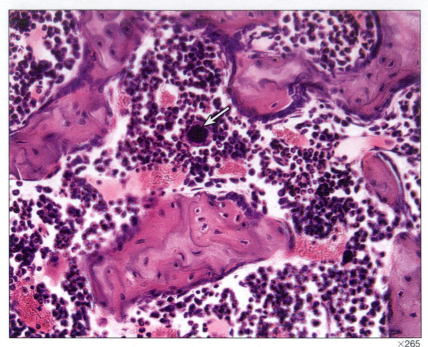

×265

6-23 **Section of Bone Marrow** ▨ Because of its size, this megakaryocyte (arrow) stands out against the marrow cells. Also see Figure 6-12b. (×265)

A Photographic Atlas of Histology

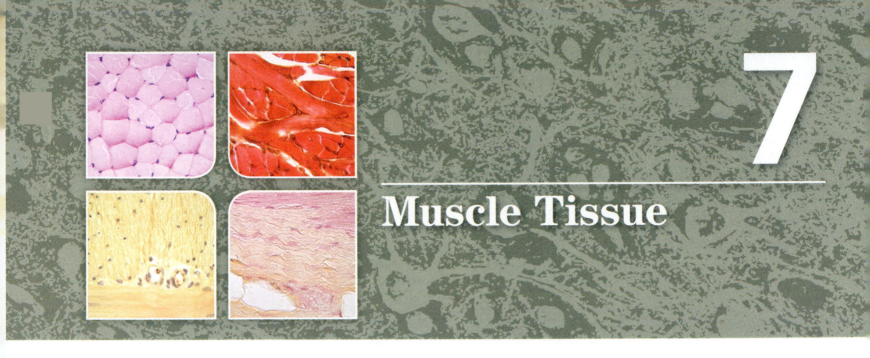

Muscle Tissue

7

:: Introduction to Muscle Tissue

Muscle tissue is a highly cellular and vascular tissue specialized for contraction. Muscle contraction results in movement of a body part, propulsion of a substance, or in some instances, stopping movement of a substance.

There are three basic types of muscle tissue: **skeletal muscle** (Figure 7-1), **cardiac muscle**, and **smooth (visceral) muscle**. The cells of all muscle tissues are long and thin, and are referred to as **muscle fibers**.

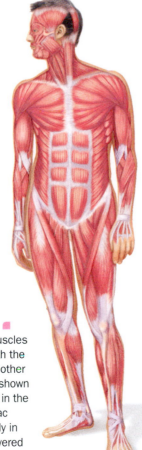

7-1 Muscular System ■
Shown are the skeletal muscles most people associate with the muscular system, but two other muscle types that are not shown are smooth muscle, found in the walls of organs, and cardiac muscle, which is found only in the heart. All three are covered in this chapter.

:: Characteristics of Skeletal Muscle

Skeletal muscle (Figure 7-2) is associated with the bones of the skeleton and is responsible for body movement. It also may be found associated with the skin (such as in the muscles of facial expression) and with some viscera (the proximal end of the esophagus, for example). In all cases, skeletal muscle is under voluntary control.

Skeletal muscle fibers are long (up to 3 cm) with a diameter between 10 and 100 μm. They are multinucleate, with their nuclei pushed to the periphery of each fiber next to the **sarcolemma** (plasma membrane) (Figure 7-3). Approximately 80% of a skeletal muscle fiber's volume is composed of **myofibrils**, which hold the contractile apparatus (Figure 7-4). The remainder is composed of mitochondria, ribosomes, storage materials (glycogen and lipid droplets), and a complex tubular system consisting of **sarcoplasmic reticulum (SR)** and **transverse (T) tubules** that wrap around the myofibrils. T tubules are invaginations of the sarcolemma and allow rapid transmission of an **action potential** (the electrical signal that says, "Contract!") to the myofibrils throughout the fiber. Sarcoplasmic reticulum, which resembles smooth endoplasmic reticulum (ER), is the site of calcium ion storage. When stimulated by an action potential, they release their calcium, which in turn activates the contractile apparatus. Two expansions of SR called **terminal cisternae** surround a T tubule in the region of the A band (see next paragraph) and form a **muscle triad**.

With the light microscope, alternating dark and light bands are visible, giving the fibers a striped or **striated** appearance (Figures 7-2 and 7-5). The dark striations are called **A bands**, whereas the lighter ones are known as **I bands**. A thin **Z disk** bisects each I band. With electron microscopy, it is seen that striations are the product of the highly organized arrangement of actin (along with associated proteins **troponin** and **tropomyosin**) and myosin filaments within each fiber (Figures 7-6 and 2-15b). These filaments form the contractile apparatus and cause fiber shortening by a mechanism known as the **sliding filament theory**. In this model, the contractile unit is the region between two Z disks and is called a **sarcomere**. During contraction, the Z disks are brought closer together. As the actin and myosin filaments slide across one another in a ratchet-like fashion, the I bands become narrower but the A bands stay the same width. Note that it is the fiber that shortens, not the filaments.

Skeletal muscle tissue is combined with connective tissues to form specific muscle organs, such as the biceps brachii or gluteus maximus. The connective tissue components of a muscle weave between the muscle fibers and bind the whole organ together. Covering the entire muscle is **epimysium** (Figures 7-7 and 7-8), a dense irregular collagenous tissue layer. Smaller extensions of epimysium penetrate the muscle as **perimysium** and surround several fibers to form a **fascicle**. Extending from the perimysium is a fine layer of reticular tissue and basal lamina called **endomysium** that surrounds each individual fiber. These connective tissue layers are all continuous with the connective tissue of the muscle's tendon, which in turn attaches to the bone's periosteum (Figures 7-9 and 7-10). In addition, many of the connective tissue fibers in the tendon are attached directly to the membranes of the muscle fibers. Thus, when a muscle contracts it pulls on its connective tissue (including its tendon), which transmits the tension to the bone, moving it.

Skeletal muscle fibers can be classified as one of three types based on diameter, amount of myoglobin (structurally similar to hemoglobin and also associated with oxygen transport), rate of contraction, and other features. The fiber types are **red slow twitch fibers, white fast twitch fibers,** and **intermediate fibers** (Figure 7-11). Red fibers are red because of their abundance of myoglobin. They have a smaller fiber diameter, a lower glycogen content, and are capable of slower and weaker contractions than white fibers, but do not fatigue as easily. White fibers have less myoglobin and more glycogen than red fibers. They also are larger, contract more rapidly and with greater strength, but fatigue easily. Intermediate fibers are intermediate between white and red fibers in these characteristics. All muscles have all fiber types, but the proportions differ depending on the primary role played by the muscle. Red fibers are abundant in postural muscles, whereas white fibers predominate in appendicular muscles.

Each skeletal muscle fiber is supplied (innervated) by a **somatic motor neuron**. The structure formed between the muscle fiber and its somatic motor neuron is a **neuromuscular junction** (Figure 7-12). Although not visible in light micrographs, there is an actual gap between the membranes of the neuron and muscle fiber called a **synaptic cleft**. When a nerve impulse reaches the end of the neuron, a chemical **neurotransmitter** (acetylcholine) is released into the synaptic cleft, diffuses across it, and stimulates the muscle cell to contract.

Muscle spindles (Figure 7-13) are sensory organs in skeletal muscles that detect stretching. They are formed from modified muscle fibers and somatic sensory neurons. If stretched, they initiate a stretch reflex that results in contraction.

▪▪ Characteristics of Cardiac Muscle

Cardiac muscle tissue (Figure 7-14) is found only in the heart where it forms the **myocardium**, the thickest layer of the heart wall. The tissue is under involuntary control and has the innate ability to contract rhythmically, although the nervous system and hormones can modify contraction rate.

Cardiac muscle fibers are striated, branched, and uninucleate (occasionally two nuclei are present), with the oval nucleus found near the fiber's center. They are less than 100 μm long and about 15 μm in diameter. Sarcomere arrangement is the same as in skeletal muscle, but there are minor differences in abundance and arrangement of T tubules and SR.

Intercalated disks (Figure 7-15), found at the junctions between cells, are seen as dark transverse lines with the light microscope. They physically bind the cells together so the force of contraction is transmitted between the linked cells. They also promote the rapid spread of electrical action potentials from cell to cell via gap junctions.

Cardiac muscle is very vascular, with abundant capillaries visible between fibers (Figure 7-16). An **endomysium** of collagenous fibers is also present.

▪▪ Characteristics of Smooth Muscle

Smooth muscle (Figure 7-17) is found in the walls of organs, so it is also known as **visceral muscle**. It is under involuntary control and is capable of slow, sustained contractions. (Think of the uterus during childbirth!) Smooth muscle fibers are long and tapered at both ends with a single, central nucleus conforming to the cell's shape. There are no striations (hence "smooth"), because the actin and myosin filaments do not show the same degree and kind of organization seen in skeletal and cardiac muscle.

Two layers of smooth muscle are often in the walls of tubular organs, with the fibers of one layer running the length of the organ and the fibers of the other layer oriented around the organ (Figure 7-18). These **longitudinal** and **circular layers** are capable of producing a specialized form of contraction in tubular organs called **peristalsis**.

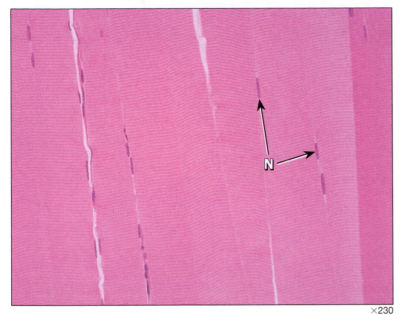

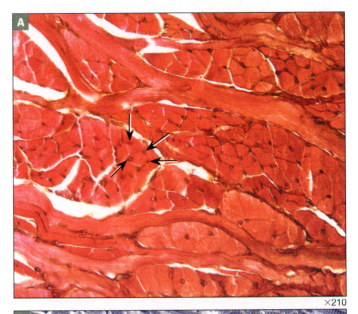

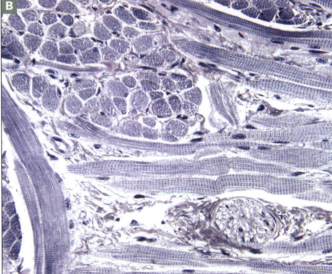

7-2 **Skeletal Muscle** ◼ Transverse striations and many peripheral nuclei (N) characterize skeletal muscle fibers. (×230)

Myofibril

Sarcoplasm

Nuclei

7-3 **Skeletal Muscle in Various Sections** ◼ These specimens from the tongue show skeletal muscle fibers sectioned in all planes. Even though the striations are not visible in cross section, the peripheral nuclei (arrows) are a useful feature for identifying this tissue. Both micrographs are ×210.

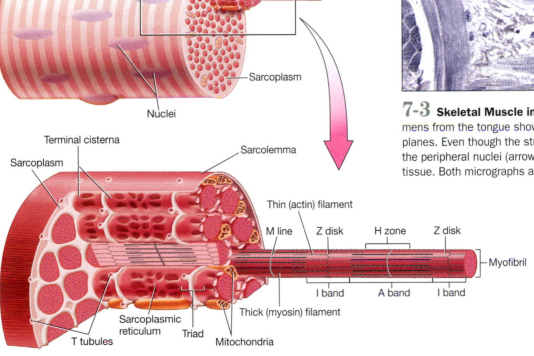

Terminal cisterna

Sarcoplasm

Sarcolemma

Thin (actin) filament

M line   Z disk   H zone   Z disk

Myofibril

I band   A band   I band

Thick (myosin) filament

Sarcoplasmic reticulum   Triad   Mitochondria

T tubules

7-4 **Muscle Fiber Structure** ◼ Sarcolemma (plasma membrane) surrounds the complex, but highly organized, interior of each fiber. Protein filaments forming the contractile machinery are found within myofibrils, which occupy the majority of a fiber's volume. Wrapped around each myofibril are two membranous systems: sarcoplasmic reticulum (SR) and T tubules. SR stores calcium ions, which are released when stimulated by an action potential carried by the T tubules from the fiber's surface to its interior (thus ensuring that all myofibrils, for all practical purposes, contract in unison). Calcium is necessary for the actin and myosin filaments to slide across one another to produce shortening of the fiber. Note the terminal cisternae of SR found on either side of T tubules, which form a muscle triad.

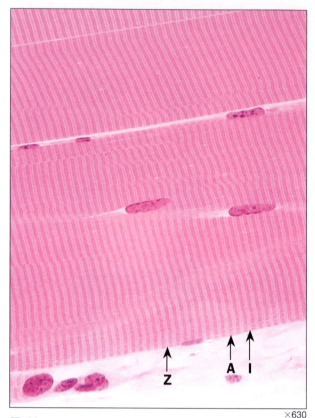

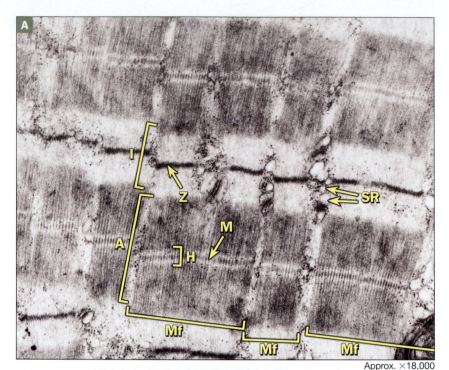

Approx. ×18,000

7-5 **Striations** ▪ In the light microscope striations are seen as thick dark stripes (A bands) and faintly visible thin dark lines (Z disks) bisecting thick light stripes (I bands). Notice that the nuclei are not in the striated part of the cell. (×630)

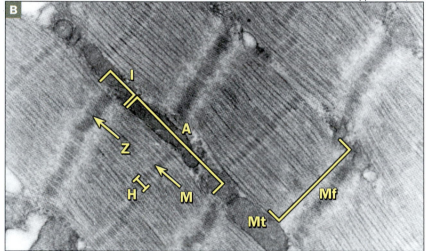

Approx. ×22,000

7-6 **The Sarcomere** ▪ While many other proteins are present, the orderly arrangement of actin and myosin filaments accounts for the striations in skeletal muscle. As you examine these TEMs, compare them to Figures 7-4 and 7-5. (**A**) This TEM of relaxed muscle clearly shows the striations. Visible are the darker A bands (A) and the lighter I bands (I). The dark part of A bands is produced by overlapping actin and myosin filaments (see below), whereas I bands are primarily actin filaments. Z lines (Z), made of multiple proteins, bisect I bands and form the boundaries of a sarcomere, the contractile unit of skeletal muscle. Light H bands (H), which are regions of myosin filaments, and darker M lines (M) are found within the A bands. Proteins that keep the myosin filament "in line" reside at the M line. Also note the nuclei (N), sarcoplasmic reticulum (SR), and myofibrils (Mf). (Approx. ×18,000) (**B**) This TEM shows a contracted muscle. Notice that the I band is relatively small. This is because most of the actin filaments' length is now overlapping with myosin filaments. A point to remember: The sarcomere shortens, the filaments don't. Note the mitochondrion (Mt). (Approx. ×22,000)   (Courtesy of UCSD Medical Center)

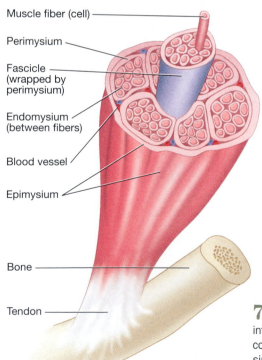

Muscle fiber (cell)

Perimysium

Fascicle (wrapped by perimysium)

Endomysium (between fibers)

Blood vessel

Epimysium

Bone

Tendon

7-7 **Skeletal Muscle Components** ▪ Binding skeletal muscles together are three layers of interwoven connective tissue, defined by their location. In order of decreasing density: epimysium covers the whole muscle, perimysium surrounds bundles of muscle fibers (fascicles), and endomysium surrounds each individual fiber. The tendon emerging from the muscle is a continuation of these connective tissue layers, especially the epimysium.

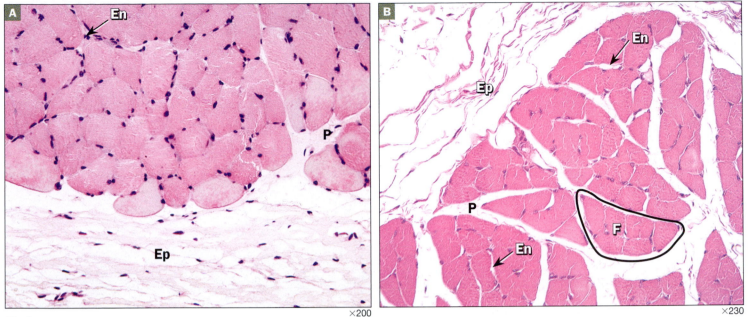

7-8 **Connective Tissue of Skeletal Muscles** ■ Muscle fibers in a skeletal muscle are held together by fibrous connective tissue. Epimysium (Ep) surrounds the entire muscle, perimysium (P) surrounds a fascicle of fibers, and endomysium (En) surrounds each individual fiber. Note the peripheral nuclei in both specimens. **(A)** A thick epimysium is seen in this muscle cut in cross section. (×200) **(B)** The fascicles in this cross-sectioned specimen have separated during preparation, but this makes the three connective tissue layers more visible and emphasizes their continuity. It also defines the fascicles (outline-F). (×230)

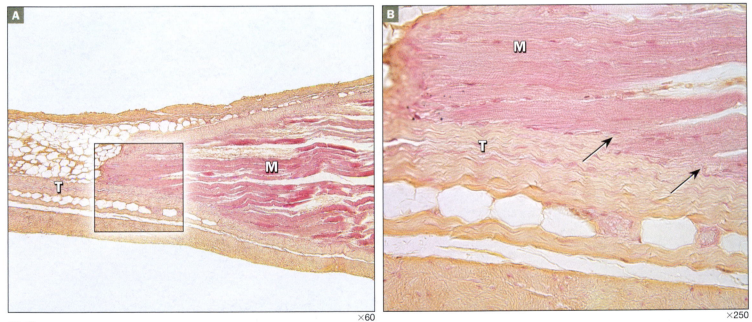

7-9 **Musculotendinous Junction** ■ **(A)** In this longitudinal section, the end of the muscle (M) and its tendon (T) are seen. (×60) **(B)** This is a higher magnification of the boxed region in **(A)**. In it you can more clearly see the continuity of the muscle's connective tissue components combining to form the tendon. Also seen are regions where the connective tissue fibers are bound to the muscle fibers' membrane (arrows). (×250)

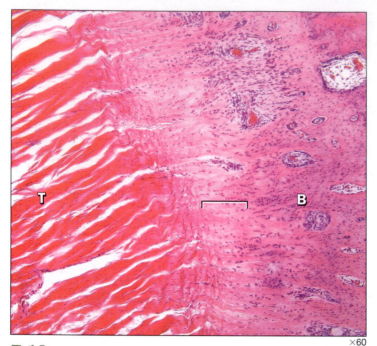

7-10 **Tendinous Attachment to Bone** ■ The collagenous fibers of the tendon (T) on the left blend with the periosteum and penetrate the bone (B) matrix to anchor the muscle firmly to the bone in the region indicated by the bracket. (×60)

×60

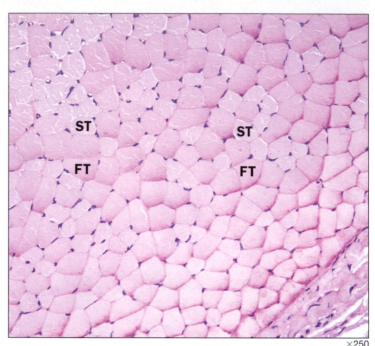

7-11 **Fast and Slow Twitch Fibers** ■ Two fiber types are identifiable in this cross section stained for glycogen (PAS reaction), which is more abundant in the larger white fast twitch fibers (FT). The fibers lacking glycogen tend to be the smaller, red slow twitch fibers (ST). (×250)

×250

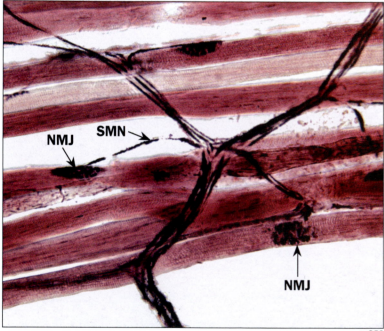

7-12 **Neuromuscular Junction** ■ The junction between a somatic motor neuron (SMN) and its muscle fiber is a complex structure known as a neuromuscular junction (NMJ). Two are seen in this whole-mount specimen. Acetylcholine is the neurotransmitter that crosses the synaptic cleft. (×250)

×250

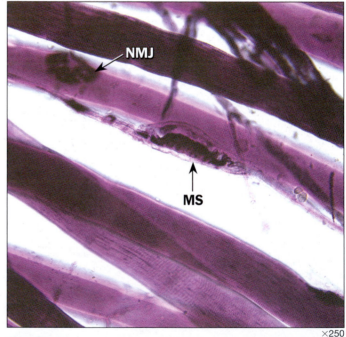

7-13 **Muscle Spindles** ■ Muscle spindles (MS) are receptors that provide sensory information about the amount of stretch placed on a muscle. A neuromuscular junction (NMJ) is also seen. (×250)

×250

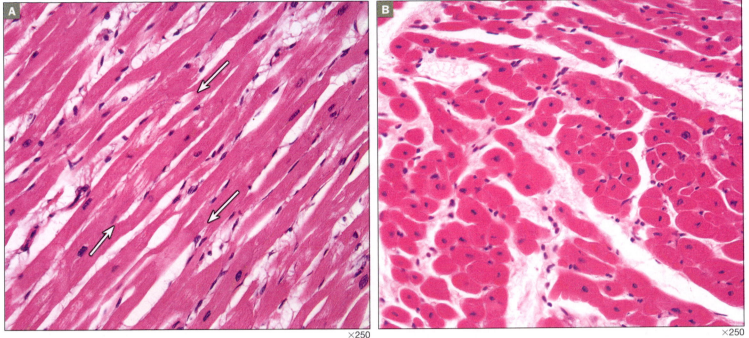

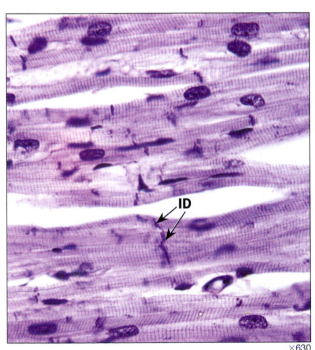

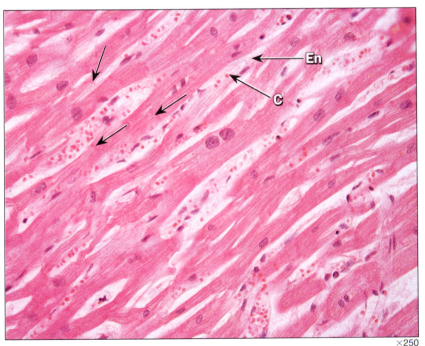

7-14 Cardiac Muscle ▪ (A) Cardiac muscle is found only in the heart, where it forms the myocardium. Its fibers are faintly striated (not visible in this micrograph of a longitudinal section), branched (arrows), and typically uninucleate. (×250) (B) The central position of the nuclei is easily seen in this cross section of cardiac muscle, but obviously, branching fibers and striations are not. (×250)

7-15 Intercalated Disks ▪ Iron-hematoxylin stain accentuates the striations and intercalated disks (ID) of cardiac muscle fibers. Membranes of adjoining cells at intercalated disks interdigitate and also possess gap junctions for impulse conduction. Fiber branching is also visible. (×630)

7-16 Capillaries of Cardiac Muscle ▪ Cardiac muscle is very vascular, as evidenced by the numerous capillaries (C) seen in this micrograph. An endomysium (En), faint intercalated disks (arrows), and branching fibers are also visible. (×250)

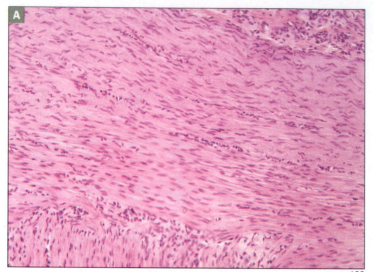

×120

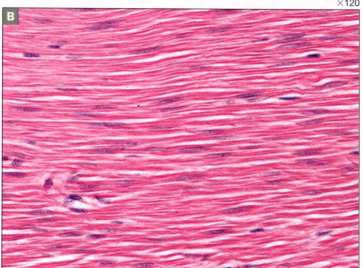

×120

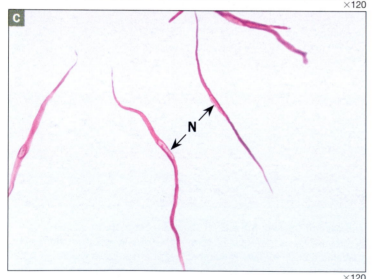

×120

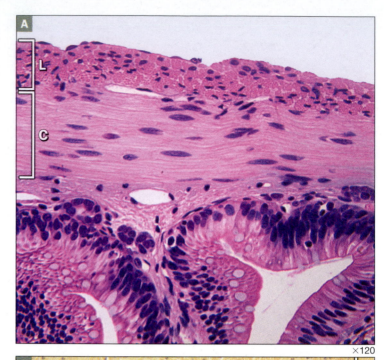

×120

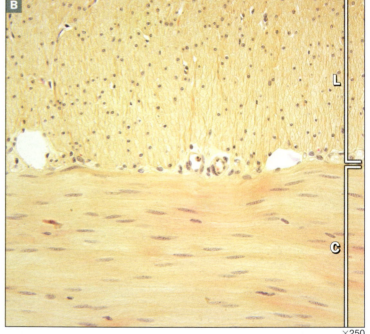

×250

7-18 **Smooth Muscle Layers** In many tubular organs, smooth muscle is found in longitudinal (L) and circular (C) layers (relative to the tube). Both specimens are cross sections of the small intestine, which means the longitudinally arranged fibers will also be cut in cross section, and the circularly arranged fibers will be cut longitudinally. It is this arrangement that moves materials through the organ by peristalsis. For histologists, it allows easy viewing of smooth muscle in longitudinal and cross sections! (**A**) ×120. (**B**) ×250.

7-17 **Smooth Muscle** (**A** and **B**) Note the absence of striations and the random distribution of nuclei throughout these sections of smooth muscle. Smooth muscle is sometimes confused with dense regular connective tissue, but in the latter, nuclei are usually in rows (compare to Figure 4-16). (**A**) (×120); (**B**) (×120). (**C**) Smooth muscle fibers are elongated with tapered ends, which are evident in these isolated cells. Notice the single nucleus (N) and absence of striations. (×120)

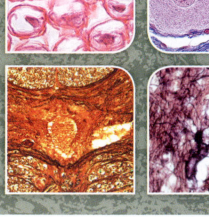

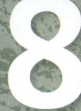

Nervous Tissue and Organs of the Nervous System

⁘ Introduction to Nervous Tissue and Organs of the Nervous System

Nervous tissue is specialized for coordinating and integrating the activities of the body's cells and organs. It accomplishes this through conduction of electrical nerve impulses and secretion of chemical neurotransmitters.

The organs of the vertebrate nervous system (Figure 8-1) are structurally classified as being part of the **central nervous system (CNS)**, which includes the brain and spinal cord; or the **peripheral nervous system (PNS)**, which includes nerves, ganglia, and sensory receptors.

Although it is beyond the scope of this book to provide a detailed description of the nervous system's functional organization, it is necessary to refer to its components (Figure 8-2). For a more detailed description of the role each part fills in the body, the reader is referred to a physiology textbook. Functionally, the nervous system can be divided into two parts: the **afferent (sensory) nervous system**, which carries information toward the CNS or up the spinal cord toward the brain, and the **efferent (motor) nervous system**, which carries information from the brain and away from the CNS. The afferent and efferent systems have **somatic** (relating to the skin and skeletal muscles) and **visceral** (relating to the internal organs) components. The visceral motor system is also known as the **autonomic nervous system**, which is structurally and functionally divided into a **sympathetic (thoracolumbar) division** and a **parasympathetic (craniosacral) division**. The former prepares the body to contend with stressful and life threatening situations, whereas the latter is involved in body maintenance during non-stressful times.

8-1 Nervous System ▪

Structurally, the nervous system can be broken down into the central nervous system (CNS), composed of the brain and spinal cord, and the peripheral nervous system (PNS), which includes nerves and ganglia.

⁘ Cells of Nervous Tissue

Nervous tissue is composed of two basic cell types: **neurons**, which are responsible for conduction and integration of nerve impulses, and **neuroglia (glial cells)**, which support neurons (Figure 8-3).

Glial Cells

Glial cells do not conduct nerve impulses. Instead, they support neurons (outnumbering them tenfold) and have many functions typically associated with cells of fibrous connective tissues. There are several types, which can be artificially divided into glial cells of the PNS and those of the CNS.

Glial cells of the CNS include **microglia, astrocytes, oligodendrocytes,** and **ependymal cells**. In H&E preparations, only their nuclei are seen, which makes all but ependymal cells difficult to identify. Each is considered briefly below.

- Microglia (Figure 8-4) are mobile phagocytic cells derived from monocytes. They are the smallest of the glial cells and have a dark-staining, elongated nucleus with little cytoplasm. Upon stimulation, their morphology and function changes to that of typical macrophages.

- Astrocytes (Figure 8-5) are large, highly branched cells (hence, "astro," referring to their "star" shape) that maintain connections with each other, blood vessels, and neurons. Their functions include inactivation of some neurotransmitters, maintaining potassium concentration in the extracellular fluid, providing structural (during embryonic development) and metabolic support for neurons, and scar tissue production. In addition, astrocytes attach to and cover the majority of the endothelial cells' basal laminae with their **perivascular feet** and participate in the development and proper functioning of the **blood-brain barrier (BBB)**. (The BBB is primarily formed by tight junctions between capillary cells that limit passage of materials between the blood and the extracellular fluid of the brain, protecting it from toxins and other injurious materials that might be in the blood.) All astrocytes possess intermediate filaments composed of the unique **glial fibrillary acidic protein (GFAP)**. As a result, astrocytes can be specifically stained with dye-bearing antibodies to GFAP. Two types of astrocytes are recognized: **fibrous** and **protoplasmic**. Fibrous astrocytes are found in white matter (see page 89), have fewer and longer **processes** (cytoplasmic extensions), and more GFAP. Protoplasmic astrocytes are the most abundant glial cells of gray matter (see page 89) and have shorter, more branched processes. Those on the surface form a permeability barrier with the basal lamina of the pia mater called the **glia limitans**.

- Oligodendrocytes are responsible for producing **myelin** (see page 89) in the CNS (Figure 8-6). Each oligodendrocyte may be associated with 50 or more different neurons. They are small cells with a dark cytoplasm and nucleus, and are the most abundant glial cells in white matter.

- Ependymal cells line the ventricles of the brain and central canal of the spinal cord (Figure 8-7). They are cuboidal to columnar in shape and join with the pia mater to form the **choroid plexus**, a vascular structure responsible for production of cerebrospinal fluid (CSF). Some cells possess cilia and microvilli.

Glial cells of the PNS include **Schwann (neurilemmal) cells, satellite cells,** and others that have more restricted distribution. Only the first two will be mentioned here and expanded upon later in this chapter.

- Schwann cells (Figure 8-8) are responsible for producing myelin in the PNS. This will be discussed in more detail later.

- Satellite cells (Figure 8-9) are associated with and support neurons in ganglia (see page 89).

Neurons

Although **neurons** come in a variety of sizes and shapes, they have many features in common (Figures 8-10 and 8-11). The portion of the neuron containing the majority of cytoplasm and the nucleus is called the **cell body**, or **perikaryon**. The nucleus often has a prominent nucleolus. The cytoplasm may show an abundance of **neurofibrils** (Figure 8-12) in it or have basophilic granules called **Nissl bodies** (Figure 8-13). The fibrils comprise the cytoskeleton, and the Nissl bodies are regions of rough endoplasmic reticulum. A pale cytoplasmic region may be visible near the nucleus. This is the site of a Golgi apparatus.

Extending from the cell body are cytoplasmic processes of two types. **Dendrites** receive impulses and conduct them to the cell body. They are usually short and highly branched. **Axons** transmit the nerve impulse away from the cell body to another neuron, a muscle, or a gland. Axons are up to a meter in length and branch at the end, forming **terminal arborizations**. The tip of each terminal arborization is expanded to form a **terminal bouton**. Depending on the type of neuron, there may be one to many dendrites, but there is always a single axon. Any long, thin neuronal process is called a **nerve fiber**, but usually the term applies to axons.

Neurons can be functionally divided into three groups. **Sensory neurons** carry impulses toward or up the CNS, whereas **motor neurons** carry impulses down or away from the CNS. **Interneurons** conduct impulses between sensory and motor neurons within the CNS.

There are three structural types of neurons (Figure 8-11). These are based on the shape of the cell body and the number and characteristics of the cytoplasmic processes. **Multipolar neurons** (Figure 8-14) are the most common. They have many short dendrites and a single long axon arising from an irregularly shaped cell body. The axon can be identified by the absence of Nissl substance at its base, the **axon hillock**. Motor neurons and interneurons are multipolar. **Bipolar neurons** have a single dendrite and a single axon emerging from opposite ends of the elongated cell body (Figure 8-15). These are not found in many places of the body. Two examples are in the olfactory and optic pathways. **Unipolar (pseudounipolar) neurons** (Figure 8-16) are derived from bipolar neurons. During development, the axon and dendrite fuse near the cell body so that only a single process emerges from it. The "dendrite" ends up being the longer of the two and is called the **peripheral process**. It carries the impulse from a sensory receptor to the cell body. The "axon" becomes the **central process**. It carries the impulse from the cell body to a neuron in the CNS. Most sensory neurons are unipolar.

Myelination

Glial cells support nerve fibers. At the very least, fibers in the PNS are nestled into depressions of Schwann cells. These typically smaller fibers are said to be **unmyelinated**. Many fibers, however, are covered with an insulating fatty material called **myelin**, and are said to be **myelinated**.

In the PNS, a fiber becomes myelinated when Schwann cells wrap around it several times (Figures 8-17 through 8-19). With each wrap, the cytoplasm is squeezed into the remainder of the cell and the two layers of cytoplasmic membrane are pressed together to form the myelin. (Imagine squeezing toothpaste from the base of the tube toward the cap.) The myelin sheath, then, is actually several double layers of cytoplasmic membrane wrapped around the fiber. (Imagine wrapping the empty part of the toothpaste tube around a stick several times.) Surrounding the myelin is the portion of the Schwann cell containing the cytoplasm. This is the **neurilemma**.[1] Although always present, cytoplasm remaining in the layers of myelin occasionally is visible as **Schmidt-Lanterman (clefts) lines** (Figure 8-20). These connect the Schwann cell's cytoplasm located next to the axon with the bulk of cytoplasm of the neurilemma.

Nodes of Ranvier (Figure 8-21) are gaps between adjacent Schwann cells where the fiber's membrane is exposed. Each myelinated segment (up to 0.1 to 1 mm; estimates vary) is called an **internode** (Figure 8-22). The activities associated with impulse production only occur at the nodes (rather than along the entire length of the fiber) and thus impulse transmission is much more rapid in myelinated fibers than in unmyelinated fibers.

In the CNS, myelination is performed by **oligodendrocytes**. Each oligodendrocyte myelinates 50 or more different fibers and, as such, does not surround each fiber with a neurilemma. Nodes of Ranvier and internodes are present in myelinated fibers of the CNS.

Gray and White Matter of the CNS

Myelin is a fatty material and has a whitish appearance. In fresh preparations, dense collections of myelinated fibers are referred to as **white matter**, whereas unmyelinated fibers and neuron cell bodies comprise **gray matter** (Figure 8-23). The region between neuron cell bodies, composed of a three-dimensional mesh of cellular processes and blood vessels, is called **neuropil**. These terms are applied to the CNS, but not the PNS.

Nerves and Tracts

Nerve fibers tend to travel together. In the PNS, collections of fibers are identifiable structures called **nerves**. Nerves are either **sensory** (containing only sensory fibers) or **mixed** (a combination of motor and sensory fibers, both somatic and visceral).

Each nerve is associated with vascular collagenous connective tissue similar in arrangement to the connective tissues of muscles (Figures 8-24 through 8-26). On the surface is **epineurium**, a fibrous covering that wraps and supports the nerve, separating it from the surrounding fascia. The **perineurium** is derived from the epineurium. It enters the nerve and forms nerve fiber bundles called **fascicles**. **Endoneurium** is a delicate connective tissue layer derived from perineurium that surrounds each fiber and Schwann cell. This arrangement weaves all the nerve fibers into a structurally sound unit.

In the CNS, fibers with a common origin and a common destination form **tracts** (Figure 8-27). Tracts do not have the connective tissue components of nerves and are difficult to identify because there are no clear boundaries between them. Tracts may either be **ascending** (sensory) or **descending** (motor), but are never mixed.

Ganglia and Nuclei

As with nerve fibers, neuron cell bodies tend to be in groups. Neuron cell bodies in the PNS are found in structures called **ganglia**. **Spinal (dorsal root) ganglia** are located on both sides of the spinal cord in association with the dorsal roots of spinal nerves (Figure 8-28). They contain unipolar (first order) sensory neuron cell bodies surrounded by **satellite cells**. **Sympathetic (prevertebral) ganglia** (Figure 8-29) are part of the sympathetic trunks on the ventral side of the vertebral column. They contain sympathetic postganglionic neuron cell bodies. The neurons are multipolar with **lipofuchsin granules** (cellular debris) and lack a well-organized layer of satellite cells. Other ganglia are found in association with the viscera (on or in organs) and contain autonomic neuron cell bodies (Figure 8-30).

A group of functionally related neurons in the CNS is called a **nucleus**. (Figure 8-31). By definition, nuclei are in the gray matter, but they are less obvious than ganglia because they lack a connective tissue covering that forms an outer boundary. There are many nuclei in the brain, especially in the thalamus and hypothalamus.

▪▪ Other Neural Structures

Meninges

Connective tissue is absent from the interior of the CNS, but it is covered with three connective tissue layers referred to as **meninges** (Figure 8-32). The innermost, the **pia mater**, is a delicate layer of collagen and elastic fibers with a basement

---
[1] Some authors restrict this term to the membrane of the Schwann cell.

membrane. The middle layer, the **arachnoid**, consists of fibrous strands that form a weblike layer continuous with the pia mater. Blood vessels pass through the **subarachnoid space**, as does **cerebrospinal fluid** (CSF). The outermost layer is made up of dense connective tissue and is called the **dura mater**. It may be visible in spinal cord preparations, but is usually absent from brain specimens since it contributes to the periosteum of the skull and is difficult to remove with the brain.

Choroid Plexus

The ependymal cells of the brain's ventricles associate with the pia mater to form highly vascular infoldings called **choroid plexus** (Figure 8-33). These are responsible for producing cerebrospinal fluid, which bathes the CNS and acts as a shock absorber, assists in maintaining chemical homeostasis, and provides buoyancy to the brain.

Synapse Structure

A **synapse** is the intercellular junction between a neuron and another cell. If the junction is formed with another neuron, it is called an **axodendritic** or **axosomatic junction**, depending on its location (Figure 8-34). If it is formed with a skeletal muscle cell, it is called a **neuromuscular junction** (Figure 8-35). In either case, the two cells involved in the junction do not actually contact one another, but rather have a 20 to 30 nm space called the **synaptic cleft** separating them. When the electrical nerve impulse reaches the end of an axon, a chemical **neurotransmitter** is released by the **presynaptic neuron** that diffuses across the synaptic cleft to bind with receptors on the **postsynaptic neuron**, or muscle cell. The consequence of a neurotransmitter binding to receptors in the postsynaptic neuron membrane may be stimulation or inhibition, depending on the neuron and the neurotransmitter. Binding of a neurotransmitter (acetyl choline) by a muscle cell causes it to contract.

■■ Organs of the Central Nervous System

Spinal Cord

The **spinal cord** is continuous with the **medulla oblongata** of the brain stem. It begins as the medulla passes through the foramen magnum at the base of the skull and continues to its own termination even with the second lumbar vertebra. In cross section (Figures 8-36 and 8-37), the white matter surrounds gray matter, which is in the shape of the letter *H*. The gray matter is divided into three or four regions, depending on the spinal cord region. The **dorsal gray horns** contain interneuron cell bodies and cell bodies of **second order sensory neurons**[2] that carry impulses to the thalamus. The dorsal horns usually extend to the surface of the cord. **Ventral gray**

horns contain somatic motor neuron cell bodies. There is considerable white matter between the ventral horns and the spinal cord's surface. **Lateral gray horns** are found in spinal cord segments involved in the autonomic nervous system, that is, T_1 through L_2 and S_2 through S_4. The former contain **sympathetic preganglionic neuron** cell bodies, whereas the latter contain **parasympathetic preganglionic neuron** cell bodies. Finally, the **gray commissure** primarily contains axons of interneurons crossing to the other side of the cord. In the middle of the gray commissure is the **central canal**. It is small, lined with ependymal cells, and carries cerebrospinal fluid.

The white matter of the cord is divided into **dorsal, lateral, and ventral funiculi**, or **columns**. The funiculi carry ascending and descending fiber tracts, but their precise locations are not identifiable due to the absence of connective tissue boundaries.

The **ventral median fissure** is a deep indentation on the ventral side of the cord along the midline. A shallower and narrower **dorsal median sulcus** is on the dorsal side.

Each spinal nerve is connected to the spinal cord by two roots. These are the **dorsal root** and the **ventral root** (Figure 8-38). Even though all spinal nerves are mixed, sensory and motor fibers segregate in the roots. All sensory fibers entering the spinal cord follow the dorsal root and have their cell bodies in the **dorsal root ganglion**, and all motor fibers leave the cord through the ventral root.

Like other parts of the CNS, the spinal cord is covered with meninges. The dura mater of the cord is continuous with the epineurium of the spinal nerve roots (Figure 8-39).

Medulla Oblongata

The **medulla oblongata** (Figure 8-40) is the most inferior part of the brain and joins the spinal cord. Its white matter is composed primarily of ascending and descending tracts. The **pyramidal tracts** carry motor fibers arising from the motor cortex of the cerebrum and are visible as the raised **pyramids** on the ventral surface of the medulla. A majority of the fibers in these tracts cross to the opposite side at the **decussation of the pyramids**. These fibers continue down into the cord to synapse with somatic motor neurons in the ventral gray horns. Medullary gray matter includes various nuclei.

Cerebellum

The **cerebellum** is composed of gray matter around white matter and has a prominently convoluted surface (Figure 8-41). The gray matter is the **cerebellar cortex** and consists of a superficial **molecular layer** and a deeper **granular layer**. The molecular layer is composed mostly of unmyelinated fibers and a few neurons, whereas the granular layer has numerous neurons. At the junction of the two layers are the distinctive **Purkinje cells**, whose dendrites project into the molecular layer and whose axons enter the white matter of the **cerebellar medulla** (Figure 8-42). The cerebellum is involved in coordinating and refining somatic motor activity. As such, it has connections to and from the motor cortex of

---

[2] First order sensory neurons have their cell bodies in spinal ganglia and transmit information from sensory receptors to second order neurons.

the cerebrum, and from **proprioceptors** in muscles, tendons, and joints.

Cerebrum

The **cerebral cortex** is the layer of gray matter on the surface of the cerebrum. The cortex is highly folded into **sulci** (depressions) and **gyri** (ridges), more commonly referred to as **convolutions**. The cerebrum is the site of higher thought processes and reasoning, as well as the location of neurons responsible for interpreting sensory input to produce various sensations, initiating voluntary motor activity, and storing memory.

In most parts of the cerebral cortex, there are six identifiable layers. These are listed below from superficial to deep (Figures 8-43 and 8-44).

I. The **molecular layer** is the most superficial layer of the cortex and is adjacent to the pia mater. It consists primarily of neuronal axons and dendrites, and scattered glial cells.

II. The **outer granular layer** consists of two neuron types: small **pyramidal cells** and granular (**stellate**) **cells**.

III. The **pyramidal cell layer** is fairly thick and contains pyramidal cells of increasing size with increasing depth.

IV. The **inner granular layer** is composed of stellate cells.

V. The **ganglionic layer** has large pyramidal cells (**Betz cells**), stellate cells, and cells of Martinotti.

VI. The **multiform cell layer** is the deepest in the cortex. It is characterized by a grouping of neurons with various shapes, including **fusiform cells**.

White matter of the cerebrum is deep to the multiform cell layer of the cortex. It is composed of **projection** (both ascending and descending), **association** (within a hemisphere), and **commissural** (connecting opposite hemispheres) **tracts**.

Nervous System				
Afferent (Sensory) System		Efferent (Motor) System		
			Visceral Motor (Autonomic)	
Visceral Sensory	Somatic Sensory	Somatic Motor	Parasympathetic (Craniosacral) Division	Sympathetic (Thoracolumbar) Division

8-2 Functional Organization of the Nervous System ◾ In spite of its complexity, there is organization to the nervous system. Shown here is the functional scheme. Learn it and then pay careful attention to the location(s) of the neuron cell bodies and fibers of each and you will see there is also structural organization.

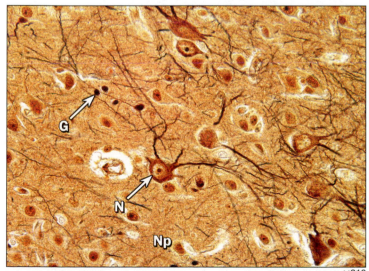

×210

8-3 Cells of Nervous Tissue ◾ Nervous tissue is made of two basic cell types: neurons (N), which are larger and conduct nerve impulses, and smaller neuroglia (glial cells) (G), which perform a variety of functions. Neurons are larger and have a complex shape that generally cannot be fully appreciated in histology specimens because they have been sectioned. Note that the nuclei are lighter staining than the nucleoli. The neuropil (Np) primarily consists of neuronal cytoplasmic processes. (×210)

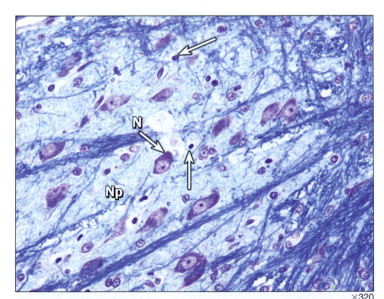

×320

8-4 Probable Microglia ◾ Microglia (arrows) are phagocytic cells of neural tissue, but are difficult to identify with a high degree of certainty in routine preparations. They are small cells with a dense and elongated nucleus. Also visible are neurons (N) and neuropil (Np). This specimen was stained using Lugol's fast blue and crystal violet. (×320)

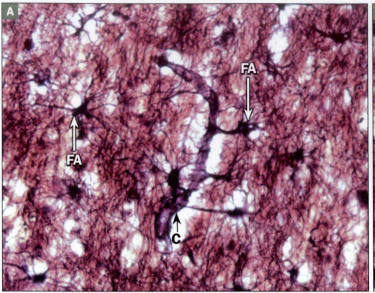

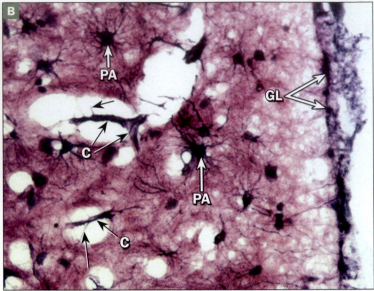

8-5 Astrocytes ◼

Astrocytes are highly branched and form connections with other astrocytes, blood vessels, and neurons. Their functions are many and varied (see text). They do not stain readily with H&E, but can be differentiated with Cajal's gold sublimate stain (**A** and **B**) or with antibody-based stains specific to glial fibrillary acidic protein (**C**). All three micrographs are sections of the brain. (**A**) These fibrous astrocytes (FA), identified based on their presence in white matter, are connected with each other, and some show connection to the capillary (C) in the center of the field. Their perivascular feet (not readily identifiable in this section) attach to the basement membrane of the capillary's endothelium. (×400) (**B**) Protoplasmic astrocytes are found in gray matter. Note the highly branched processes in the labeled cells (PA) and the connections (arrows) to capillaries (C). Also note the staining density on the surface. These are the astrocytes participating with the pia mater to form the glia limitans (GL). (×320) (**C**) These protoplasmic astrocytes were stained with antibodies specific to their glial fibrillary acidic proteins. Notice the shorter length and higher degree of branching of their processes compared to the fibrous astrocytes in (**A**). (×400)

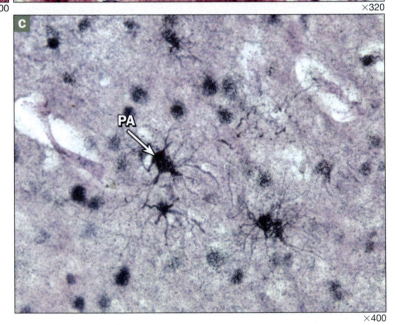

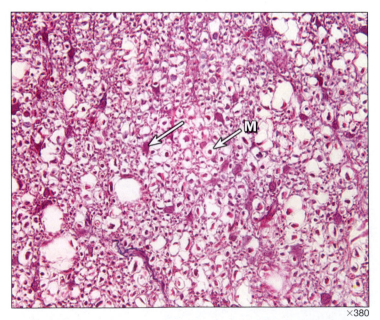

8-6 Oligodendrocytes ◼

The most abundant glial cell of white matter is the oligodendrocyte (arrow). These cells are responsible for producing myelin (M) in the CNS. (×380)

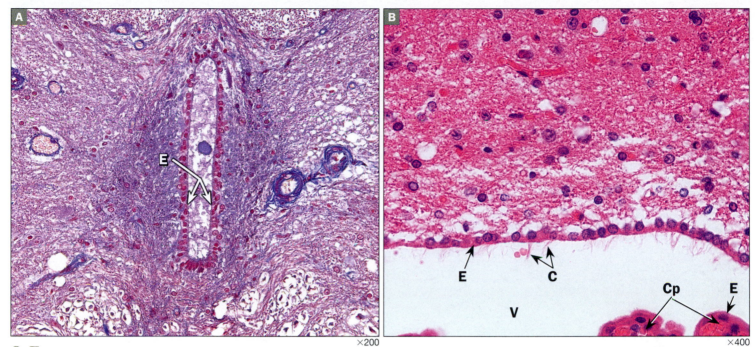

×200

×400

8-7 **Ependymal Cells** ■ The ventricles of the brain and the central canal of the spinal cord are lined with an epithelium-like layer of ependymal cells. (**A**) Shown is the central canal of the spinal cord. Note the single layer of cuboidal to columnar ependymal cells (E). (×200) (**B**) In this section of the brain, the ependymal cells (E) show cilia (C). The white space is the ventricle (V). At the bottom of the field are pieces of the choroid plexus (Cp), which is lined with modified ependymal cells and is responsible for producing cerebrospinal fluid (see Figure 8-33). (×400)

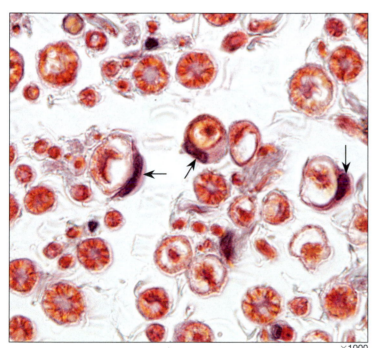

×1000

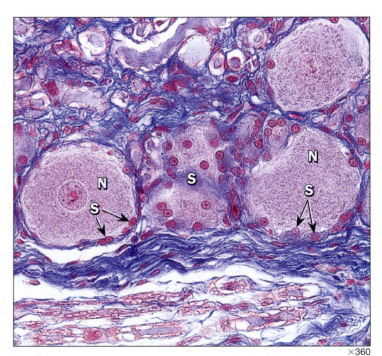

×360

8-8 **Schwann Cells** ■ Myelin in the PNS is produced by Schwann cells (arrows). At this magnification of a nerve cross section, the Schwann cell nucleus and cytoplasm (neurilemma) is visible. However, at lower magnification, Schwann cells may only be identified by their dark-staining, crescent-shaped nuclei. (×1000)

8-9 **Satellite Cells** ■ Satellite cells surround neurons in ganglia. They maintain the environment around neurons and provide insulation for synapsing neurons in autonomic ganglia. These neurons (N) are from the dorsal root ganglion and are surrounded by satellite cells (S). The satellite cells form an obvious covering of the neurons on the left and right. The cell on the left was sectioned through its nucleus; the one on the right was not. In the center you see that the plane of section passed through the satellite cell layer of the neuron (which isn't visible). (×360)

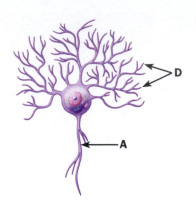

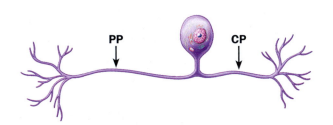

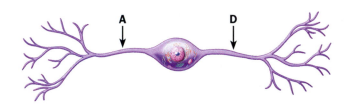

8-10 **Neuron Structure** ◼ Shown are the three structural types of neurons. At the top is a multipolar neuron with numerous, short, and highly branched dendrites (D) and a single, long axon (A), which also may be branched. Motor neurons and interneurons are multipolar. In the center is a bipolar neuron, with a single axon and dendrite. These are found in some sensory pathways. At the bottom is a unipolar (or pseudounipolar) neuron with a single branched process formed from the fusion of the axon and dendrite. Sensory neurons entering the spinal cord are unipolar, with the peripheral process (PP) carrying information from the sensory receptor and the central process (CP) entering the spinal cord.

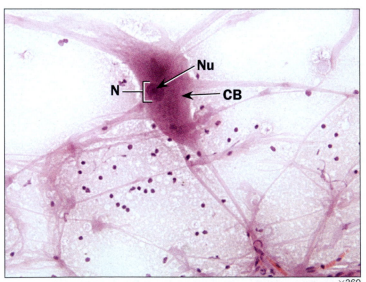

×360

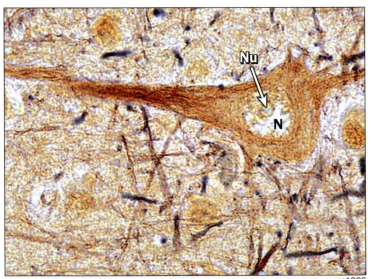

×1000

8-11 **A Typical Neuron** ◼ This micrograph is a whole-mount smear of spinal cord tissue. The neuron shown here exhibits typical features: large, irregular shape; one axon; and one to many dendrites but in this cell it is not possible to distinguish between them (see Figure 8-12). Different stains are used to highlight different neuronal structures, but generally the nucleus (N) is lighter staining than the prominent nucleolus (Nu). The cytoplasm surrounding the nucleus is called the cell body (CB), or perikaryon. The material surrounding the neuron is the neuropil and the majority of small, dark nuclei in it belong to glial cells. Note also the tangle of axons and dendrites in the left and lower portions of the field. Most don't belong to the neuron shown. (×360)

8-12 **Neurofilaments** ◼ The cytoskeleton of neurofilaments (dark lines) is often visible in neurons. Notice the large nucleus (N) with its darker nucleolus (Nu). This specimen is a silver-stained section of brain. (×1000)

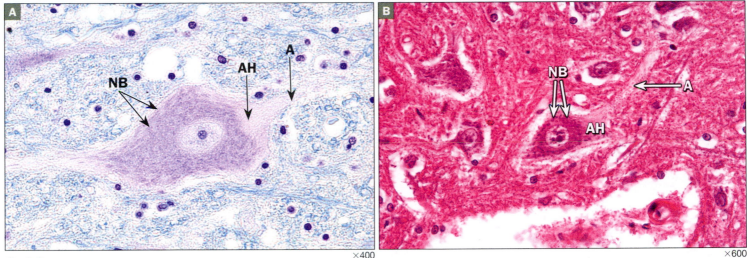

8-13 Nissl Bodies in Neurons ■ With proper staining, Nissl bodies (NB) are visible in the cytoplasm of some neurons as granular material. Electron micrographic studies have shown the Nissl substance to be rough endoplasmic reticulum. The Nissl substance is absent from the base of the axon, the axon hillock (AH), making it possible to identify the axon (A) without seeing its entire length. Of course, if the section doesn't pass through the axon hillock you won't be able to identify the axon. Both (**A**, ×400) and (**B**, ×600) are sections of multipolar neurons.

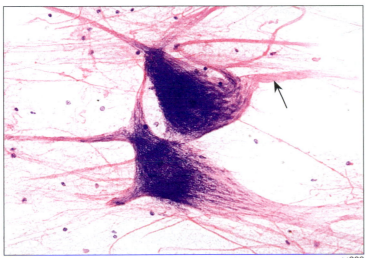

8-14 Multipolar Neuron ■ This is a smear of neural tissue. Notice the multiple cytoplasmic processes of these neurons. It is not clear which is the axon in each, but the arrow indicates a likely candidate in the upper cell. The others are dendrites. (×200)

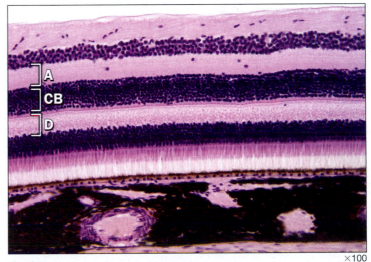

8-15 Bipolar Neurons of the Retina ■ Bipolar neurons have a single axon and dendrite (also see Figure 8-10). In this section of the retina, their parts are organized into layers. Cell bodies are in the layer labeled "CB" with the axons (A) and dendrites (D) extending into the layers on either side. In addition to the retina, bipolar neurons are found in the auditory pathway. (×100)

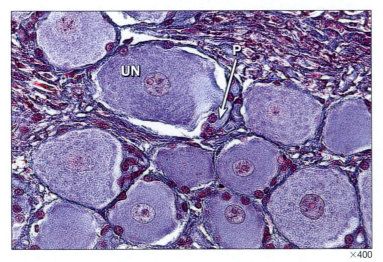

8-16 Unipolar (Pseudounipolar) Neurons ■ Unipolar neurons (UN) have a single process (P) that divides into a peripheral process, which comes from a sensory receptor, and a central process, which leads to the CNS. The cell body is spherical. This specimen was taken from a dorsal root ganglion. (×400)

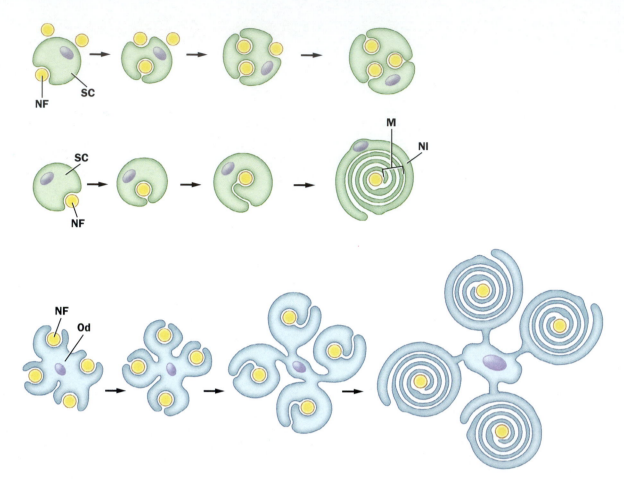

8-17 Myelin Sheath 🔲 (Center) In the peripheral nervous system, myelin (M) is produced by compressed modified cytoplasmic membrane of a Schwann cell as it wraps around a nerve fiber (NF). The neurilemma (Nl) is composed of the Schwann cell (SC) wrapped around the myelin. (**Top**) Unmyelinated fibers (above) are also associated with Schwann cells, but notice that it doesn't wrap around them. (**Bottom**) In the central nervous system, oligodendrocytes (Od) myelinate several different fibers at once. Notice the oligodendrocyte cytoplasm doesn't wrap around the myelin, and so there is no neurilemma.

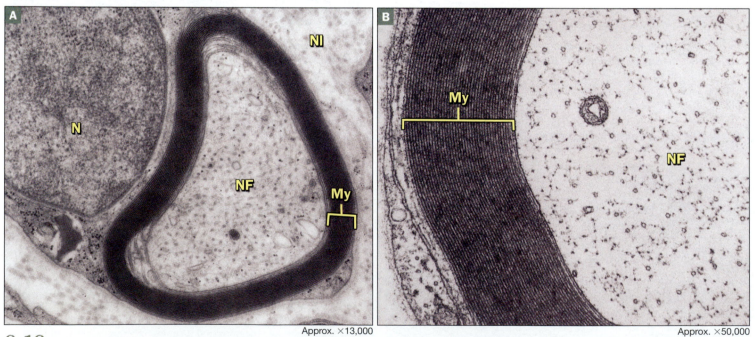

Approx. ×13,000   Approx. ×50,000

8-18 Myelin Sheath 🔲 (**A**) This transmission electron micrograph shows the myelin sheath (My) as multiple wraps of the modified Schwann cell membrane. The neurilemma (Nl), Schwann cell nucleus (N), and nerve fiber (NF) are also visible. (Approx. ×13,000) (**B**) The layers of membrane are visible in this higher magnification of myelin. (Approx. ×50,000)

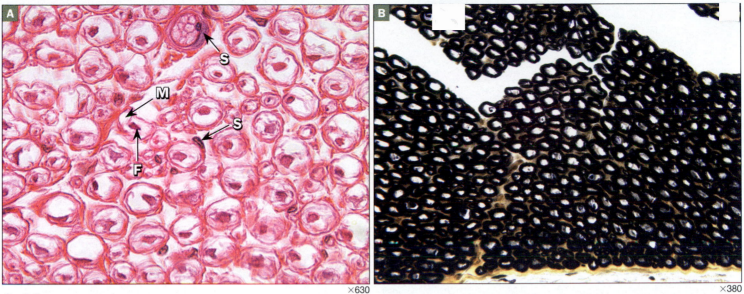

×630   ×380

8-19 **Myelinated Fibers** ▪ **(A)** In this nerve cross section, the myelin sheaths (M) surround nerve fibers (F), but are not uniformly seen due to slide preparation. Schwann cell nuclei (S) are also visible. (×630) **(B)** This nerve cross section was prepared with an osmium stain that stains fat black and thus highlights the myelin. (×380)

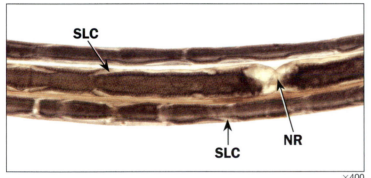

×400

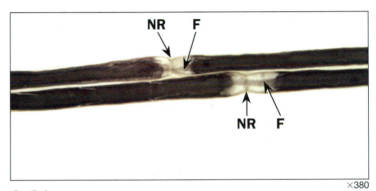

×380

8-20 **Schmidt-Lanterman Clefts** ▪ During myelination, some cytoplasm is trapped in the myelin sheath and is visible as Schmidt-Lanterman clefts (SLC). A node of Ranvier (NR) is also visible. (×400)

8-21 **Nodes of Ranvier** ▪ Gaps in the myelin sheath between adjacent Schwann cells are called nodes of Ranvier (NR). The electrical activity associated with impulse transmission only occurs at the nodes of a myelinated fiber rather than its entire length, as in unmyelinated fibers. This results in faster impulse conduction. The fiber (F) is visible as a gray line crossing the node. (×380)

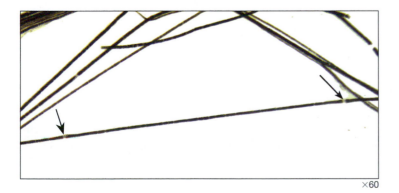

×60

8-22 **Internodes** ▪ Two nodes of Ranvier are indicated with arrows; the region in between is known as the internode. Since internodes are not involved in impulse transmission and they constitute the majority of the fiber, impulse transmission is more rapid in myelinated fibers than in unmyelinated ones. (×60)

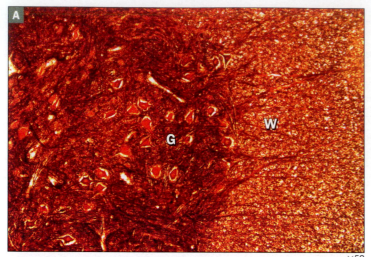

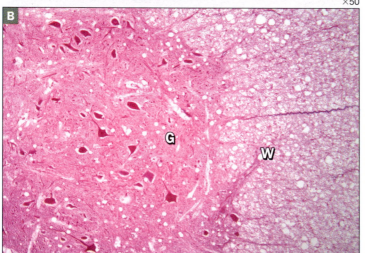

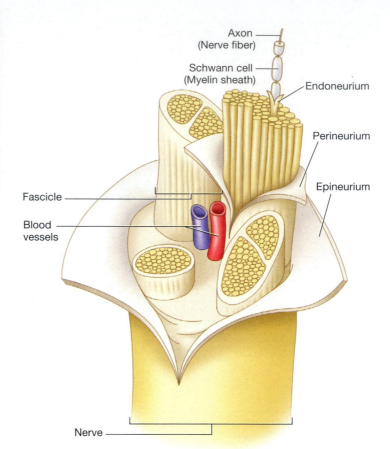

8-24 **Nerve Structure** ▰ Nerves are made of nerve fibers and connective tissue. Each nerve is surrounded by a connective tissue epineurium. The perineurium surrounds fascicles of fibers, and the endoneurium surrounds each individual fiber.

8-23 **Gray and White Matter** ▰ In the CNS, regions of myelinated fibers have a whitish appearance and are known as white matter (W). The main cells of white matter are oligodendrocytes. Gray matter (G) is composed of neuron cell bodies, glial cells, and unmyelinated fibers (though a few myelinated fibers may be found). Both specimens are from the spinal cord. (**A**) Silver stain, ×50. (**B**) H&E stain, ×50.

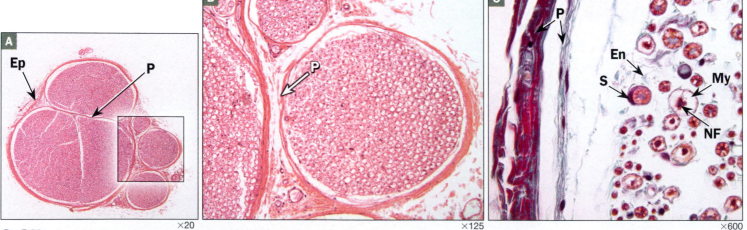

8-25 **Connective Tissue Components of a Nerve** (**A**) This is a cross section of a small nerve. It is covered with epineurium (Ep), which penetrates the nerve as perineurium (P) and forms bundles of nerve fibers called fascicles. Four fascicles are present; the white circles within each are myelinated nerve fibers. (H&E stain, ×20) (**B**) This is an enlargement of the boxed area in (**A**) showing one fascicle. (×125) (**C**) This section of a nerve was stained with Masson stain, which makes connective tissue blue. The endoneurium (En) and part of the perineurium (which was separated during preparation) are visible. Also seen are Schwann cells (S), myelin (My), and fibers (NF). (×600)

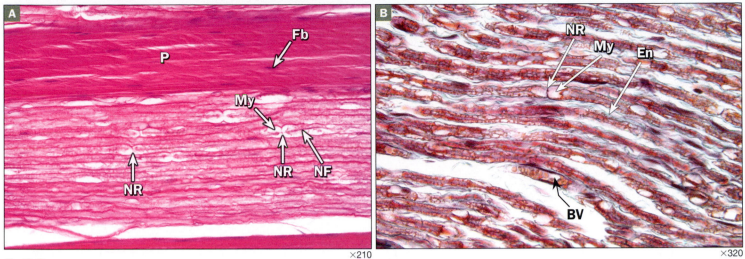

8-26 Longitudinal Sections of a Nerve ■ (A) The perineurium (P) with fibroblast nuclei (Fb) is obvious, but the endoneurium is difficult to discern in this H&E preparation of a nerve cut in longitudinal section. Myelin (My), nerve fibers (NF) and nodes of Ranvier (NR) are also visible. (×210) (B) This longitudinal section of a nerve prepared with Masson stain clearly illustrates the endoneurium (En). A blood vessel (BV) is also visible. Other structures are labeled as in (A). (×320)

8-27 Tracts ■ Collections of myelinated nerve fibers in the CNS are called tracts, and they comprise the white matter. Although the general location of each tract is known, their precise boundaries are unclear due to the absence of connective tissue or any other landmark around them. For instance, in this spinal cord specimen, the lateral (L) spinothalamic and anterior (A) spinocerebellar tracts are adjacent, but there is no clear boundary between them. (×20)

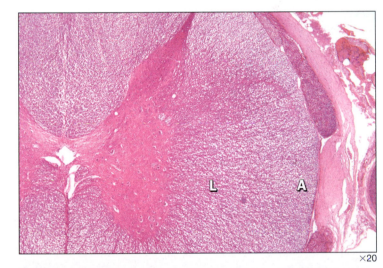

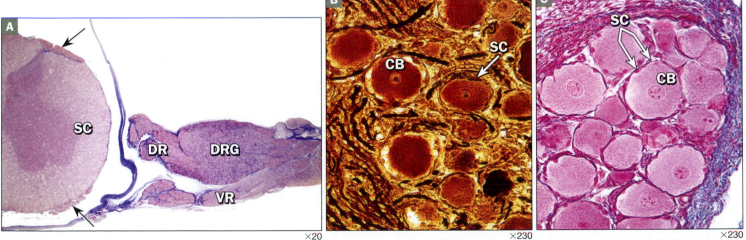

8-28 Dorsal Root Ganglion ■ Neuron cell bodies in the PNS are found in ganglia. Shown here are three examples of dorsal root ganglia, which are located in the dorsal root of each spinal nerve and contain sensory neuron cell bodies. (A) The dorsal root ganglion (DRG) is seen as an expanded region of the dorsal root (DR). The ventral root (VR) is also visible. It contains motor fibers. The plane of this section did not pass completely through the dorsal and ventral roots, and so each appears to be separated from the spinal cord (SC). However, because each spreads out in the immediate vicinity of the spinal cord, pieces of their attachments are visible on the surface of the cord (arrows). (×20) (B and C) The unipolar neuron cell bodies (CB) and satellite cells (SC) surrounding them are seen in these micrographs. (Both ×230)

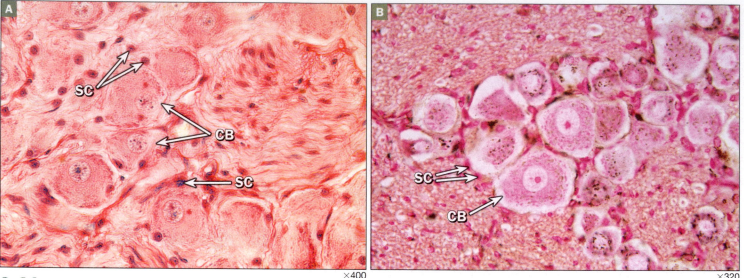

8-29 Autonomic Ganglia ■ (A) Sympathetic postganglionic neuron cell bodies (CB) are seen in this sympathetic ganglion. The neurons are multipolar and satellite cells (SC), while present, are fewer in number than in dorsal root ganglia. (×400) (B) In addition to the features visible in (A), the neurons in this ganglion show brown lipofuchsin granules, which are breakdown products from lysosome activity. They increase in number with age. (×320)

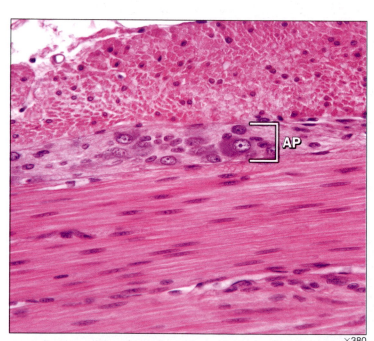

8-30 Auerbach's Plexus ■ Some ganglia are embedded in other organs. Neurons serving the musculature of the digestive tract are located between muscle layers in the digestive organs and form Auerbach's plexus (AP). A second plexus, the submucosal (Meissner's) plexus, is also present in these organs and is responsible for regulating glandular activity, but is not shown here. Also see Figure 14-13. (×380)

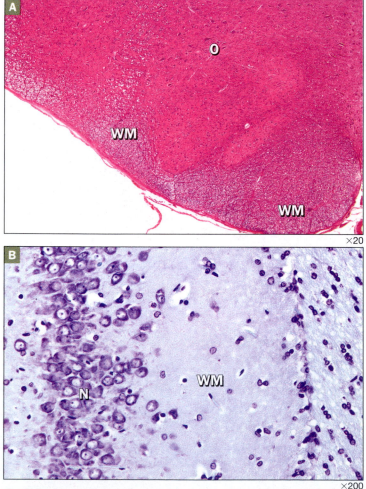

8-31 Nuclei in the CNS ■ Groups of functionally related neuron cell bodies in the CNS are called nuclei and they form gray matter, which stands out against the white matter (WM). (A) Shown is the olivary nucleus (O) of the medulla oblongata. (×20) (B) Part of an unidentified nucleus (N) in the brain stained with Lugol's fast blue and crystal violet is shown in this micrograph. (×200)

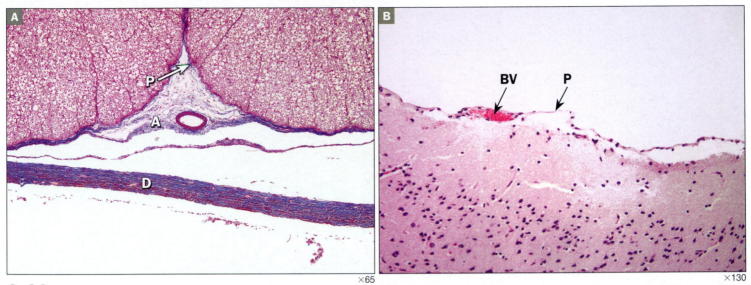

×65

×130

8-32 Meninges ◼ **(A)** The three meningeal layers are visible in this spinal cord specimen. The outermost dura mater (D) has pulled away from the arachnoid (A) during preparation. The pia mater (P) is visible as a blue line on the surface of the cord. (×65) **(B)** A blood vessel (BV) is visible in the pia mater (P) of this cerebrum specimen. The other meningeal layers have been removed. (×130)

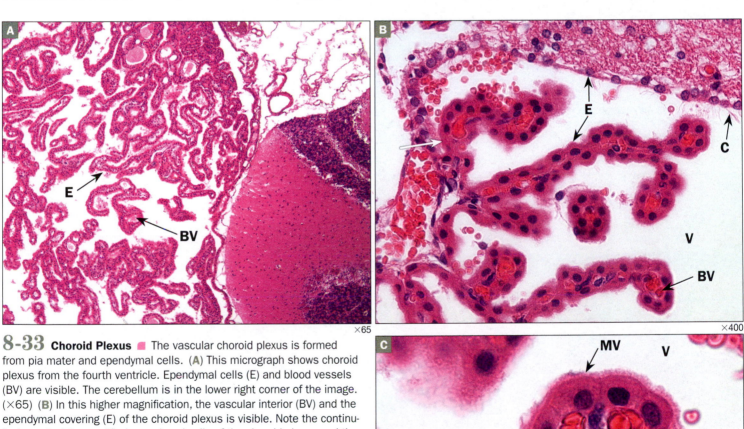

×65

×400

×1000

8-33 Choroid Plexus ◼ The vascular choroid plexus is formed from pia mater and ependymal cells. **(A)** This micrograph shows choroid plexus from the fourth ventricle. Ependymal cells (E) and blood vessels (BV) are visible. The cerebellum is in the lower right corner of the image. (×65) **(B)** In this higher magnification, the vascular interior (BV) and the ependymal covering (E) of the choroid plexus is visible. Note the continuity (arrow) of the modified ependymal cells of the choroid plexus and the ependymal cells lining the ventricle (V), which are ciliated (C). Blood cells in the ventricle are an artifact of preparation. Ventricles are normally filled with cerebrospinal fluid, which lacks blood cells. (×400) **(C)** Note the microvilli (MV) on the surface of the ependymal cells. As in **(B)**, the blood cells in the ventricle (V) are artifacts of preparation. (×1000)

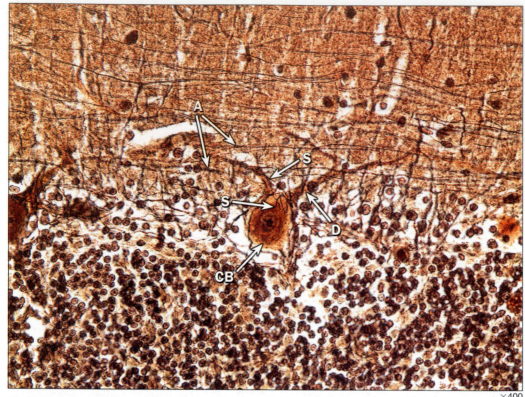

8-34 **Synapses** ▪ The synapses (S) between several axons (A, thin black lines) and the cell body (CB) (axosomatic) and dendrites (D, thick golden processes) (axodendritic) of a Purkinje cell in the cerebellum are shown in this micrograph. Note that this is a section. An axon that "ends" on the dendrite is not necessarily the site of a synapse; it may just be where the axon was cut. The value of this micrograph lies in showing all the axons that are located in the neighborhood of the large neuron and likely form synapses with it. Also see Figure 8-42. (×400)

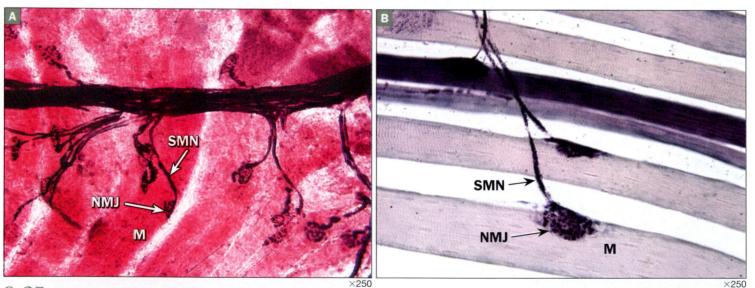

8-35 **Neuromuscular Junctions** ▪ Neuromuscular junctions (NMJ) contain the synapse between a somatic motor neuron (SMN) and a skeletal muscle fiber (M). They are complex structures made from the membranes of both cells. (Both ×250)

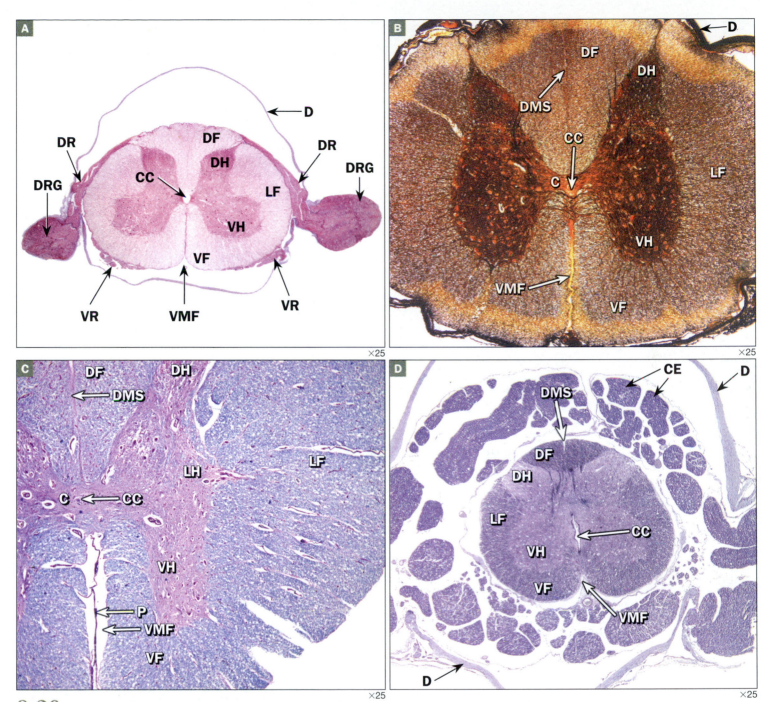

8-36 Spinal Cord in Cross Section ▪ These four micrographs are of spinal cords from different specimens and regions. Specimens (**A**) and (**C**) are from the thoracic region. Specimens (**B**) and (**D**) are from the cervical and lumbar regions, respectively. The gray objects surrounding the lumbar cord (**D**) are spinal nerves of the cauda equina. All were magnified ×25.

Key to symbols used

C = central commissure

CC = central canal

CE = spinal nerves of cauda equina

D = dura mater

DF = dorsal white funiculus (column)

DH = dorsal gray horn (with interneuron cell bodies)

DMS = dorsal median sulcus

DR = dorsal root (with sensory fibers)

DRG = dorsal root ganglion (with visceral and somatic sensory neuron cell bodies)

LF = lateral white funiculus (column)

LH = lateral gray horn (with autonomic—in this case, sympathetic—preganglionic neuron cell bodies)

P = pia mater

VF = ventral white funiculus (column)

VH = ventral gray horn (with somatic motor neuron cell bodies)

VMF = ventral median fissure

VR = ventral root (with motor fibers)

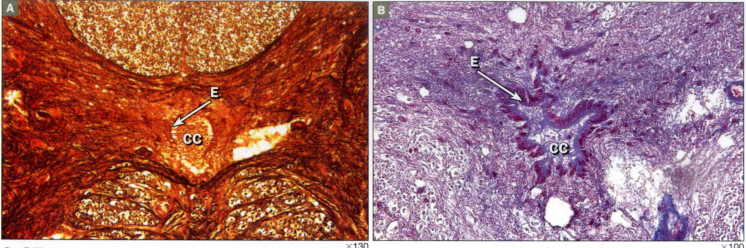

8-37 **Central Commissure and Central Canal of Spinal Cord** ▰ (**A**) The central commissure is gray matter, but fibers (black lines) crossing from one side of the cord to the other are also present. The central canal (CC) is lined with ependymal cells (E) and contains cerebrospinal fluid. (×130) (**B**) The central canal. (×100)

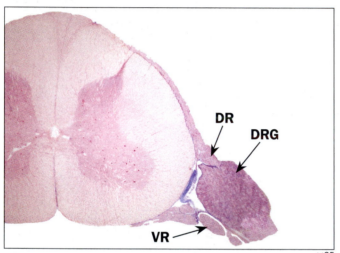

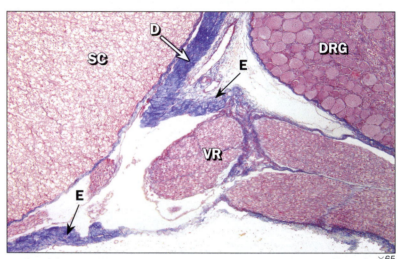

8-38 **Spinal Nerve Roots** ▰ Each spinal nerve is attached to its segment of the spinal cord by two roots. The dorsal root (DR) carries sensory fibers entering the cord. The cell bodies of these sensory neurons are located in the dorsal root ganglion (DRG). The ventral root (VR) carries motor fibers out of the cord. (×25)

8-39 **Dura Mater and Epineurium** ▰ The dura mater (D) and epineurium (E) form a continuous layer where the nerve roots join the spinal cord. The ventral root (VR), dorsal root ganglion (DRG), and spinal cord (SC) are shown. (×65)

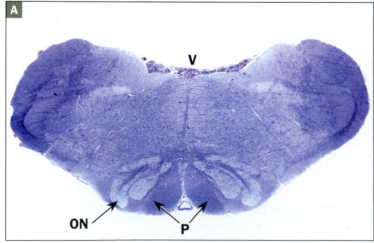

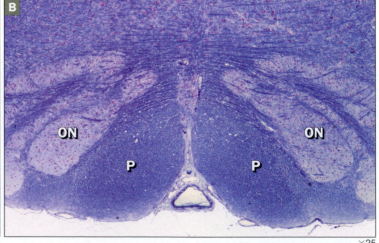

8-40 **Medulla Oblongata** ▰ The medulla oblongata houses ascending (sensory) and descending tracts (motor), and several nuclei. (**A**) This is a panoramic view of the medulla magnified ×6. The fourth ventricle (V) is at the top. At the bottom are the pyramids (P), which are major descending tracts. The olivary nucleus (ON) is also visible. (**B**) This is a higher magnification of the olivary nuclei and the pyramids. (×25)

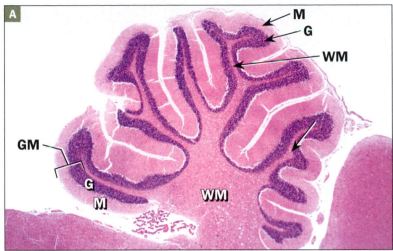

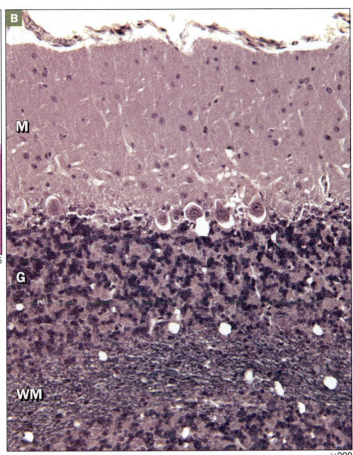

8-41 Cerebellum ■ The cerebellum is involved in coordinating motor functions. (**A**) Shown is a section of the cerebellum of a small mammal. Its convolutions and organization of gray matter (GM) around white matter are apparent. The gray matter is the cerebellar cortex and is divided into a superficial molecular layer (M) and a deeper granular layer (G). The white matter (WM) carries fibers entering and leaving the cerebellum. (×35) (**B**) This micrograph was magnified ×200 and shows the layers in the cerebellum.

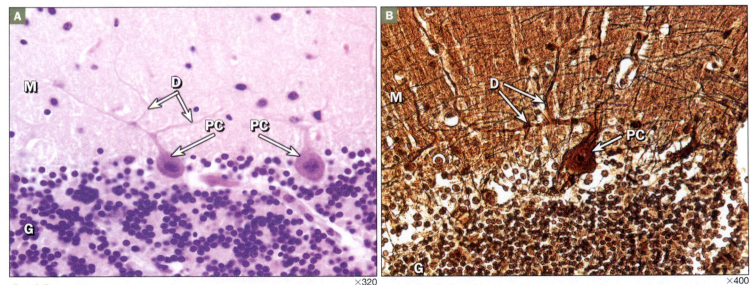

8-42 Purkinje Cells ■ The most distinctive cells of the cerebellum are the Purkinje cells (PC), which are found at the junction of the molecular (M) and granular (G) layers. They have highly branched dendrites (D) that enter the molecular layer. Their single axon (not shown in these sections) penetrates the granular layer. (**A**) This micrograph illustrates the branched dendrites of Purkinje cells. (×320) (**B**) The horizontal axons in the molecular layer are visible as black lines in this specimen stained with Woelke's stain and nuclear fast red stain. Also note the prominent nucleolus in the Purkinje cell. (×400)

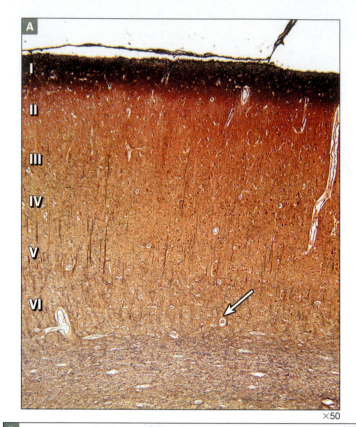

×50

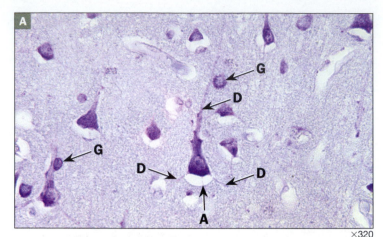

×320

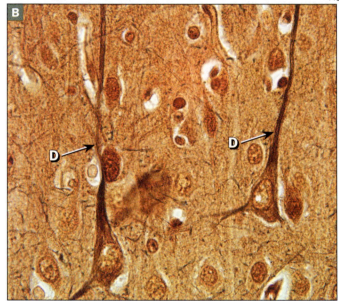

×530

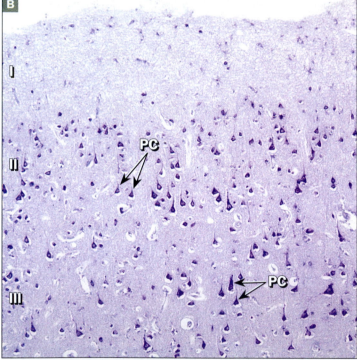

×100

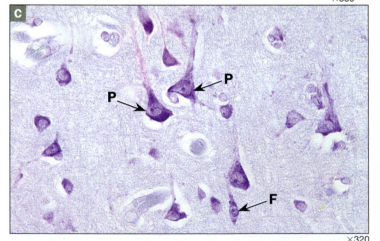

×320

8-43 **Cerebral Cortex** ▣ The cerebral cortex is a thin layer of gray matter on the surface of the cerebrum. In most parts of the cerebrum, it is divided into six layers. (**A**) From superficial to deep: (I) molecular (plexiform) layer, (II) outer granular layer, (III) pyramidal cell layer, (IV) inner granular layer, (V) ganglionic layer, (VI) multiform cell layer. (×50) (**B**) This is a higher magnification of a crystal violet-stained section of cerebral cortex, showing layers I, II, and III. Layer I is composed of fibers that run parallel to the surface, glial cells, and a few neurons. The division between layers II and III is not as distinct as that separating layers I and II. Pyramidal cells (PC) are in both, but are larger in layer III. Other neurons called granular (stellate) cells are abundant in layer II (and IV). (×100)

8-44 **Cells of the Cerebral Cortex** ▣ (**A**) The most distinctive cells of the cortex are the pyramidal cells. Their apex is pointed toward the surface. The axon (A) emerges from the other end. Dendrites (D) are found at the apex and at the corners of the base. Pyramidal cells are found in most levels, with the larger ones being deeper in the cortex. Two probable granular cells (G) are also shown. (×320) (**B**) Two pyramidal cells are seen in this specimen stained with a silver stain. (×530) (**C**) Fusiform cells (F) have a single axon emerging from the side and dendrites coming off both tapered ends. Pyramidal cells (P) are also seen in this specimen. (×320)

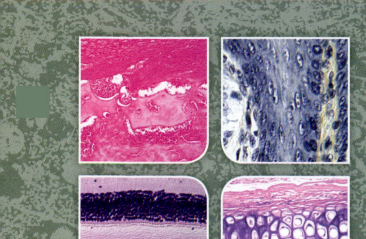

9

Special Sensory Organs

Introduction to the Senses

Sensory receptors receive and respond to stimuli arising either from within the body or from the external environment. They are divided into receptors of the **general senses** and the **special senses**.

General sensory receptors are simple in construction and are widely distributed in the body. Examples include touch receptors (**Meissner's corpuscles**) and pressure receptors (**Pacinian corpuscles**) of the skin, which are covered in Chapter 11. Other general sensory receptors are covered in their respective chapters.

The special senses (Figure 9-1) include taste, smell, vision, hearing, and balance and equilibrium. Their receptors are more complex in construction and are more localized. They are the topic of this chapter.

Olfactory Receptors

The receptors for olfaction are the simplest of the special senses. Olfactory epithelium covers the upper nasal cavity and superior nasal conchae (Figure 9-2). It is a modified pseudostratified ciliated columnar (PSCC) epithelium that contains the **olfactory receptor cells**, which are bipolar neurons. The end of the dendrite is dilated to form an **olfactory vesicle**, from which extend one or two dozen nonmotile cilia.

The actual chemical mechanism of how olfactory sensations are produced is beyond the scope of this book, but basically it amounts to this: membrane-bound proteins of the cilia bind to specific **odorant molecules** and initiate an action potential in the olfactory cell, which travels down the axon. Axons from olfactory cells form relatively small groups (collectively referred to as the **olfactory nerve, cranial nerve I–CN I**) that pass through a foramen in the cribriform plate to synapse with second order neurons in the **olfactory bulb**. From there, the impulse is carried to the hypothalamus,

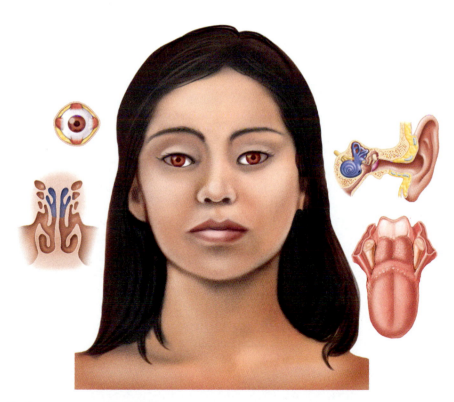

9-1 Special Sensory Organs ■ Organs of the special senses include those of vision, hearing, balance and equilibrium, taste, and smell. They are more complex in structure than those of the general senses and are highly localized in the body.

limbic system, and olfactory cortex in the temporal lobe of the cerebral cortex where the sensation of smell is produced.

Two other cells are located in the olfactory epithelium. **Basal cells** are small and located near the basement membrane. These stem cells can produce new olfactory receptor cells (whose life span is approximately one month—note, this is an example of neuron regeneration!) and **supporting cells.** The tall supporting (**sustentacular**) cells have microvilli and provide physical and nutritive support to the receptor cells, filling a role not unlike that of glial cells.

The three cell types are difficult to differentiate in H&E-stained specimens, but nucleus location provides a high percentage basis for identification. The nuclei of basal cells are located in the lower third of the epithelium, and nuclei of sustentacular cells are near the surface. The nuclei of olfactory receptor cells are in the middle.

The connective tissue of the deep olfactory mucosa (**lamina propria**) contains **Bowman's glands**. These serous glands produce a watery secretion that dissolves odoriferous chemicals and makes them more able to bind to and stimulate the receptors.

Taste Buds

Taste buds (Figure 9-3) are found in the epithelium of the tongue as well as other parts of the oral mucosa and house the chemoreceptor cells for the sensation of taste. They are oval-shaped with an opening at the surface called the **taste pore.** Internally, lighter-staining **taste (gustatory) cells** and darker **sustentacular cells** have long microvilli that project into the taste pore. The former are the chemoreceptor cells, but are of epithelial origin, not neural (as with olfactory receptors). **Basal cells**, which are stem cells that produce the other two cell types, are also present.

There are five basic taste stimuli: sour, salty, sweet, bitter, and umami (a Japanese word meaning "savory"). **Tastant molecules** of the sour and salty types stimulate taste cells by affecting ion channels in the microvilli membranes. The other three tastants stimulate by binding to membrane receptors in the microvilli membranes. In each case, the result is an action potential. Depending on their location on the tongue, taste cells form a synapse with sensory fibers of one of three cranial nerves (**facial–CN VII, glossopharyngeal–CN IX**, or **vagus–CN X**), which transmit the signal to neurons in the medulla oblongata. From there, the pathway leads to the thalamus, and on to the cerebral cortex in the insula.

The Eye

The eyeball (Figure 9-4) is the site of photoreceptors responsible for vision. It is composed of three basic layers (Figure 9-5). From external to internal, they are the **fibrous tunic**

(**tunica fibrosa**), the **vascular tunic (tunica vasculosa)**, and the **neural tunic (tunica nervosa)**. In addition, there are two cavities (Figure 9-4) in the eye. The **anterior cavity** is anterior to the lens and contains the watery **aqueous humor**, which supplies oxygen and nutrients to the avascular lens and cornea. The **posterior cavity** is posterior to the lens and occupies the greatest volume of the eye. It contains the gel-like, refractive **vitreous body**.

Fibrous Tunic

The fibrous tunic is mostly composed of the **sclera**, with the anterior one-sixth forming the **cornea**. The sclera is made of densely arranged collagen fibers, which accounts for its white appearance. It is an attachment site for the extraocular muscles and is continuous with the dura mater of the optic nerve.

The cornea (Figure 9-6) is transparent and avascular with five distinct layers. On the anterior, the **corneal epithelium** is a thin, highly innervated, nonkeratinized stratified squamous epithelium that is continuous with the **conjunctival epithelium** of the inner eyelid (**palpebral conjunctiva**). Deep to the corneal epithelium is **Bowman's membrane**, a thin basal lamina made of collagen. The **stroma** is the thickest layer and is composed of approximately 60 to 70 lamellae of collagen fibers. The fibers in each lamella are parallel, but are arranged at 90° angles in adjacent layers. Thin sheets of **keratocytes** are found between lamellae. The **canal of Schlemm** is found in the stroma at the **sclerocorneal junction** (Figure 9-7). **Descemet's membrane** is a thick basement membrane between the stroma and the **corneal endothelium**, which is a simple squamous or cuboidal epithelium that lines the posterior of the cornea. Among other functions, the corneal endothelium keeps the stroma dehydrated to maintain its transparency by actively transporting Na ions to the anterior chamber, with water following by osmosis.

Vascular Tunic

Deep to the fibrous tunic is the vascular tunic. It is composed of the choroid, ciliary body, and iris. The **choroid** (Figure 9-8) is made of loose connective tissue. It is highly vascular and contains an abundance of **melanin**, a black pigment.

The **ciliary body** (Figure 9-9a) is a circular expansion of the vascular tunic even with the lens. **Ciliary processes** (Figure 9-9b) extend from the ciliary body and produce **aqueous humor**, which occupies the anterior cavity of the eye (see page 109). **Suspensory ligaments of the lens** also extend from the ciliary processes and insert on the lens capsule. Smooth **ciliary muscle** within the ciliary body adjusts tension on the suspensory ligaments and in turn on the lens, thus changing its shape and allowing it to focus light on the retina.

The **iris** (Figure 9-10) is the colored part of the eye. It separates the **anterior chamber** and the **posterior chamber** of the anterior cavity. The opening in its center is the **pupil**. On the posterior surface of the iris is a layer of pigmented epithelium. The **stroma** of the iris is on its anterior surface and extends into the interior. Rather than epithelium, fibroblasts and **melanocytes** (cells that produce the black pigment melanin) form an irregular covering of the deeper, highly vascular loose connective tissue. The heavily pigmented posterior is composed of two layers: the superficial **posterior pigment epithelium** (in contact with the posterior chamber) and the deeper **anterior pigment myoepithelium.** As a consequence of these densely pigmented layers, light only enters the eye through the pupil. These pigmented layers also contribute to eye color, but not in the way you might expect. It is the number of stromal melanocytes and the amount of melanin they possess that determine eye color; there are not different pigments for each. The abundance of collagen also plays a role. With few melanocytes and limited melanin, light reflecting off the black pigment layers of the posterior of the iris appears blue. Successively darker eye colors correspond to greater abundance of melanocytes and melanin in the stroma.

Regulation of light entering the eye occurs through the action of two muscles—the **dilator pupillae muscle** and the **sphincter pupillae muscle**—which open and close the iris, respectively. Extensions of the pigmented myoepithelial cells are oriented radially around the pupil and comprise the former. Smooth muscle cells oriented circularly around the pupil comprise the latter.

Aqueous humor is derived from capillaries in the ciliary processes. It flows from the posterior chamber, through the pupil, into the anterior chamber, and is returned to the blood by the canal of Schlemm. Aqueous humor supplies the lens and cornea with oxygen and nutrients.

The lens (Figure 9-11) is an avascular, biconvex, transparent disk derived from embryonic epithelium. Its flexibility allows it to change shape (as a result of changes in tension brought about by contraction and relaxation of the ciliary muscle) and bring images into focus on the retina. It consists of three layers. On the surface is a transparent, collagenous **lens capsule** to which the suspensory ligaments attach. The second layer is a simple cuboidal **subcapsular epithelium** that lies deep to the capsule on the anterior surface. Finally, up to 3,000 elongated and hexagonal **lens fibers** make up the greatest portion of the lens. Derived from subcapsular epithelium throughout life they elongate along the anteroposterior axis of the lens and lose their organelles as they mature. The fibers' refractive ability derives from the various accumulated protein **crystallins** contained in them.

Neural Tunic

The **retina** is a complex structure composed of several types of neurons and other supporting cells. Modified neurons called **rods** and **cones** act as the **photoreceptors.** It is estimated that 7 million cones and 120 million rods occupy each retina.

Rods and cones have a complex shape. There is a **nuclear region**, which contains the nucleus, and an **inner fiber** extending anteriorly that forms synapses with other neurons of the retina. Extending posteriorly are **inner** and **outer segments** joined by a short **connecting stalk.** The inner segment produces pigment(s) for the outer segment and houses organelles consistent with such production (e.g., ribosomes and mitochondria). The outer segment has either a cylindrical shape (in rods) or a conical shape (in cones) and is the basis for naming each cell type. Within the outer segment of each are layers of membrane that house the pigments for light absorption. Connecting the two segments is a short stalk that contains a cilium derived from a basal body located in the inner segment. This suggests that the outer segment is actually a modified cilium!

Functionally, rods and cones differ in the amount of light necessary to stimulate them. Rods are stimulated in low light intensity and are responsible for monochromatic ("black and white") vision. Cones are only stimulated by higher light intensities and are responsible for color vision.

The **retina** (Figure 9-12) consists of 10 layers. With their complex shapes and their orientation perpendicular to the retina, different parts of rods and cones show up in several of the layers. The layers are listed below from outside (adjacent to the choroid) to inside (adjacent to the vitreous humor).

- A **pigmented epithelium** (retinal pigment epithelium—RPE) abuts the choroid. It is composed of short columnar cells that accumulate melanin. This pigment absorbs light that has not been absorbed by the rods and cones and prevents reflection back into the eye. The pigment cells also surround the rod and cone segments and form the **blood-retina barrier.**

- The **photoreceptive layer** contains the rod and cone segments.

- The thin, acidophilic **external limiting membrane** is not a membrane at all. It is a region of tight junctions between **Müller cells** (large glial cells—see the next page) and the rods and cones.

- The **outer nuclear layer** consists of densely packed rod and cone cell bodies and their nuclei.

- The **outer plexiform layer** is a region of axodendritic synapses between the rods and cones and the next layer of bipolar and other neurons.

- The **inner nuclear layer** contains cell bodies of **bipolar neurons**, other neurons, and Müller cells.

- The **inner plexiform layer** is a region of axodendritic synapses between bipolar neurons and the neurons (ganglion cells) of the next layer as well as other neurons.

- The **ganglion cell layer** contains cell bodies of multipolar **ganglion cells**, whose axons form the **optic tract.**

- The **optic nerve fiber layer** is composed of ganglion cell axons that converge at the optic disk and emerge as the **optic tract**. (Because the neural tunic is an outgrowth of the brain, the optic nerves are more appropriately referred to as "tracts.")

- The innermost retinal layer is the **inner limiting membrane**. It is the basal lamina of long glial cells called Müller cells that extend from the inner limiting membrane to the outer limiting membrane, where they form tight junctions with the rods and cones. Müller cells physically and metabolically support rods and cones.

Where the optic tract emerges from the eye, there are no photoreceptor cells. This is the **blind spot** (Figure 9-13). A few millimeters lateral and slightly inferior to it is a small pit in the retina where visual acuity is greatest. This is the **fovea centralis**. In its center, long, thin cones are the only photoreceptors. Their shape allows a higher density, which, not unlike high-resolution monitors with more pixels, allows greater visual acuity. At its periphery, the other retinal layers are absent or greatly reduced.

Eyelid, Conjunctiva, and Lacrimal Glands

The **eyelid** (Figure 9-14) derives structural support from a plate of fibroelastic tissue called the **tarsus** and skeletal muscle fibers from the **orbicularis oculi** and **levator palpebrae** (in the upper eyelid) **muscles**. Anteriorly, it is covered with a thin skin. Posteriorly, it is covered by the **palpebral conjunctiva,** a mucous membrane with a stratified columnar epithelium with goblet cells. The palpebral conjunctiva reflects and covers the exposed portion of the sclera as the **bulbar conjunctiva**. The mucous secretions lubricate the eyelids and eye surface. The majority of secretions lubricating and cleansing the eyes, however, come from the tubulo-acinar lacrimal glands located at the superior and lateral aspect of each eyeball. **Meibomian (tarsal) sebaceous glands** are located at the free edge of each eyelid and produce an oily secretion that prevents the eyelids from sticking together and reduces the evaporation rate of the tears.

■■ The Ear

The external ear consists of the **pinna (auricle)** and the **external auditory meatus**. The pinna (Figure 9-15) is composed of a framework of elastic cartilage covered with skin. It collects sound waves and funnels them through the external auditory meatus to the eardrum. The proximal part of the external auditory meatus is formed from elastic cartilage; the distal portion is bone. Both are lined with skin containing glands that secrete **cerumen** (earwax). The fibrous **tympanic membrane** forms the partition between the external and middle ear.

Middle Ear

The **middle ear cavity** is a space within the temporal bone and is lined with simple cuboidal to simple squamous epithelium. It opens into the nasopharynx via the **auditory (Eustachian) tube**. The **ossicles** are three small bones (**malleus, incus,** and **stapes**) that link the tympanic membrane to the oval window of the inner ear. Sound waves cause vibrations in the tympanic membrane and are amplified by the ossicles.

Internal Ear

The internal ear is made up of small cavities and channels hollowed out of the temporal bone. Collectively, these constitute the **osseous (bony) labyrinth**. The **membranous labyrinth** is contained within and conforms (more or less) in shape to the osseous labyrinth. Both are filled with fluid. The osseous labyrinth contains **perilymph**, whereas the membranous labyrinth contains **endolymph**. There are three regions in the internal ear—the vestibule, the semicircular canals, and the cochlea.

The **vestibule** (Figure 9-16) is the middle portion of the osseous labyrinth. Within it are the **utricle** and **saccule**. Both are made of membranous labyrinth. They are lined with a simple cuboidal epithelium and each contains a **macula** (Figure 9-17). The maculae are oriented at right angles to one another and are composed of receptor cells used in maintenance of balance and equilibrium. The actual receptors are **sensory hair cells** that have stereocilia and a single cilium (**kinocilium**) projecting into a gelatinous layer of glycoprotein called the **otolithic membrane. Otoliths (otoconia)**, made of calcium carbonate and protein, are also embedded in the glycoprotein. Head movements result in bending of the stereocilia and stimulation of the hair cells. This mechanical stimulation of hair cells is converted into action potentials carried by the vestibular branch of the vestibulocochlear nerve (**CN VIII**) to various parts of the brain. The brain processes this information and determines the position of the head in space and initiates compensatory motor reflexes, if necessary.

Extending posteriorly from the vestibule are three **semicircular canals** arranged at right angles to one another. **Semicircular ducts** made of membranous labyrinth are in each canal, both ends of which open into the utricle. The **ampulla** is a dilation at one end of each duct. It contains the **crista ampullaris** (Figure 9-18), which has **sensory hair cells** similar to those of the maculae. The **cupula** is a gelatinous glycoprotein layer that overlies each crista. Body movements result in inertia in the endolymph, which pushes on the cupulae and stimulates the hair cells. Sensory fibers in the vestibular branch of **CN VIII** carry this information to the brain where the complex pattern of hair cell stimulation is interpreted as movement in a particular direction at a particular rate.

The **cochlea** (Figures 9-16 and 9-19) contains the receptors for hearing. It consists of a spiral canal extending anteriorly from the vestibule. The bony labyrinth is divided into two separate canals by the membranous **scala media (cochlear duct)**, which is filled with endolymph. The **scala vestibuli (vestibular duct)** and **scala tympani (tympanic duct)** are on either side of the scala media and contain perilymph. Because the scala media does not extend the entire length of the cochlea, the scala vestibuli and scala tympani are continuous at the apex of the cochlea. The **modiolus** forms the bony axis of the cochlea.

In cross section, the scala media looks triangular, with the **vestibular** and **basilar membranes** separating it from the scala vestibuli and scala tympani, respectively. The outer wall is composed of the endolymph-secreting stria vascularis, which rests upon the connective tissue spiral ligament.

(Figure 9-19). Resting on the basilar membrane is the **organ of Corti** (Figure 9-20), which contains **hair cells** and **support cells**. The hair cells are the actual sound receptors and have stereocilia embedded in the **tectorial membrane** that overlies them. Vibrations of a particular frequency (related to the wavelength of the sound that caused it) result in movement of a particular part of the basilar membrane. This stimulates the hair cells, which in turn stimulate the sensory bipolar neurons that occupy the **spiral ganglion** (Figure 9-21). Their axons form the auditory branch of the vestibulocochlear nerve (**CN VIII**). The auditory cortex interprets the information as sound of a particular pitch.

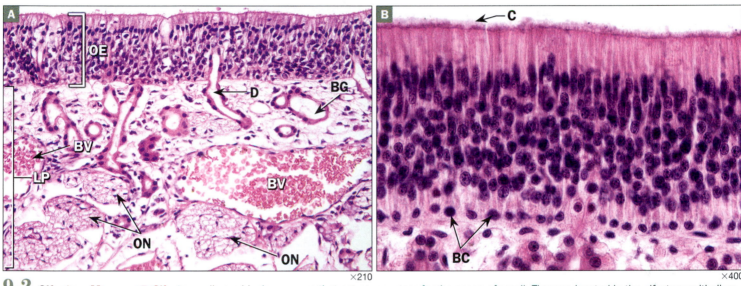

9-2 **Olfactory Mucosa** ▪ Olfactory cells are bipolar neurons that act as receptors for the sense of smell. They are located in the olfactory epithelium (OE), a modified PSCC in the nasal cavity. It is difficult to identify the three cell types of this epithelium with H&E-stained preparations, but nucleus location provides a means of making good guesses. Basal cells have nuclei located in the lower third, whereas the nuclei of olfactory cells and sustentacular cells are located in the middle and upper portions, respectively. (**A**) In this micrograph, Bowman's glands (BG), which produce a watery secretion that dissolves odorants, and their ducts (D) are visible in the lamina propria (LP). Also visible are blood vessels (BV) and olfactory nerves cut in cross section (ON). (×210) (**B**) In this higher magnification, basal cells (BC) and cilia (C) are clearly visible. The dense nuclear layer is made up of olfactory and sustentacular cells. (×400)

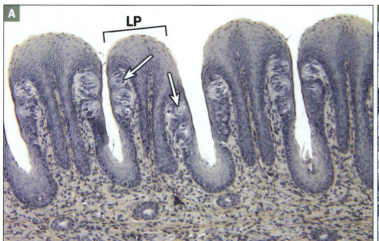

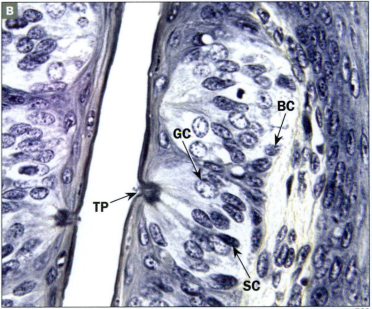

9-3 **Taste Buds** ▪ Chemoreceptors for the sensation of taste are located in taste buds found in the epithelium lining the oral cavity. (**A**) Taste buds (arrows) on lingual papillae (LP). (×130) (**B**) Detail of taste buds; visible are the taste pores (TP), gustatory cells (GC) with light-staining nuclei, sustentacular cells (SC) with darker nuclei, and basal cells (BC). (×760)

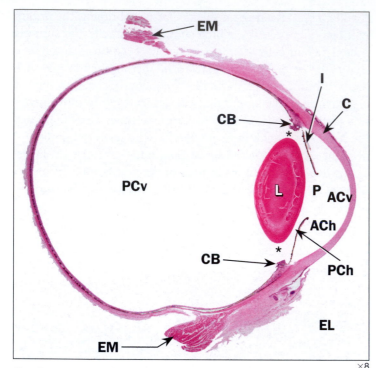

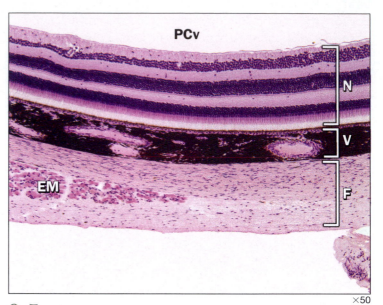

9-4 **Panorama of an Eyeball in Section** 🔲 Shown is a sagittal section of an eyeball. The following features are labeled: anterior cavity (ACv), which is made of the anterior chamber (ACh) and posterior chamber (PCh) and is filled with aqueous humor (not seen); posterior cavity (PCv), which is filled with the vitreous body (not seen); cornea (C); iris (I); pupil (P), which connects the anterior and posterior chambers; lens (L); ciliary body (CB); extrinsic muscles (EM), which move the eyeball; and eyelids (EL). The suspensory ligaments that support the lens and separate the anterior and posterior cavities are missing from this preparation (*). (×8)

9-5 **Layers of the Eyeball** 🔲 The three layers of the eyeball, from outside in, are the fibrous tunic (F), vascular tunic (V), and neural tunic (N). An extrinsic ocular muscle (EM) and the posterior cavity (PCv) are also visible in this specimen. (×50)

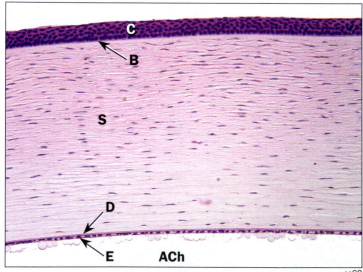

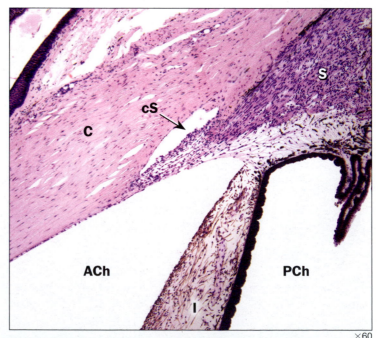

9-6 **Cornea** 🔲 The transparent anterior portion of the fibrous tunic is the cornea. There are five layers in the cornea. On the anterior surface is the corneal epithelium (C), a nonkeratinized stratified squamous epithelium. Bowman's membrane (B) is a collagenous basal lamina deep to the epithelium. Stroma (S) comprises the bulk of the cornea and is made of highly organized collagen fiber layers. Lastly, the simple squamous corneal endothelium (E) and Descemet's membrane (its basal lamina) (D) are posterior to the stroma. The anterior chamber (ACh) is also labeled. (×60)

9-7 **Canal of Schlemm** 🔲 A venous sinus known as the canal of Schlemm (cS) is at the junction of the cornea (C) and sclera (S). It returns aqueous humor from the anterior chamber (ACh) to the bloodstream. The posterior chamber (PCh) and iris (I) are also labeled. (×60)

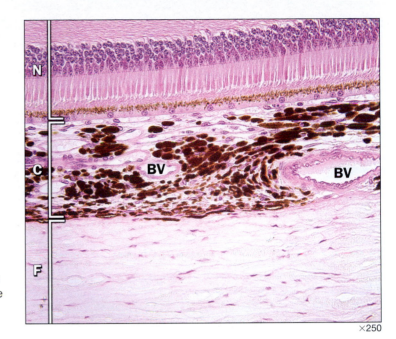

×250

9-8 **Choroid** ◼ The vascular tunic is made up of the choroid (C), a pigmented layer between the fibrous (F) and neural (N) tunics. Note the blood vessels (BV). (×250)

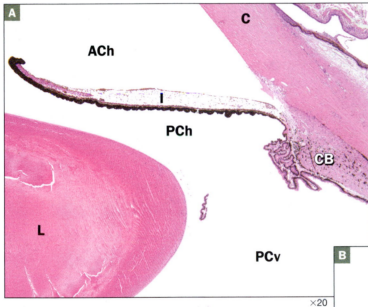

×20

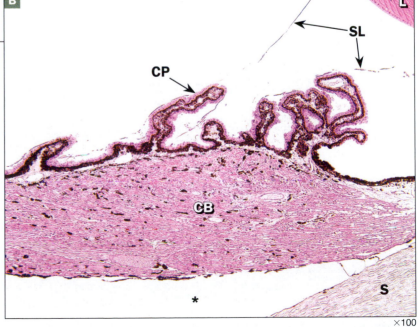

×100

9-9 **Ciliary Body** ◼ (A) In the anterior of the eye, the vascular tunic is expanded to form the ciliary body (CB). Also visible are the cornea (C), iris (I), lens (L), anterior and posterior chambers (ACh and PCh), and posterior cavity (PCv). The suspensory ligaments holding the lens to the ciliary body were not preserved in this preparation. (×20) (B) Ciliary processes (CP) are extensions of the ciliary body (CB) that produce aqueous humor. Remnants of suspensory ligaments (SL) are also visible, as is part of the lens (L). The space (*) is an artifact of preparation where the sclera (S) has separated from the ciliary body. (×100)

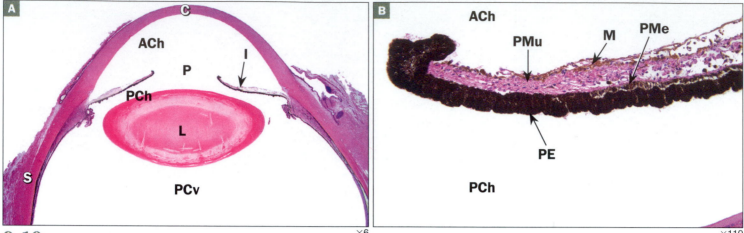

×6   ×110

9-10 **Iris** ■ **(A)** The iris (I) divides the anterior cavity into an anterior chamber (ACh) and a posterior chamber (PCh). Also visible are the lens (L), pupil (P), sclera (S), cornea (C), and the posterior cavity (PCv), which holds the vitreous body (not seen). (×6) **(B)** This micrograph shows the iris in detail. Visible are the layers of pigmented posterior epithelium (PE); pigmented myoepithelium (PMe), the junction of which is largely indistinguishable in this specimen; and the pupillary muscle (PMu) within. Brownish regions in the anterior are melanocytes (M). (×110)

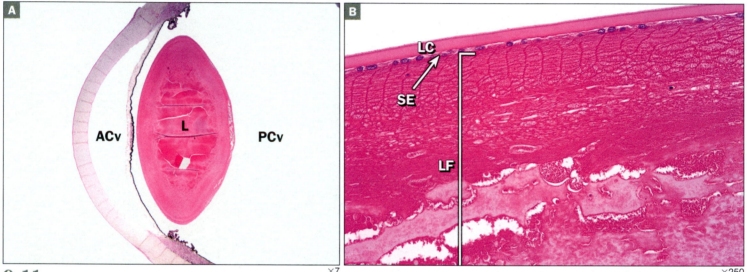

×7   ×250

9-11 **Lens** ■ **(A)** The lens (L) divides the eye into anterior (ACv) and posterior cavities (PCv). In this micrograph, suspensory ligaments are not visible. The iris also appears to lack a pupil, but this is due to the plane of the section. (×7) **(B)** In this higher magnification of the lens, the lens capsule (LC), subcapsular epithelium (SE), and lens fibers (LF) are visible. (×250)

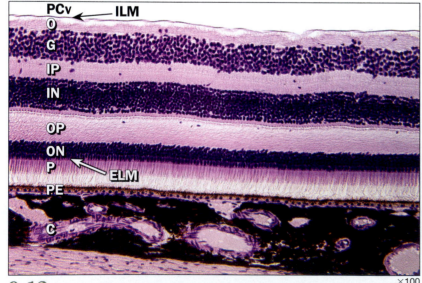

×100

Key to the 10 layers of the retina

ILM	=	inner lining membrane
O	=	optic nerve fiber layer
G	=	ganglion cell layer
IP	=	inner plexiform layer
IN	=	inner nuclear layer
OP	=	outer plexiform layer
ON	=	outer nuclear layer
ELM	=	external limiting membrane
P	=	photoreceptive layer (rod and cone segments)
PE	=	pigmented epithelium

9-12 **Retina** ■ The posterior cavity (PCv) is at the top of this micrograph and the choroid (C) is at the bottom. In between is the retina. (×100)

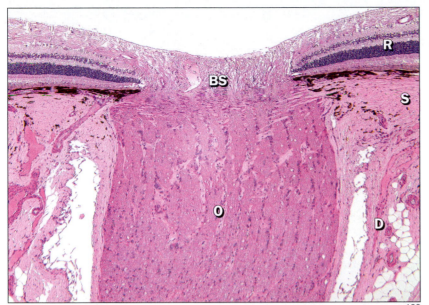

9-13 **Optic Nerve** ■ The optic nerve (O) is composed of ganglion cell fibers, glial cells, and blood vessels. Note the absence of photoreceptor cells where the optic nerve leaves the posterior of the eye. This results in a blind spot (BS) in each eye. Notice the typical multilayered retina (R) on either side of the blind spot. Also note that the sclera (S) is continuous with the dura mater (D) of the optic nerve. (As an outgrowth of the brain, the optic nerve is better referred to as the optic tract, so it is covered with dura mater, not epineurium.) (×100)

×100

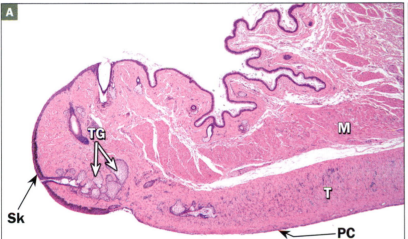

×25

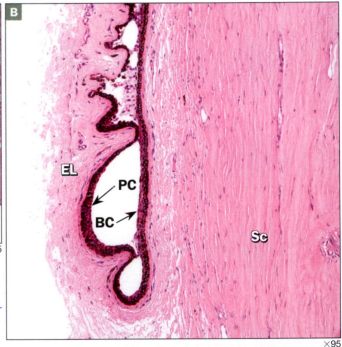

×95

9-14 **Eyelid** ■ (A) The eyeball in this micrograph would be at the bottom. The eyelid is covered with a highly folded thin skin (Sk) on its anterior and a stratified columnar epithelium, the palpebral conjunctiva (PC), on its posterior. The skeletal muscle (M), fibrous tarsal plate (T), and tarsal (Meibomian) glands (TG) are also visible. (×25) (B) This section of an eyelid (EL) shows the continuity of the palpebral conjunctiva with the bulbar conjunctiva (BC) lining the sclera (Sc). (×95)

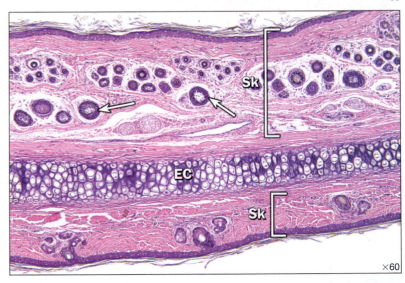

×60

9-15 **Pinna** ■ The external ear is covered with skin (Sk) that is tightly bound to an internal framework of elastic cartilage (EC). Numerous hair follicles cut in cross section are also visible (arrows). (×60)

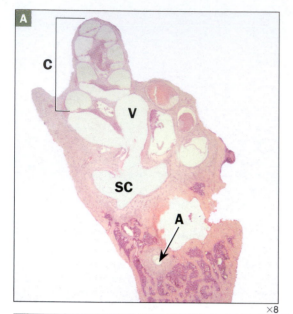

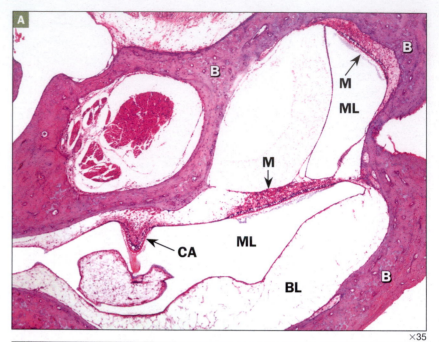

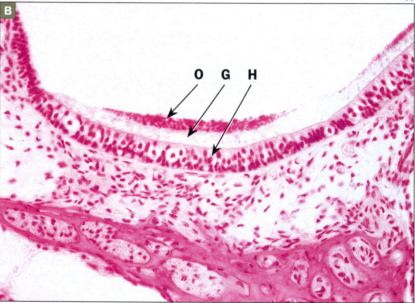

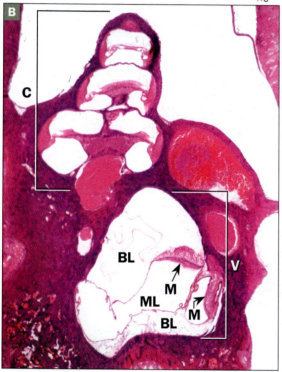

9-16 **Internal Ear** ▮ These sections of temporal bone show much of the internal ear. Shown are the spiral cochlea (C), semicircular canals (SC), and vestibule (V). (**A**) Also visible in this specimen is the auditory tube (A). (×8) (**B**) The two maculae (M) are visible within the vestibule of this specimen, as are membranous (ML) and bony labyrinth (BL). (×30)

9-17 **Macula of the Utricle and Saccule** ▮ The vestibule of the inner ear houses the membranous utricle and saccule, each with a macula. (**A**) The two maculae (M) are oriented at right angles, as shown in this micrograph. Bone tissue (B), bony labyrinth (BL) and membranous labyrinth (ML) are labeled. Also visible is a crista ampullaris (CA) from one of the semicircular canals. (×35) (**B**) This detail of one macula shows the calcium carbonate otoliths (O) embedded in a glycoprotein (G) layer (or what's left of it) that covers the mechanoreceptor hair cells (H). The maculae provide sensory information about head position. (×250)

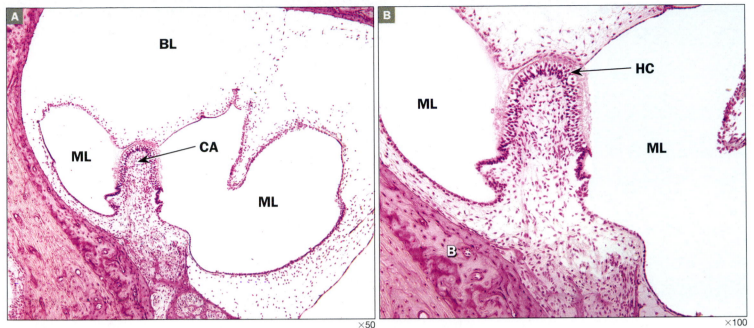

9-18 **Ampulla of a Semicircular Canal** ◼ The membranous labyrinth in each of the three semicircular canals, called semicircular ducts, has a dilated end called the ampulla. Within each ampulla is the crista ampullaris, a receptor organ that provides sensory information about body movement. (A) The bony (BL) and membranous (ML) labyrinths of the ampulla are labeled in this micrograph. In their natural states, bony labyrinth is filled with perilymph and membranous labyrinth is filled with endolymph. Note that the membrane is unnaturally collapsed due to preparation of the specimen. The crista ampullaris (CA) is also visible. (×50) (B) In this detail of the crista ampullaris, the hair cell layer (HC) is visible, but much of the cupula (the glycoprotein layer covering the crista) is missing. Bone tissue (B) forming the wall of the bony labyrinth is labeled. (×100)

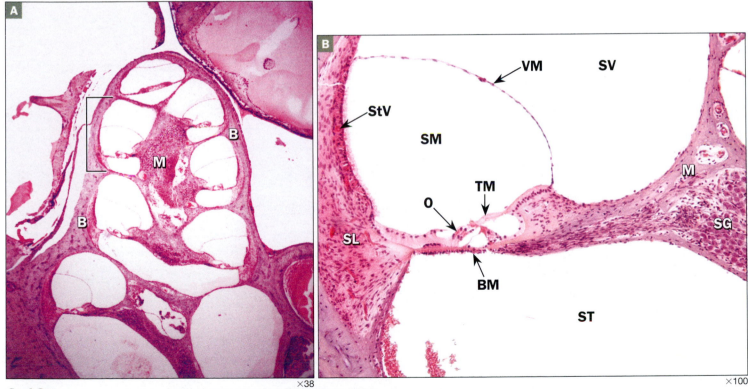

9-19 **Cochlea** ◼ (A) Shown is the entire cochlea in vertical section. Its edges and center (the modiolus–M) are made of bone (B). The modiolus houses bipolar neurons of the cochlear branch of the vestibulocochlear nerve (CN VIII). The bracket indicates one turn of the cochlea and corresponds to the enlarged micrograph in (B), but is from a different specimen. (×38) (B) The membranous labyrinth is represented by the scala media (SM, also known as the cochlear duct), which is separated from the bony labyrinth by the vestibular membrane (VM) and basilar membrane (BM). The bony labyrinth consists of the scala vestibuli (SV) and scala tympani (ST, which are also known as the vestibular and tympanic ducts, respectively). The organ of Corti (O) rests on the basilar membrane. Also shown are the tectorial membrane (TM), stria vascularis (StV), which produces endolymph, spiral ganglion (SG), modiolus, and connective tissue spiral ligament (SL). (×100)

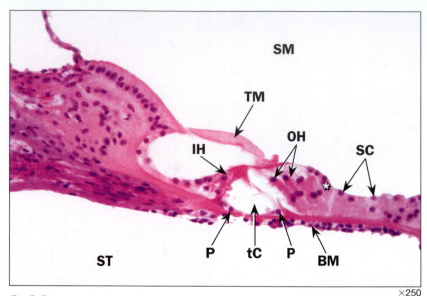

9-20 **Organ of Corti** ▪ The organ of Corti is the receptor for the sensation of hearing. The actual receptors are hair cells, of which there are two types: an inner hair cell (IH) and outer hair cells (OH). Other parts of the organ of Corti, such as pillar cells (P), other support cells (SC), inner tunnel of Corti (tC), basilar membrane (BM), and the tectorial membrane (TM) are also visible. The outer tunnel of Corti is not seen in this preparation, but would be located near the asterisk (*). The scala media (SM) is above the organ of Corti and the scala tympani (ST) is below it. (×250)

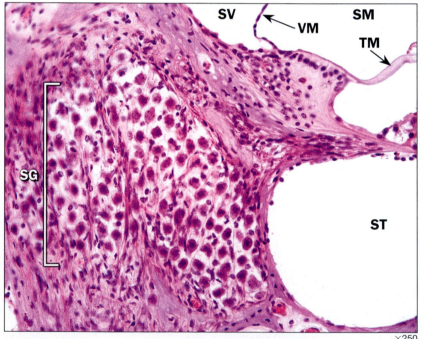

9-21 **Spiral Ganglion** ▪ The bipolar neuron cell bodies whose axons form the cochlear branch of the vestibulocochlear nerve (CN VIII) are located in spiral ganglia (SG) within the modiolus. They transmit sensory impulses from the hair cells to the cerebral cortex to produce the sensation of hearing. (×250)

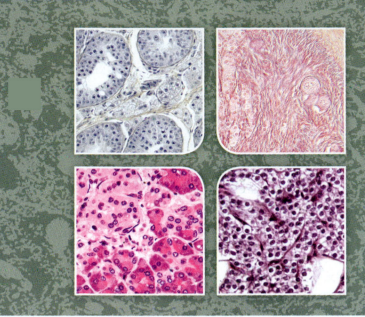

10

Endocrine System

Introduction to the Endocrine System

The endocrine system is composed of **endocrine glands** and **endocrine cells**. The former are multicellular organs, and the latter are cells dispersed within organs having more than an endocrine function.

Endocrine glands (Figure 10-1) are typically epithelial in origin and are produced as a result of surface cells growing down into deeper tissues. Unlike exocrine glands, which maintain their connection with the surface (by way of their duct), the connection of endocrine glands is lost during development

Pituitary gland

Thyroid gland

Adrenal gland

Pancreas

Ovary

10-1 Endocrine System
Shown are major endocrine glands of the body. In addition to those shown, this chapter covers the pineal gland of the brain and the testes of the male. Each gland produces one or more hormones that are carried by the blood and have an effect on one or more target organs.

and the glands are **ductless**. Each gland produces one or more amino acid, peptide, polypeptide, glycoprotein, or lipid hormone, which are secreted into the bloodstream. For this reason, endocrine glands are very vascular. The hormones have a physiological effect on specific **targets**, cells in organs elsewhere in the body. In this way, the endocrine system regulates activities in concert with the nervous system.

Research into chemical signaling in the body has revealed mechanisms that can be considered "endocrine" in function, though they don't fit the traditional definition. **Paracrine cells** deliver their secretion into surrounding tissues directly or through local blood vessels. **Autocrine cells** produce a secretion in which they (or cells like them) are the targets. **Juxtacrine cells** display their secretion on their surface and exert their effect when target cells contact them.

Endocrine glands are structurally diverse, but they do have some general features in common. The secretory cells are referred to as **parenchyma**. There is also often a connective tissue **capsule** and, of course, the numerous capillaries into which hormones are secreted.

Endocrine glands covered in this chapter are the pituitary gland, thyroid gland, parathyroid glands, adrenal glands, pineal gland, pancreas, testes, and ovaries.

Pituitary Gland (Hypophysis)

The pituitary gland is located inferior to the hypothalamus and occupies the sella turcica of the sphenoid bone. It is about the size of a garden pea. The pituitary is divided into two parts: the **adenohypophysis** (**anterior pituitary**, or **anterior lobe**), which is formed from an out-pouching of embryonic pharyngeal ectoderm (**hypophyseal**, or **Rathke's, pouch**) and the **neurohypophysis** (**posterior pituitary**, or **posterior lobe**), which is a downgrowth from the hypothalamus. Both begin to form in the third embryonic week. As is typical of endocrine glands, the adenohypophysis loses its connection with the surface, but the neurohypophysis retains its connection to the hypothalamus via the **infundibular stalk**. What we see in the fully formed pituitary gland is actually an organ formed from the fusion of very different embryonic structures and tissues, and this is reflected in how each functions (Figure 10-2).

Adenohypophysis (Anterior Pituitary)

The adenohypophysis is composed of three parts: the **pars distalis**, which is the largest, the **pars intermedia**, which is found between the adenophypophysis and neurohypophysis, and the **pars tuberalis**, which wraps around the infundibulum. Hormones of the adenohypophysis and their functions are listed in Table 10-1.

Two main cell types are recognized in the adenohypophysis using traditional staining methods. These are the easily stained **chromophils** and the poorly staining **chromophobes** (Figure 10-3). Chromophils are further differentiated into **acidophils** and **basophils**, depending on their affinity for acidic and basic stains, respectively. Immunohistochemical techniques and electron microscopy have resulted in categorizing these cells based on their secretions. **Somatotropes** and **mammotropes** secrete growth hormone (GH) and prolactin, respectively, and are acidophils. The basophilic **corticotropes**, **thyrotropes**, and **gonadotropes** secrete adrenocorticotropic hormone (ACTH), thyroid stimulating hormone (TSH), and follicle stimulating hormone (FSH) and luteinizing hormone (LH), respectively. Most chromophils produce only one kind of hormone, though gonadotropes may produce both FSH and LH, and corticotropes produce two hormones—ACTH and β–lipotrophic hormone (β–LPH)—derived from cleavage of the same precursor molecule. All chromophil types are found in the pars distalis.

Chromophobes are chromophils that have discharged their secretory granules (i.e., degranulated) or are stem cells.

The pars intermedia (Figure 10-4) consists of chromophobic and basophilic cells located between the anterior and posterior pituitary and is visible in some specimens. While its overall function is unclear in humans (most studies have been done in animals), the pars intermedia houses chromophobes and what appear to be corticotropic cells. There is some evidence that they produce melanocyte stimulating hormone (MSH) and α- and β-endorphins. It has distinctive colloid-filled cysts, which are remnants of the hypophyseal pouch.

The pars tuberalis houses gonadotropic cells that produce FSH and LH and corticotropic cells that produce ACTH.

Secretion by the five tropic cell types in the adenohypophysis is under the control of releasing and inhibiting factors produced by neurons in hypothalamic nuclei. Their secretions are carried by veins of the **hypothalamic-hypophyseal portal system**[1] to the capillaries of the adenohypophysis, where they exert their effect on the appropriate chromophils. For example, gonadotropin-releasing hormone (GnRH) from the hypothalamus stimulates gonadotropic cells in the adenohypophysis to release FSH and LH.

Neurohypophysis (Posterior Pituitary)

The neurohypophysis (Figure 10-5) is composed of unmyelinated axons of **neurosecretory cells** located in two hypothalamic nuclei (supraoptic and paraventricular). It is these neurons that synthesize **antidiuretic hormone** (ADH, also known as **vasopressin**) and **oxytocin**, which are then transferred in vesicles down the axons and into the neurohypophysis for storage. In some axons, vesicle accumulation may cause a dilation called a **neurosecretory**, or **Herring, body**. An action potential causes their release into the neurohypophyseal capillaries and subsequently into general circulation. Table 10-2 summarizes the hormones of the neurohypophysis and their functions.

Cells, such as mast cells and fibroblasts, may be found in the neurohypophysis, but glial cells called **pituicytes** are the most abundant. They perform a supporting role for the axons, not unlike astrocytes of the CNS.

▪▪ Thyroid Gland

The **thyroid gland** (Figure 10-6) is found anterior to the larynx in the neck. It is composed of two lobes and is surrounded by a thin **capsule**. Connective tissue **septa** divide the thyroid gland into **lobules**. Table 10-3 summarizes the hormones of the thyroid and their functions.

The **thyroid gland** is composed of hundreds of thousands (to millions) of microscopic cavities called **follicles**. Each follicle is formed by a simple epithelium, ranging in height from squamous to low columnar, with the taller epithelia associated with higher follicle activity. The thyroid gland is unusual in that it stores its secretion extracellularly in colloid, a thick fluid found in the interior of each follicle. Follicular cells secrete **thyroglobulin**, an inactive precursor of thyroid hormone, into the colloid where it becomes **iodinated** (iodines are added to it). The iodinated thyroglobulin is then endocytosed by the follicle cells and digested into the active forms of **thyroxine**, T_3 and T_4, which are subsequently secreted into capillaries for distribution throughout the body. Both hormones control metabolic rate and growth (including fetal), among several other functions.

Parafollicular (clear) cells also occupy the thyroid follicles. They are larger, less abundant, and stain lighter than follicular cells. They produce **calcitonin**, which lowers blood calcium levels.

▪▪ Parathyroid Glands

The four **parathyroid glands** are located on the posterior of the thyroid gland. Each is enclosed by a fibrous **capsule** that

---

[1] A portal system is an arrangement of blood vessels that carries blood from one capillary bed to another capillary bed without first going through the heart. In this case, the two capillary beds are in the infundibular stalk and the adenohypophysis, and are joined by veins.

sends **septa** into the gland and divides it into **lobules** (Figure 10-7). **Parathyroid hormone** (PTH) is involved in regulating blood calcium and phosphate levels. Table 10-4 summarizes PTH and its functions.

The parenchyma is composed of hormone-secreting **chief cells** and **oxyphil cells** of unknown function. Chief cells are small with round, centrally positioned nuclei and pale, eosinophilic cytoplasm. Oxyphils are larger with an abundance of eosinophilic cytoplasm.

Adrenal Glands

The **adrenal (suprarenal) glands** are located superior to each kidney. They consist of a fibrous **capsule** surrounding the parenchyma, which is divided into an outer **cortex** and an inner **medulla** (Figures 10-8a and 10-8b). The adrenal hormones and their actions are summarized in Table 10-5.

The adrenal cortex is divided into three layers. The **zona glomerulosa** (Figure 10-8c) is a thin layer deep to the capsule. Its cells are in rounded clusters and have dense-staining nuclei. They secrete the mineralocorticoid hormone aldosterone, which increases blood pressure by increasing sodium reabsorption in the kidney tubules. The **zona fasciculata** (Figure 10-8d) is deep to the zona glomerulosa and is the thickest of the three cortical layers. Its cells, called **spongiocytes**, are arranged in rows and have abundant cytoplasmic lipids typical of steroid-secreting cells. The main hormone is cortisol, which raises blood glucose levels, among other metabolic effects. The **zona reticularis** (Figure 10-8e) is the innermost cortical layer. The nuclei and cytoplasm of its cells stain more intensely than the spongiocytes. These cells secrete small amounts of sex hormones.

The adrenal medulla (Figure 10-9) is essentially a ganglion of the sympathetic nervous system. Occupying it are **chromaffin cells**, which are homologous (having the same embryonic origin) to sympathetic postganglionic neurons and produce one of two hormones: either **norepinephrine** or its derivative, **epinephrine (adrenalin)**. The two hormones act in concert with direct sympathetic innervation to prepare the body for dealing with stressful situations.

Chromaffin cells retain some neuronal features, but they differ in some ways, too. Structurally, they lack the axon and dendrites of "typical" neurons, but they still receive neural stimulation from sympathetic preganglionic fibers. When stimulated, they release a chemical (the hormone) by exocytosis, but they release it *into the blood*, not a synapse like "typical" neurons do with neurotransmitters. Consistent with this, the adrenal medulla is richly supplied with capillaries.

Pineal Gland

The **pineal gland** is a small outgrowth from the roof of the third ventricle (Figure 10-10 and Table 10-6) covered with pia mater. Modified neurons called **pinealocytes** secrete the hormones **melatonin** and **serotonin**, and are characterized by large, irregularly shaped nuclei with prominent nucleoli. **Interstitial cells**, which are structurally and functionally similar to astrocytes, are found surrounding clusters of pinealocytes. **Brain sand (corpora arenacea)**, made of calcium phosphate and calcium carbonate, becomes more abundant with age, but is of unknown function. The pineal gland regulates **circadian rhythm** by receiving information about light and dark from the retina. When the retina is stimulated by light, melatonin production by the pinealocytes is inhibited. In the absence of light, the inhibition is removed and melatonin production increases. Variation in melatonin plasma levels (which correspond to light and dark periods of the 24-hour day) affects activity of the pituitary gland, hypothalamus, and other organs.

Pancreas

The **pancreas** has endocrine and exocrine components. **Islets of Langerhans** comprise the endocrine portion (Figure 10-11). The majority of cells (up to 70%) in an islet are the **insulin**-secreting **ß cells**. The **glucagon**-secreting **ß cells** are toward the periphery of the islet and comprise about 20% of the cells. These hormones decrease and increase blood sugar levels, respectively. The hormone **somatostatin**, whose function is unclear, is produced by ∂-cells. It is known to inhibit insulin and glucagon secretion and to be chemically identical to GnRH from the hypothalamus. Table 10-7 summarizes the major pancreatic hormones and their functions.

There are (at least) four other cell types found in small quantities in the islets that produce hormones of less significance (or, probably more correctly: less well understood). Typical histological stains do not distinguish between the seven different cells that manufacture and secrete each hormone, but they can be differentiated with immunocytochemical stains specific for their secretions.

Testes

The testes have a cytogenic function (sperm production) and an endocrine function. The **interstitial cells of Leydig** are located in the vascular connective tissue between seminiferous tubules of the testes (Figure 10-12). These cells have a round nucleus with one or two eccentric nucleoli and lipids (typical of steroid-secreting cells) in the cytoplasm. They are responsible for secretion of testosterone, the male sex hormone. Its functions are summarized in Table 10-8. For more information about the testes, see Chapter 17.

Ovaries

Like the testes, ovaries have a cytogenic and an endocrine function. As ovarian follicles develop (Figure 10-13), the ovum undergoes meiosis and the surrounding follicle cells proliferate. The **thecal cells** of developing ovarian follicles produce an androgen, which is converted to estradiol (an estrogen; a female sex hormone) by **granulosa cells.** To a lesser extent, thecal cells produce a precursor that the granulosa cells convert to progesterone. After ovulation, the ovarian follicle undergoes changes and develops into a **corpus luteum** (Figure 10-14). The follicular granulosa cells differentiate into **granulosa lutein cells** that form the bulk of the corpus luteum. The theca interna cells differentiate into **theca lutein** cells, which are somewhat smaller and tend to be located near the surface. Progesterone is the primary hormone, but some estrogen continues to be produced. If pregnancy occurs, the corpus luteum continues growing and secreting hormones for the first trimester, after which it degenerates and the placenta assumes the role of hormone production. If pregnancy does not occur, the corpus luteum degenerates within approximately two weeks of ovulation. See Table 10-9 and Chapter 17 for more about ovarian hormones and their actions.

Table 10-1 Hormones of the Adenohypophysis (Anterior Pituitary Gland)

Source	Hormone	Target(s) and Action(s)
Thyrotropic cell (basophil)	Thyrotropic hormone (TSH); also known as thyrotropin	Stimulates growth of thyroid follicle cells and their production of thyroglobulin (the precursor of thyroid hormone, see below)
Corticotropic cell (basophil)	Adrenocorticotropic hormone (ACTH)	Nurtures and stimulates adrenal cortex to produce hormones (see below)
Somatotropic cell (acidophil)	Growth hormone (GH); also known as somatotropin	Multiple effects (and many poorly understood), but indirectly stimulates growth of cartilage in epiphyseal plates of bone
Mammotropic cell (acidophil)	Prolactin (PRL)	Mammary gland development and milk production/secretion
Gonadotropic cell (acidophil)	Follicle stimulating hormone (FSH)	Stimulates ovarian follicle development and estrogen secretion in females; stimulates sperm production in males
Gonadotropic cell (acidophil)	Luteinizing hormone (LH)	Promotes ovarian follicle maturation, corpus luteum development and maintenance, ovulation, and progesterone secretion in females; nurtures interstitial cells and promotes androgen secretion by them in males

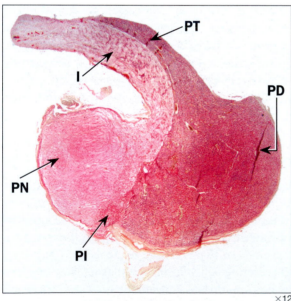

×12

10-2 Pituitary Gland (Hypophysis) ◼ The drastically different appearances of the anterior pituitary gland (adenohypophysis) and posterior pituitary gland (neurohypophysis, or pars nervosa) are consistent with their different embryonic origins. The former is derived from oral ectoderm, whereas the latter is an outgrowth of the hypothalamus. The adenohypophysis (AH) is divided into the pars distalis (PD), pars tuberalis (PT), and pars intermedia (PI). The neurohypophysis (NH) is divided into the pars nervosa (PN) and the infundibular stalk (I), which carries nerve fibers from the hypothalamus. (×12)

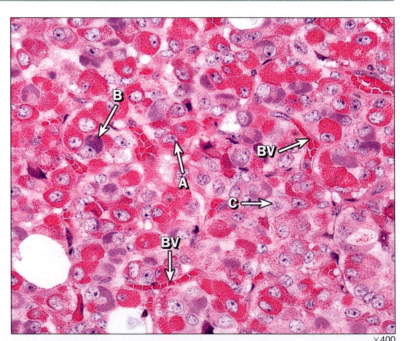

×400

10-3 Adenohypophysis (Anterior Pituitary Gland) ◼ The secretory cells of the adenohypophysis gland can be differentiated with H&E stain into chromophils, which stain intensely, and chromophobes (C), which don't. The former can further be differentiated into reddish acidophils (A) and purplish basophils (B). Further identification requires immunohistochemical staining for the specific hormones. Note the numerous blood vessels (BV) surrounding the secretory cells. (×400)

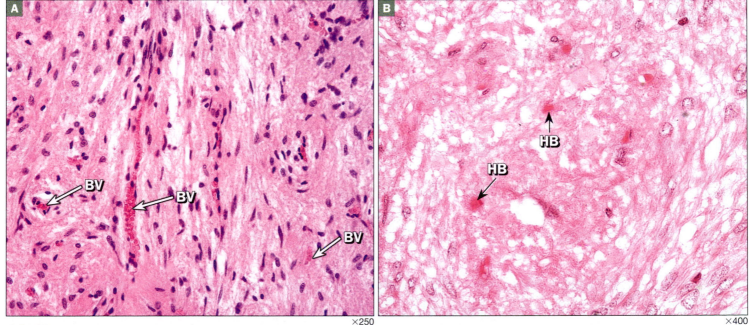

10-4 **Pars Intermedia** ■ The pars intermedia (PI) is located between the pars nervosa (PN) and pars distalis (not shown in this section). Its general appearance resembles the pars distalis, but can be distinguished by its colloid-filled cysts (C). Note the blood vessels (BV) in both the pars nervosa and pars intermedia.

×200

Table 10-2 Hormones of the Neurohypophysis (Posterior Pituitary Gland)		
Source	**Hormone**	**Target(s) and Action(s)**
Hypothalamic neurons	Antidiuretic hormone (ADH); also known as vasopressin	Increases water retention by the renal collecting ducts, thus reducing urine volume
Hypothalamic neurons	Oxytocin	Stimulates contraction of uterine muscle and of mammary gland myoepithelial cells

×250

×400

10-5 **Pars Nervosa (Posterior Pituitary)** ■ (A) The bulk of the pars nervosa is composed of unmyelinated fibers (seen as pink strands in this micrograph) from neurons in the hypothalamus. Most nuclei in this field belong to glial-like pituicytes. Note the blood vessels (BV). (×250) (B) Stored hypothalamic secretions (ADH and oxytocin) often produce swellings at the ends of axons called Herring bodies (HB). Note the "webby" texture of this specimen, which is indicative of nerve fibers in the CNS. (×400)

Table 10-3 Hormones of the Thyroid Gland

Source	Hormone	Target(s) and Action(s)
Follicular cells	Thyroxine (T$_3$ and T$_4$); (Thyroglobulin is an inactive precursor)	Necessary for growth and regulates metabolic rate
Parafollicular cells (clear cells)	Calcitonin	Lowers blood calcium levels

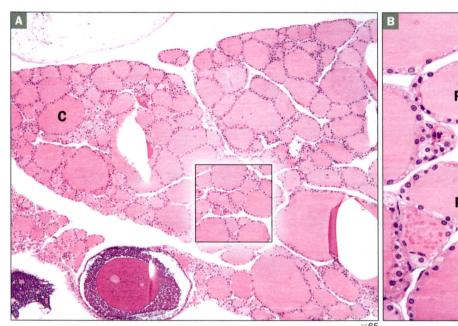

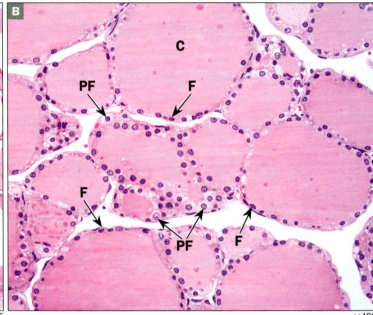

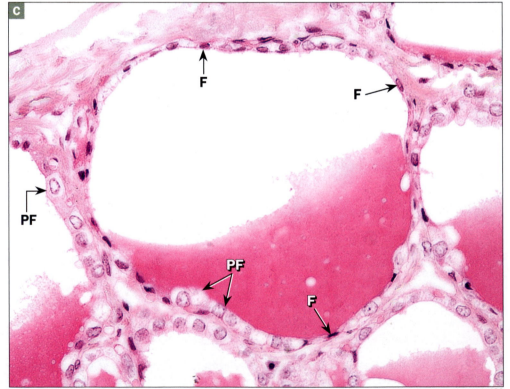

10-6 **Thyroid Gland** ▪ (**A**) The follicular nature of the thyroid gland is apparent in this micrograph. The pink material inside each follicle is colloid (C). (×65). (**B**) This is a higher magnification of the boxed region in (**A**). Each follicle is made up of simple cuboidal follicular cells (F) that secrete thyroglobulin (the inactive precursor of thyroid hormones) into the cavity where it gets iodinated. It comprises the majority of colloid material. Also visible are parafollicular (clear) cells (PF). (**C**) Also in the follicle walls (and sometimes between them) are parafollicular (clear) cells. They secrete calcitonin, a hormone involved in regulating blood calcium levels. Note the difference in the appearance of follicular and parafollicular cell nuclei. (×400)

Table **10-4** Hormones of the Parathyroid Glands

Source	Hormone	Target(s) and Action(s)
Chief (principal) cells and possibly oxyphil cells	Parathyroid hormone (PTH)	Increases blood calcium levels by increasing bone resorption and by increasing calcium recovery by the kidneys

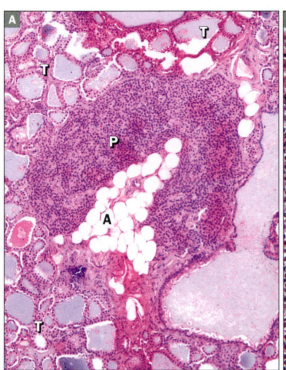

×100

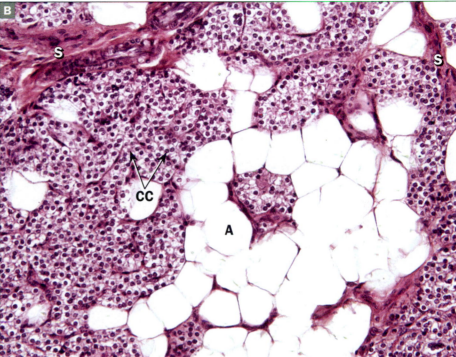

×200

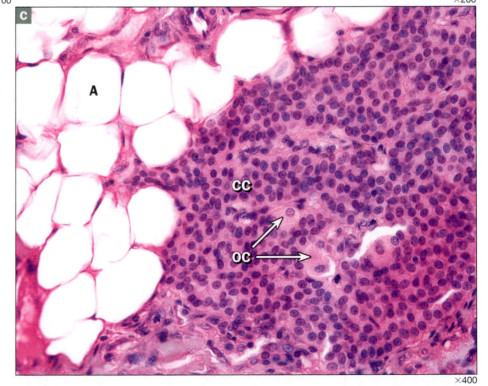

×400

10-7 **Parathyroid Gland** ◾ (**A**) The four parathyroid glands are located on the posterior of the thyroid gland, with two on each side. In this micrograph, one parathyroid (P) is surrounded by thyroid gland tissue (T). Colloid is bluish and the white patches are adipocytes (A). (×100) (**B**) The parathyroid secretory chief cells (CC) are organized into clusters or strands. They are small with round nuclei and pale cytoplasm, and comprise the majority of cells in this specimen. Portions of two connective tissue septa (S) are seen. These project into the gland from its thin, fibrous capsule. Also visible are adipocytes (A), which become more abundant with age. (×200) (**C**) Scattered among the chief cells (CC) are oxyphil cells (OC) of unknown function. They increase with age. Adipocytes are also seen. (×400)

Table 10-5 Hormones of the Adrenal Glands

Source	Hormone	Target(s) and Action(s)
Adrenal cortex	Aldosterone (and other mineralocorticoids)	Regulates ion (sodium and potassium) and water levels by affecting activity of the distal tubules of kidney, sweat glands, and gastric mucosa
Zona glomerulosa		
Zona fasciculata	Coritsol (and other glucocorticoids)	Regulates glucose formation and polymerization into glycogen in the liver and other tissues, and promotes oxidation of fats
Zona reticularis	Glucocorticoids and a weak androgen (dehydroepiandrosterone)	Glucocorticoids (see above); Dehydroepiandrosterone is converted to testosterone in other cells
Adrenal medulla	Norepinephrine and epinephrine (also known as adrenalin)	Prepare body for physical challenges by increasing blood glucose levels, increasing availability of fatty acids, causing vasoconstriction and vasodilation in appropriate organs, increasing heart and breathing rates, and much more
Chromaffin cells		

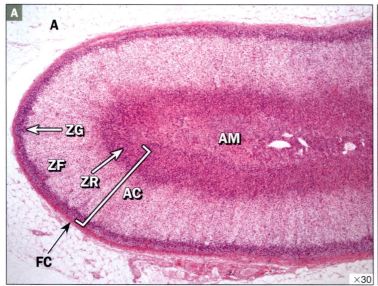

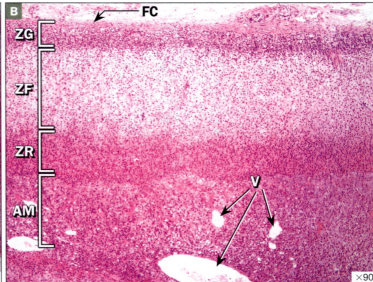

10-8 Adrenal Cortex ■ (**A**) Shown is the complete thickness of an adrenal gland. Around the gland is adipose tissue (A), and on its surface is the fibrous capsule (FC). The next three layers comprise the adrenal cortex (AC). They are: the zona glomerulosa (ZG), zona fasciculata (ZF), and zona reticularis (ZR). In the center is the adrenal medulla (AM). The symmetrical layering of the cortex and medulla is obvious in this specimen, but because of the gland's irregular shape, and depending on the location of the section, you may see preparations where layers are absent or repeated. (×30) (**B**) This higher magnification shows the zona glomerulosa, zona fasciculata, zona reticularis, and adrenal medulla. The staining properties of the cells in each layer easily distinguish between them. Note the distinctive large veins (V) in the adrenal medulla. (×90) (**C**) This micrograph is from a different specimen than (**A**) and (**B**), and its primary subject is the clustered cells of the zona glomerulosa, which secrete aldosterone. Also visible are the fibrous capsule and zona fasciculata. (×200) *(continues)*

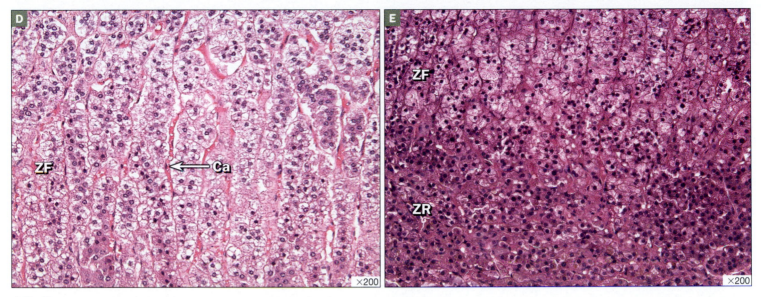

×200   ×200

10-8 **Adrenal Cortex** *(continued)* ■ **(D)** This is from the same specimen as **(C)** and it shows the zona fasciculata, whose cells are arranged in columns and secrete cortisol. Notice their pulpy appearance due to lipid droplets, a characteristic of steroid-secreting cells. Capillaries (Ca) are also seen. (×200) **(E)** This micrograph shows the zona fasciculata and zona reticularis of the same specimen as in **(C)** and **(D)**. The zona reticularis cells stain more deeply than the zona fasculata cells. They secrete small amounts of sex hormones. (×200)

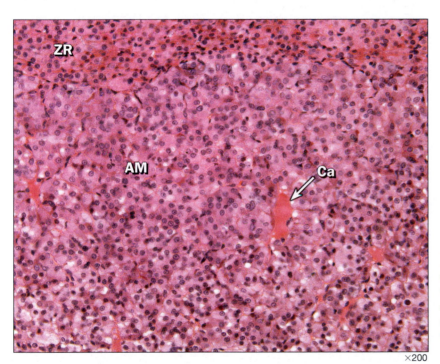

×200

10-9 **Adrenal Medulla** ■ The cells of the adrenal medulla (AM) are undifferentiated sympathetic postganglionic neurons that secrete epinephrine and norepinephrine. It is found at the core of the adrenal gland. Large sinusoidal capillaries (Ca), characteristic of the adrenal medulla, are visible. Also note the zona reticularis (ZR) at the top of the field. (×200)

Table 10-6   Hormones of the Pineal Gland

Source	Hormone	Target(s) and Action(s)
Pinealocytes	Melatonin (primarily)	Responsible for circadian rhythm in many organs

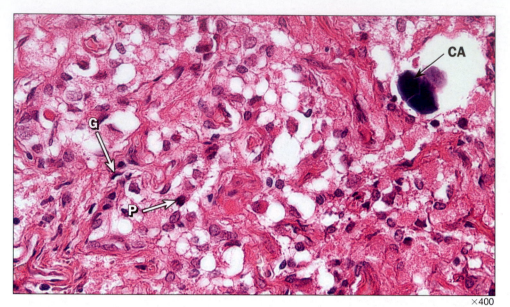

×400

10-10 **Pineal Gland** ▰ Pinealocytes (P) are modified neurons with round nuclei and prominent nucleoli. They are arranged in clusters associated with capillaries (which are difficult to sort out in this preparation). Also present are glial cells (G), which comprise about 5% of pineal cells. They are identifiable by dark, elongated nuclei. A calcium phosphate crystal (CA) is also seen. Collectively, these crystals are called corpora arenacea, or brain sand. Their function is unknown. (×400)

Table 10-7 Hormones of the Pancreas

Source	Hormone	Target(s) and Action(s)
α (A) cells	Glucagon	Stimulates glucose production from amino acids, breakdown of glycogen, and secretion of glucose into the blood
β (B) cells	Insulin	Increases uptake of blood glucose by the liver, skeletal muscle, and adipose tissue
δ (D) cells	Somatostatin	Identical to hypothalamic GnRH and inhibits glucagon and insulin secretion; other functions are unclear

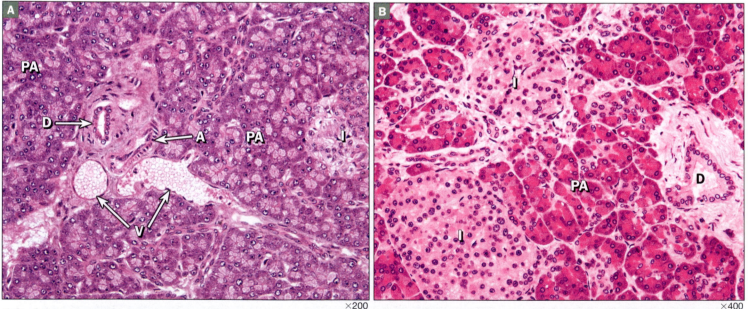

×200   ×400

10-11 **Pancreas** ▰ (**A**) This thin section provides a panoramic view of the pancreas and shows most of the structures you will encounter when viewing a slide. The bulk of the pancreas is composed of exocrine acini (PA), which produce pancreatic juice (see Chapter 14). The endocrine portion is made of islets of Langerhans (I), and one is visible in this field. These cells generally stain more lightly and are smaller than the acinar cells. If staining doesn't allow you to identify them, look for patches of small cells where the nuclei are closer together than most of the specimen. Also visible in this field are venules (V), an arteriole (A), and a duct of the exocrine acini (D). (×200) (**B**) This higher magnification of a different thin section shows two islets. Two main cell types—α, or A, cells; and β, or B, cells—occupy the islet, and they are difficult to identify in standard H&E preparations, but can be demonstrated using immunocytochemical methods. α cells secrete glucagon and tend to be located near the periphery of the islet, whereas β cells secrete insulin and are located more centrally. There are at least five other cell types in the islet. Notice not only the difference in color between the acini and the islets, but also their overall textures. Also visible is a duct. (×400)

Table 10-8 Hormones of the Testes

Source	Hormone	Target(s) and Action(s)
Testicular interstitial (Leydig) cells	Testosterone and other androgens	Promote development of maleness in fetus; promote pubertal and post-pubertal development and maintenance of secondary male sex characteristics and sperm production, and other actions

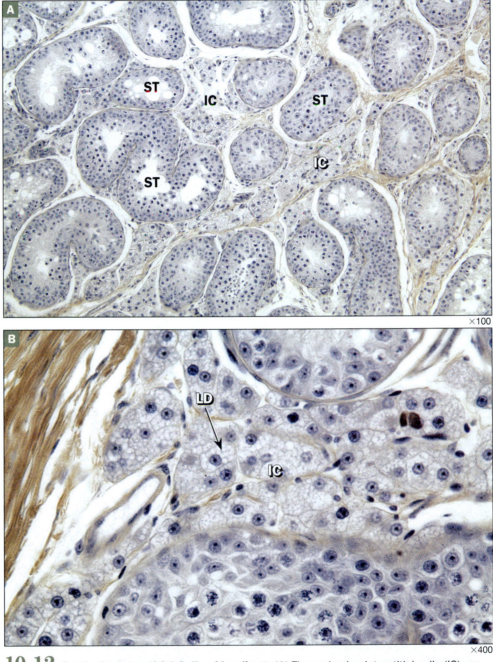

10-12 Testicular Interstitial Cells of Leydig ◼ **(A)** The endocrine interstitial cells (IC) are found between sperm-producing seminiferous tubules (ST). (×100) **(B)** Interstitial cells secrete testosterone and can be identified based on their location between seminiferous tubules and their obvious cytoplasmic lipid droplets (LD) typical of steroid-secreting cells. (×400)

Table 10-9 Hormones of the Ovaries

Source	Hormone	Target(s) and Action(s)
Ovarian follicle and corpus luteum	Estrogens	Promote development of secondary female sex characteristics and follicle and endometrium development during menstrual cycle, and many other actions
Corpus luteum and placenta (some from ovarian follicle)	Progesterone	Continued development and maintenance of the endometrium, cyclic development of mammary gland ducts and lobules

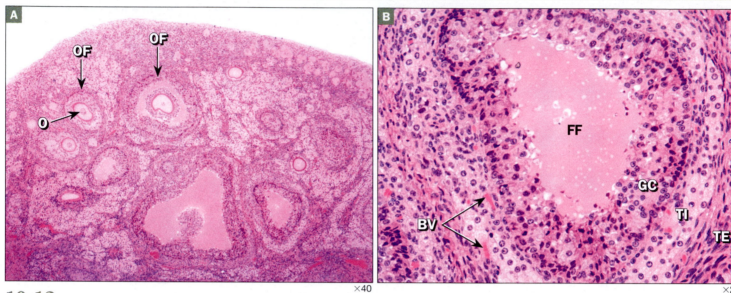

×40   ×200

10-13 **Ovary and Ovarian Follicles** ■ (A) This mammalian ovary illustrates numerous ovarian follicles (OF), each of which contains a developing ovum (O), which are not always seen in the plane of section and layers of surrounding cells. It is the surrounding cell layers that produce the hormones estrogen and progesterone. (×40) (B) A single follicle is shown in this higher magnification of the same specimen. Follicular fluid (FF) fills the follicle's hollow center. Layers forming the follicle wall (from inside to outside) are granulosa cells (GC), theca interna (TI), and theca externa (TE). Granulosa cells convert precursors made by the theca interna cells into estradiol and progesterone. Note the typically pulpy appearance of the steroid-secreting theca interna cells. Also note how vascular (BV) the theca interna is. Once the hormones are made by granulosa cells, they are transported back to the theca interna and are distributed by the blood throughout the body. (×200)

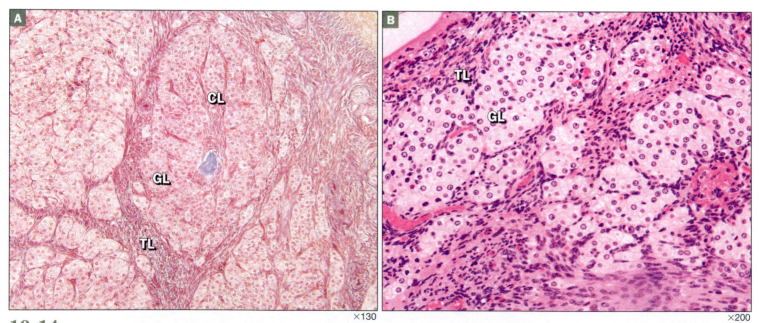

×130   ×200

10-14 **Corpus Luteum** ■ After ovulation, the follicle cells remaining in the ovary develop into a corpus luteum (CL), an endocrine gland responsible for secreting progesterone and some estrogen. (A) This is a corpus luteum after ovulation. The majority of cells are granulosa lutein (GL) cells. Theca lutein (TL) cells are also visible. (×130) (B) In this higher magnification, the pulpy cytoplasm of the granulosa lutein cells is visible. This is due to the numerous lipid droplets composed of the steroid hormone progesterone. If pregnancy does not occur, it will degenerate. (×200)

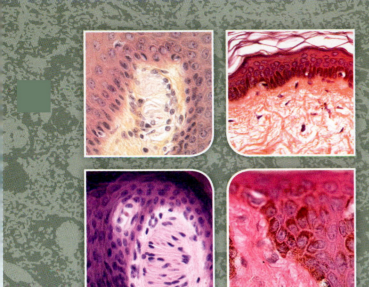

11

Integumentary System

Introduction to the Integument

The integumentary system (Figure 11-1) consists of the skin and its appendages, such as hair, nails, and various glands. It functions as a covering for the entire body. In this role, it protects against mechanical damage and presents a barrier to penetration by chemicals and infectious agents. It also is involved in sensation, thermoregulation (through sweat glands and regulating blood flow), vitamin D synthesis, and immunity.

It is the largest organ in the body, comprising up to 20% of its mass. The average thickness of the skin is about 1 to 2 mm, but it tends to be thicker on dorsal surfaces than on ventral surfaces (the palms of the hands and soles of the feet are exceptions to this, because they are thick ventral surfaces).

Layers of the Integument

The skin is composed of two layers: the superficial **epidermis** and the deeper **dermis** (Figures 11-2 and 11-3). Deep to the dermis is the **hypodermis**, also known as **superficial fascia**. Where it is replaced with adipose tissue, it is known as **subcutaneous fat**. Although the hypodermis is not part of the integument, it will be covered in this chapter, because it is visible on most skin slides and some epidermal appendages penetrate it.

Epidermis

The epidermis is derived from ectoderm and is composed of **keratinized stratified squamous epithelium**. Its thickness ranges from 0.1 mm (over most of the body) to 1.4 mm (on the soles of the feet). **Thick skin** (Figure 11-4a) is found on the palms of the hands and soles of the feet. The rest of the body is covered with **thin skin** (Figure 11-4b).

The main epidermal cells are called **keratinocytes**. The basal cells are the healthiest because of their proximity to the dermal capillaries. It is in this layer that epidermal stem cells are found. As they undergo mitosis, they push preceding generations of cells toward the surface and down the oxygen concentration gradient. Eventually, the keratinocytes occupy a position where they can't get enough oxygen to satisfy their metabolic needs and they die. This process involves degeneration of the nucleus and other organelles, and accumulation of the protein **keratin**. It is the progression from healthy to dying to dead cells that produces the layers seen histologically in the epidermis.

The epidermis of thick skin presents five distinct layers (Figure 11-5), whereas in thinner skin only three are generally

11-1 Integumentary System ■
The integumentary system consists of the skin and its appendages, such as hair, nails, and sweat glands.

visible. From deep to superficial (which coincides with the stages of development), these are the stratum basale, stratum spinosum, stratum granulosum, stratum lucidum, and stratum corneum. The **stratum basale (stratum germinativum)** is the deepest layer of the epidermis. It is composed of healthy (due to their proximity to the dermal capillaries) cuboidal to low columnar cells, many of which undergo mitosis. The **stratum spinosum** is the thickest layer. It is characterized by the "prickly" appearance of its cells due to the desmosomes that attach adjacent cells and to shrinkage during preparation. The deeper cells continue mitotic activity, but this ability is lost in the more superficial layers. The **stratum granulosum** is characterized by cells containing dark-staining keratohyalin granules, an indication that they have begun to keratinize. It is usually about five cells thick. Secretion of a lipid material by these cells makes the epidermis waterproof. The **stratum lucidum** is characterized by cells that have lost their nuclei and have accumulated keratin. It is only seen in thick skin, but not in all preparations. The most superficial layer of the epidermis is the **stratum corneum**. It consists of dead, flattened, anucleate cells that have accumulated abundant keratin. As these cells approach the surface, they lose their intercellular attachments (desmosomes) and are sloughed off. The life span of a keratinocyte depends on the age of the individual and its location, but common estimates are between 15 and 30 days.

Besides keratinocytes, other cells are seen in the epidermis. **Langerhans cells** (Figure 11-5c) are a component of the immune system and function as antigen-presenting cells. They originate in bone marrow and are characterized by a dark-staining nucleus with pale cytoplasm and numerous cytoplasmic extensions (hence their other name, **dendritic cells**). They are found in many places, but are most abundant in the stratum spinosum. Epithelial tactile (**Merkel**) cells are found in the stratum basale of fingertips and oral mucosa, and have indented nuclei. They act as mechanoreceptors and are best seen in electron micrographs.

Melanocytes (Figure 11-6) are pale-staining cells derived from neural tissue and are found in the stratum basale. They produce the brown to black pigment melanin in membrane-bound structures known as **melanosomes** that are deposited in the cytoplasm of keratinocytes of the stratum basale and stratum spinosum. The melanin accumulates near the nucleus on the side closest to the surface, where it protects the nucleus by absorbing ultraviolet radiation. Each melanocyte serves a handful of keratinocytes and forms a structural unit called an **epidermal-melanin unit**. Differences in skin color are not due to density differences of these units, but rather are due to the rate of melanin production, how widely distributed it is (primarily through the stratum spinosum), and how much is accumulated in each of the keratinocytes. The environment can also affect skin color. Exposure to sunlight results in darkening of the skin (tanning), which is a consequence of increased melanocyte activity and darkening of existing melanin. Figure 11-6 shows pigmented skin.

Dermis

The dermis is deep to the epidermis and is the connective tissue component of the skin. The surface in contact with the epidermis is highly folded into elongated **dermal ridges** or conical **dermal papillae** (Figure 11-7) that interlock with epidermal projections. This anchors the epidermis to the dermis and resists separation of the two layers when subjected to shearing forces. Dermal ridges are seen on the surface of the palm and sole as "**fingerprints**."

The portion of the dermis in contact with the epidermis and comprising the dermal papillae is a looser and finer connective tissue and forms the **papillary layer**. The papillae contain capillary loops (see next paragraph) and tactile receptors called **Meissner's corpuscles** (Figure 11-8). The majority of the dermis is composed of a vascular dense irregular connective tissue. This is the **reticular layer** (Figure 11-7). Fibroblasts are the most common cell, but most cells of fibrous connective tissue are present. Large blood vessels, nerves, and epidermal appendages are present in the reticular layer. Pressure receptors called **Pacinian corpuscles** may also be seen (Figures 11-2 and 11-9).

The skin plays a major role in thermoregulation. Its large surface area (roughly 1.5 to 2 m^2) in contact with the environment makes it especially suited for elimination of excess body heat by conduction and radiation, but it also can be a liability in cold conditions when body heat needs to be retained. One mechanism for temperature regulation involves the blood vessels in the papillary layer of the dermis. **Arteriovenous (AV) shunts**, or **anastomoses**, (see Chapter 12) allow blood to flow directly from arterioles to venules without passing through capillaries. When body temperature falls below normal, these shunts open and the blood bypasses the capillaries in the dermal papillae (especially in the fingers and toes), which limits heat loss to the environment by conduction and radiation. These same shunts close to allow greater blood flow near the skin's surface if excess heat must be removed from the body.

Hypodermis

The hypodermis consists of loose connective tissue and anchors the skin to the underlying tissues without binding it too tightly. This allows free movement of underlying muscles without pulling on the skin. The loose connective tissue may be replaced by fat, which acts as an insulating layer (Figure 11-10). Hair follicles, Pacinian corpuscles, and sweat glands may be seen in the hypodermis as well as in the dermis.

⬛ Appendages of the Skin

The epidermis gives rise to a variety of appendages. These are nails, hair follicles, and sweat glands.

Hair and Hair Follicles

The **hair follicle** (Figures 11-2 and 11-11) is an angular downgrowth of the epidermis into the dermis or hypodermis. It in innervated by sensory nerve fibers. The base of the follicle is dilated to form the **hair root,** which is penetrated by a **dermal papilla** that houses capillaries. Together, the root and papilla form the **hair bulb**. The follicle is surrounded by a thick basement membrane called the **glassy (hyaline) membrane,** which itself is wrapped in dense connective tissue.

The **hair** is made of keratinized cells. It is produced by dividing cells at the base of the follicle called the **hair matrix,** which is the functional equivalent of the stratum basale of the epidermis. Thus, the hair grows from its base, not its tip. Cells become keratinized in a mechanism similar to that seen in the epidermis. The portion of the hair above the skin's surface is called the **hair shaft**. Frequently, the hair falls out of the follicle during slide preparation, so all that is seen is the follicle and associated structures.

Two types of hairs are present in humans. **Vellus hairs** are short, fine, and microscopic. These comprise the majority of hairs on the human body. **Terminal hairs** are larger and coarser. These are the hairs everyone recognizes as hairs, such as those of the scalp.

In cross section, the hair and follicle present several layers (Figure 11-12). These are described from the interior of the hair to the outermost part of the follicle.

- The **medulla** is at the center of the hair. It is most obvious in the root; in the shaft the cells are cornified or completely absent.

- The **cortex** makes up the bulk of the hair. In the root, the cortex is made up of cuboidal cells, but in the shaft the cells are flattened and keratinized. Pigment granules and air spaces between the cortical cells produce hair color.

- The **cuticle** of the hair is made up of hard keratin and surrounds the cortex.

- The **internal root sheath** is part of the follicle and extends from its base to where the sebaceous gland enters. It consists of three layers. The **cuticle of the internal root sheath** is similar in construction to the cuticle of the hair and its cells interdigitate with it. **Huxley's layer** consists of a couple of layers of flattened cells. **Henle's layer** is a single row of flattened rectangular cells.

- The **external root sheath** is composed of several cell layers. The single layer of cells in contact with the connective tissue sheath is columnar; the remaining cells are polygonal in shape. These cells are derived from the outermost part of the matrix and are separated from the connective tissue sheath by the glassy membrane. It is an extension of the stratum basale and stratum spinosum of the epidermis. The external root sheath houses a population of **epidermal stem cells** capable of division and that serve as a source of sebaceous gland and follicle cells. They also contribute epidermal cells after injury.

- The external root sheath is surrounded by its thick basement membrane, called the glassy membrane (mentioned above).

- External to the glassy membrane, but derived from the dermis, is a sheath of connective tissue (mentioned above).

Sebaceous Glands

Hair follicles are associated with simple or branched acinar **sebaceous glands** (Figures 11-11b and 11-13). Gland cells near the follicle disintegrate (so the gland is holocrine) and release the oily substance **sebum** into the follicle, which moisturizes and lubricates the hair. Division of cells at the base of the gland replaces these cells. Because they are thicker than their respective follicle, sebaceous glands are often seen in sectioned specimens without their follicles.

Arrector Pili Muscles

Arrector pili muscles (Figures 11-11b and 11-14) are smooth muscles that insert on the follicle's connective tissue sheath. They are positioned in the obtuse angle formed by the follicle and the skin surface. Their contraction straightens the hair, which in other mammals causes the fur to form a thicker insulating layer, but in humans only produces "goose bumps." The sebaceous gland is found in the angle formed between the arrector pili muscle and the follicle.

Sweat Glands

Sweat glands are downgrowths of the epidermis. They are simple, coiled tubular glands of two types. **Eccrine sweat glands** (Figure 11-15) are more numerous and produce a watery secretion that has a cooling effect on the body as it evaporates. The coiled secretory portion is made up of simple cuboidal epithelium and the lumen is small. The relatively straight duct leading to the surface is made up of two cell layers and eventually stains darker than the secretory layer. **Apocrine sweat glands** (Figure 11-16) are found in the axillary and groin regions. The lumen of the secretory portion is wider than in eccrine glands and the secretion is more viscous. Both eccrine, specifically those in the palms and soles of the feet, and apocrine glands produce secretions in response to emotional stress.

Nails

Nails (Figure 11-17) are made of keratinized cells that form a hard plate on the dorsal and distal sides of the fingers and toes. The main part of the nail is the **nail plate**, which ends distally as the **free edge**, the part that gets trimmed. At the proximal end is the **nail root**, which lies beneath a fold of skin. The nail rests on an epidermal layer (corresponding to the stratum basale and stratum spinosum) called the **nail bed**. At the proximal end, the nail bed is thickened to form the **nail matrix**. It is responsible for producing the nail in a process similar to hair production. The stratum corneum folds over the proximal end of the nail plate as the **eponychium** and under the free edge as **hyponychium**.

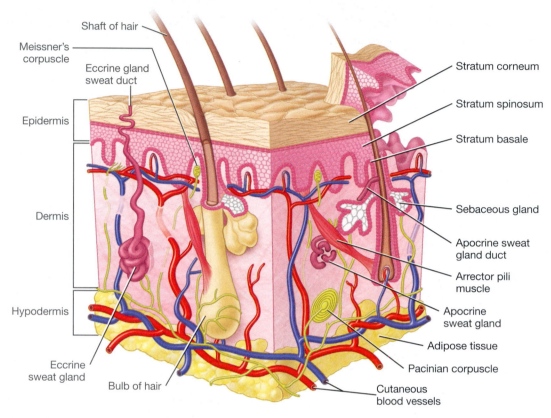

11-2 **Structures of the Integument** ■ Refer to this figure as you read about the layers and structures of the integumentary system.

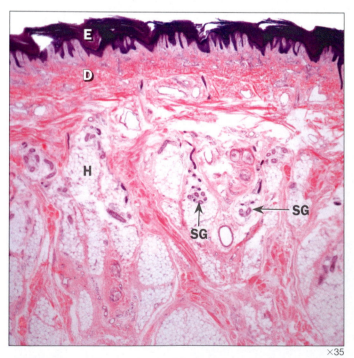

×35

11-3 **The Integument** ■ The integument consists of the superficial epidermis (E), a keratinized stratified squamous epithelium, and the deeper dermis (D), mostly a dense irregular connective tissue. The hypodermis (H) is deep to the dermis and is largely adipose tissue in this specimen, though a few sweat glands (SG) are present. (×35)

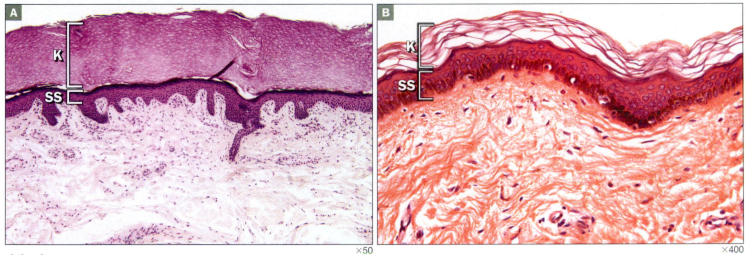

11-4 **Thick and Thin Skin** ◼ As you examine these specimens, be mindful of the difference in magnification. (**A**) This specimen is from the sole of the foot and is representative of thick skin. Note the thick keratinized layer (K) on the surface of the other epidermal layers, mostly stratum spinosum (SS). (×50) (**B**) Thin skin has a much thinner keratinized layer that appears shredded. Note the pigmentation in the basal epidermal layers. (×400)

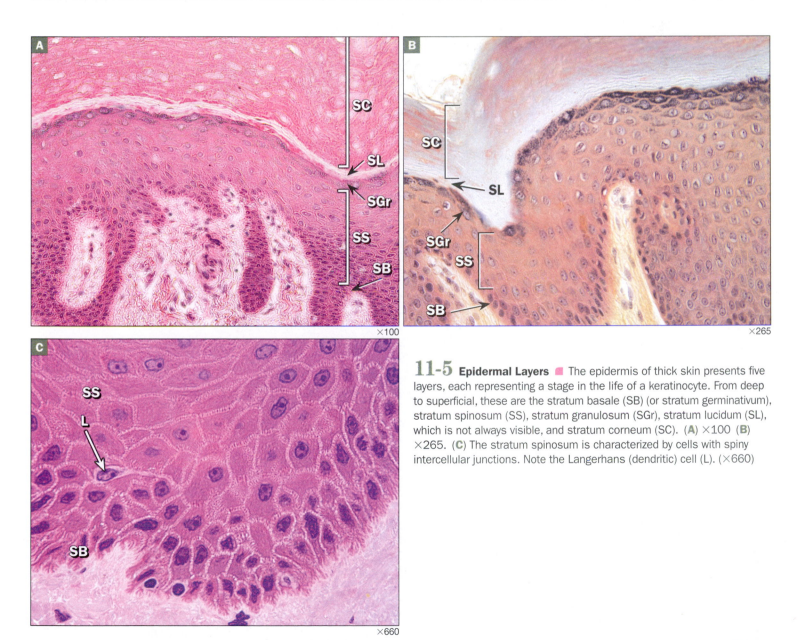

11-5 **Epidermal Layers** ◼ The epidermis of thick skin presents five layers, each representing a stage in the life of a keratinocyte. From deep to superficial, these are the stratum basale (SB) (or stratum germinativum), stratum spinosum (SS), stratum granulosum (SGr), stratum lucidum (SL), which is not always visible, and stratum corneum (SC). (**A**) ×100 (**B**) ×265. (**C**) The stratum spinosum is characterized by cells with spiny intercellular junctions. Note the Langerhans (dendritic) cell (L). (×660)

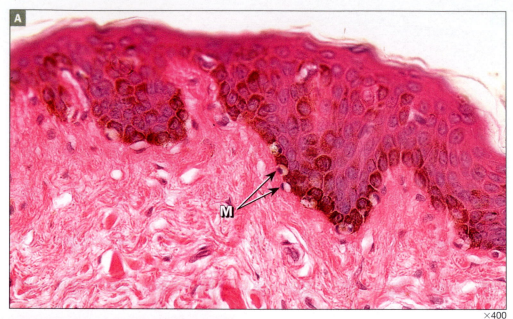

×400

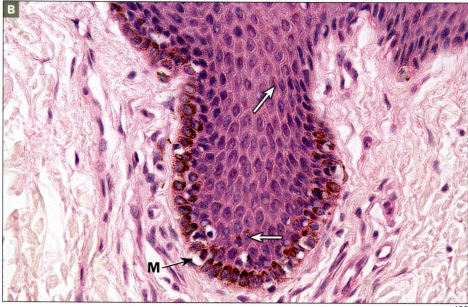

×400

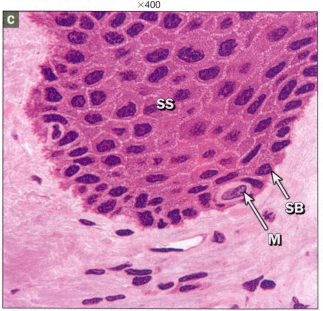

×765

11-6 **Pigmented Thin Skin** ■ Skin accumulates a brown to black pigment called melanin, which is produced by melanocytes (M). Differences in the amount of melanin are responsible for relative darkness of the skin. (**A**) Shown is a specimen of pigmented thin skin. Note the abundance of melanin in the basal layer of the epidermis and that it tends to be most dense on the side of the nucleus exposed to the sun. (×400) (**B**) The same features are shown in this micrograph of thin skin as in (**A**), but also notice that melanin has been deposited in some cells of the stratum spinosum (arrows). (×400) (**C**) Melanocytes are large, pale-staining cells found in the basal layers of the epidermis, and are also visible in micrographs (**A**) and (**B**). Also note the spiny cells of the stratum spinosum (SS). (×765)

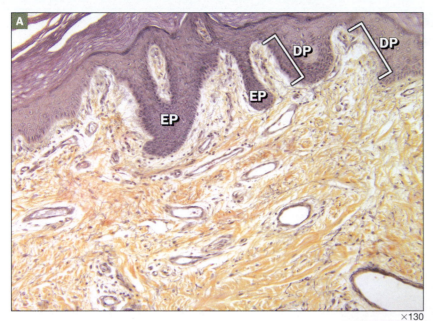

×130

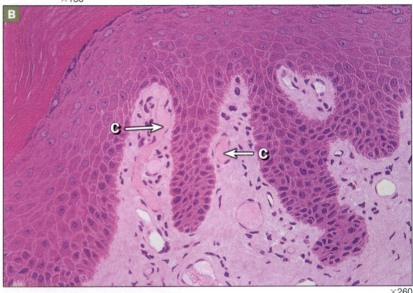

×260

11-7 **Dermis** 🔷 (A) Dermal papillae (DP) project into and interdigitate with the epidermal pegs (EP) of the epidermis. The irregular margin between the two layers increases surface area and limits separation due to shearing forces. (×130) (B) This micrograph shows capillaries (C) in the dermal papillae of a thin section of skin. (×260) (C) The papillary layer (P) of the dermis is in contact with the epidermis and is made of a loose connective tissue. The deeper reticular layer (R) is thicker and is a dense irregular connective tissue. The difference in texture is obvious in this micrograph. (×100)

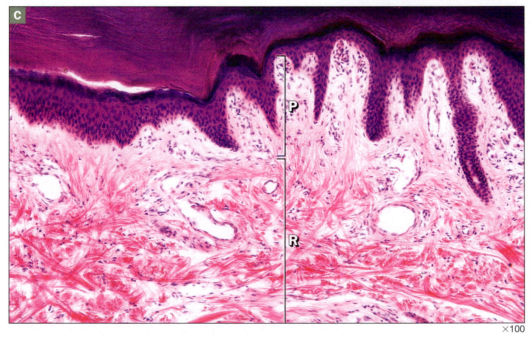

×100

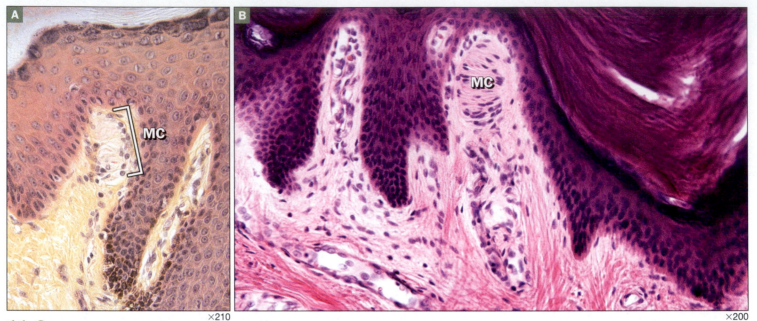

×210

×200

11-8 Meissner's Corpuscles ◼ Meissner's corpuscles (MC) are receptors for light touch found in dermal papillae. They are especially densely distributed in fingertips, palms, and the soles of feet, but are not seen in every papilla. The corpuscle is oval shaped. Look for the elongated nuclei of fibroblasts wrapping it transversely. (**A**) ×210 (**B**) ×200

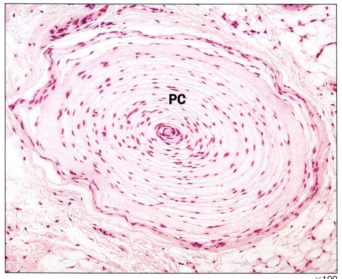

×100

11-9 Pacinian Corpuscles ◼ These pressure receptors (PC) look like a sliced onion in section and are found in the dermis and hypodermis, as in this example. (×100)

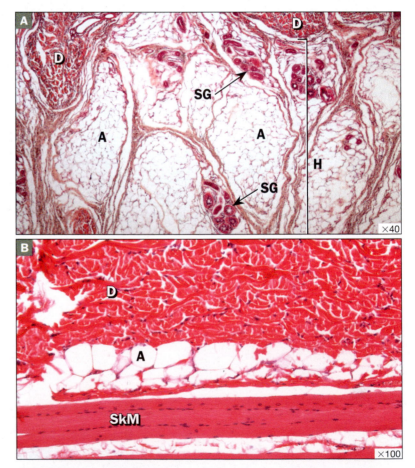

×40

×100

11-10 Hypodermis ◼ Deep to the dermis (D), the hypodermis (H) is a layer of loose connective tissue or adipose tissue (A) that loosely binds the integument to the underlying structures. It allows free movement of muscles without pulling on the skin. (**A**) This micrograph shows adipose tissue and numerous sweat glands (SG) in the hypodermis. (×40) (**B**) In this specimen, the hypodermis (H) is reduced to a few layers of adipocytes lying between the dermis (D) above the skeletal muscle (SkM) below. (×100)

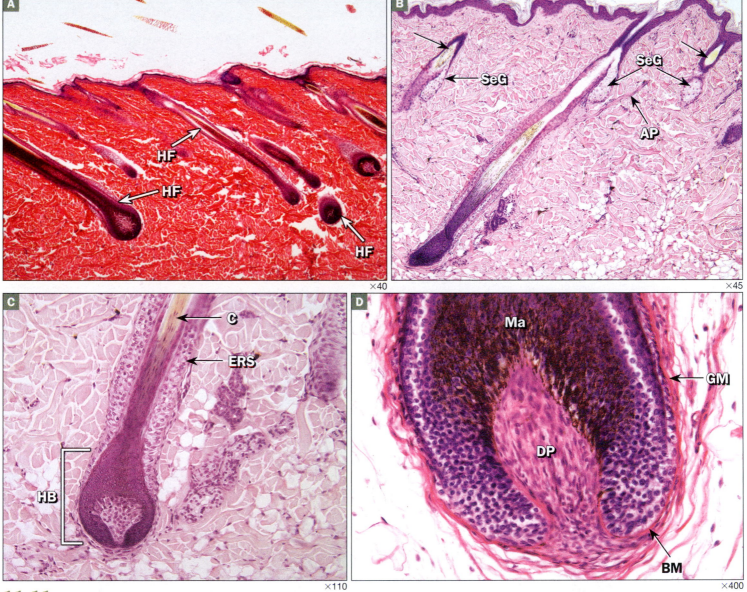

11-11 **Hair Follicle** ▪ (**A**) Hair follicles (HF) are epidermal invaginations into the dermis. They form an angle with the surface and rarely are seen in their entirety because the sections are so thin. This means you will likely have to piece together the entire structure from fragments in the specimen. (×40) (**B**) This shows a fairly complete hair follicle, but pieces of other follicles are also visible (arrows). Sebaceous glands (SeG) and an arrector pili muscle (AP) can also be seen. Note the position of the gland relative to the muscle. (×45) (**C**) The deepest part of the follicle is dilated and forms the hair bulb (HB). Also visible are the cortex (C) and external root sheath (ERS). (×110) (**D**) Each follicle has a dermal papilla (DP) that has capillaries and a nerve. It is separated from the hair root cells by a basement membrane (BM), which is continuous with the glassy membrane (GM) on the outside of the follicle. Note the large amount of pigment in the hair matrix cells (Ma), which are responsible for hair growth. (×400)

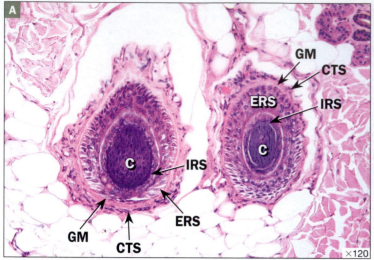

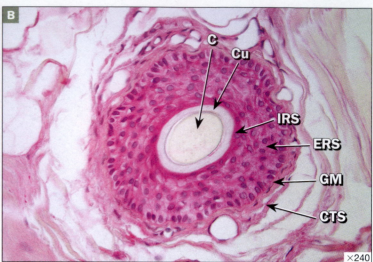

11-12 Hairs in Cross Section ■ (A) This cross section of two hair follicles was made at the level of the hypodermis. (×120) (B) This section was made higher in the dermis. Symbols used are the same as in (A). (×240)

Key to symbols used

C	=	cortex	**ERS**	= external root sheath
CTS	=	connective tissue sheath	**GM**	= glassy membrane
Cu	=	cuticle	**IRS**	= internal root sheath

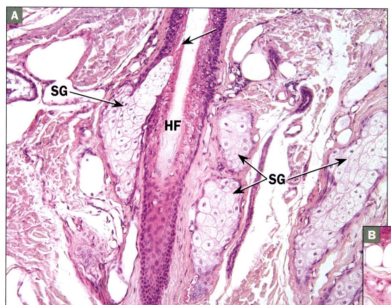

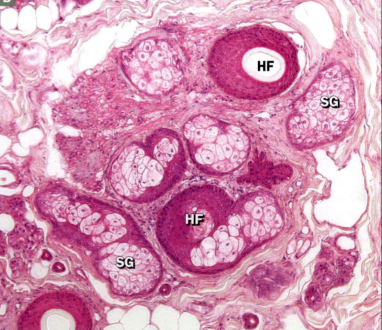

11-13 Sebaceous Glands ■ Cells of sebaceous glands (SG) are large and often have a foamy appearance. Because they are larger than their associated follicle (HF), sebaceous glands are often seen with no follicle in the section. Both sections were made at the level of the dermis. (A) The sebaceous gland on the left is seen to empty into the follicle (arrow near the top of the micrograph). The ducts of the others are out of the plane of section. (×120) (B) Shown here are follicles cut in cross section. Most of the sebaceous glands show no connection with them except for the one at the bottom center (×100)

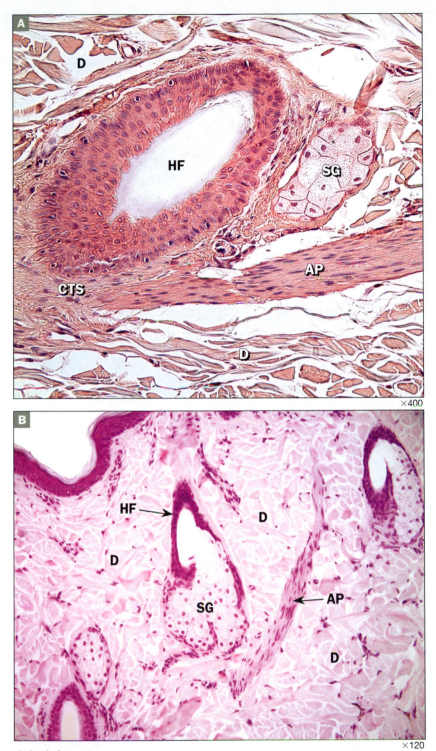

11-14 **Arrector Pili Muscles** ■ Contraction of an arrector pili muscle causes the hair to stand erect. (**A**) This micrograph shows an arrector pili (AP) muscle attached to the connective tissue sheath (CTS) of a follicle cut in oblique section through the dermis (D). Note how the sebaceous gland (SG) is positioned between the arrector pili muscle and the hair follicle (HF). (×400) (**B**) It is very difficult to find a perfectly sectioned hair follicle, so one has to make do with what is available. In this micrograph, only a very small piece of the follicle (HF) is present, but the sebaceous gland (SG) and arrector pili muscle are seen in the dermis. (×120)

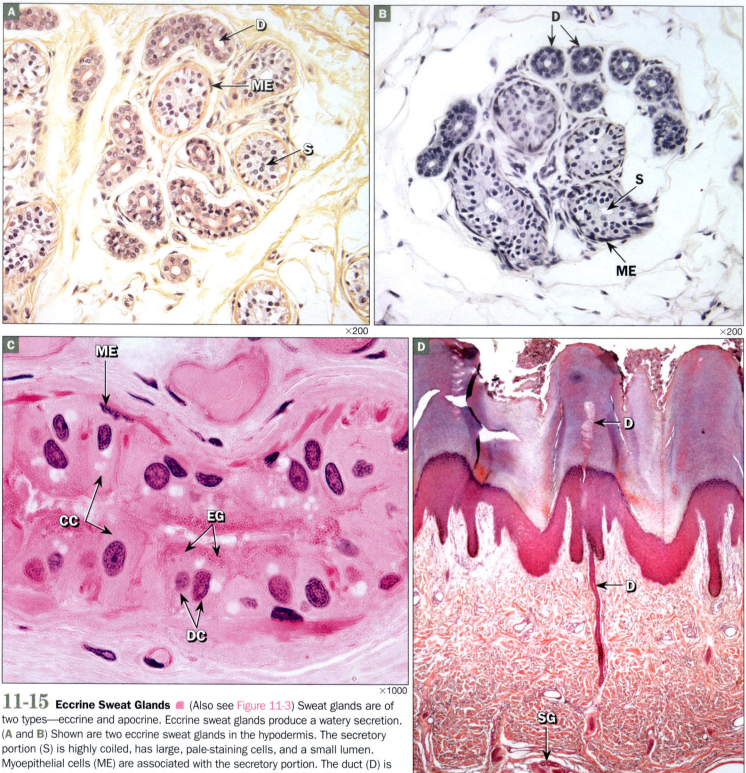

11-15 **Eccrine Sweat Glands** ▪ (Also see Figure 11-3) Sweat glands are of two types—eccrine and apocrine. Eccrine sweat glands produce a watery secretion. (A and B) Shown are two eccrine sweat glands in the hypodermis. The secretory portion (S) is highly coiled, has large, pale-staining cells, and a small lumen. Myoepithelial cells (ME) are associated with the secretory portion. The duct (D) is lined with two layers of darker-staining cells. (×200) (C) Three cell types are seen in this thin section of an eccrine sweat gland. Clear cells (CC) contact the basement membrane and produce the sweat. Dark cells (DC) do not reach the basement membrane. They produce antibacterial chemicals that are released from eosinophilic granules (EG) into the lumen. Myoepithelial cells (ME) are the third cell type. (×1000) (D) This micrograph shows a sweat gland duct (D) as it passes from the hypodermis, where the glands (SG) are, through the dermis and into the epidermis. (×40)

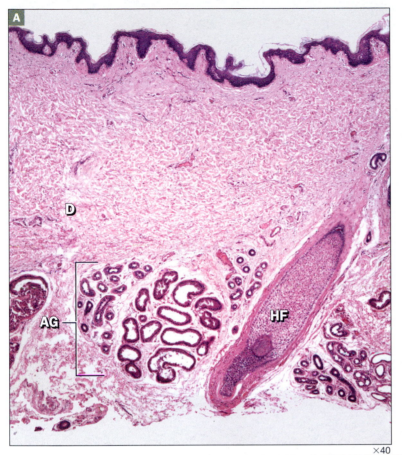

11-16 **Apocrine Sweat Glands** 🔴 Apocrine sweat glands are found in the axillary and genital regions of the body. Their secretion is more viscous than that of eccrine sweat glands due to the presence of proteins, which when digested by skin microbes produces an odor. (**A**) Shown is an apocrine gland (AG) from the axilla. It is located in the dermis (D) next to a hair follicle (HF). (×40) (**B**) The secretory portion (S) of apocrine sweat glands is coiled and tubular, and is lined by a simple cuboidal to simple columnar epithelium. Its large lumen (L) makes distinguishing these from eccrine glands relatively easy. The ducts empty into hair follicles just above the sebaceous gland. (×400)

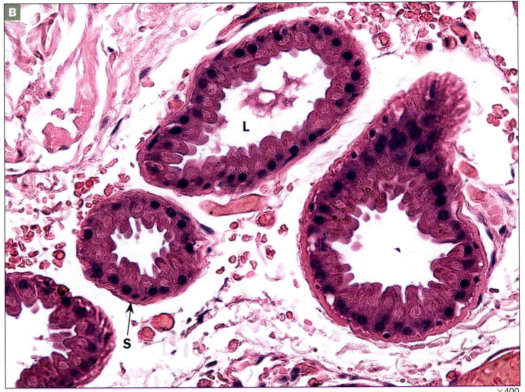

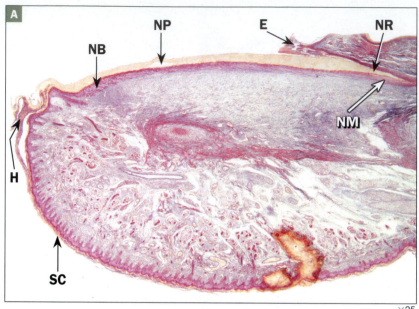

×25

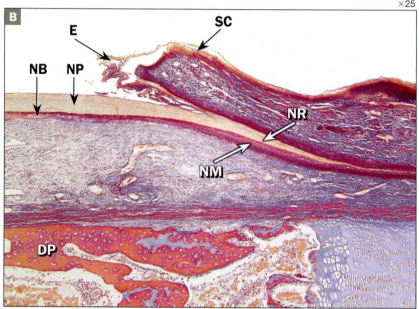

×65

11-17 **Nails** ■ (**A**) This micrograph is of a fetal finger cut in sagittal section. Notice the continuity of the stratum corneum with the eponychium and hyponychium. (×25) (**B**) This micrograph shows greater detail of the nail root. (×65)

Key to symbols used

DP	= distal phalanx	**NM**	= nail matrix
E	= eponychium	**NP**	= nail plate
H	= hyponychium	**NR**	= nail root
NB	= nail bed	**SC**	= stratum corneum

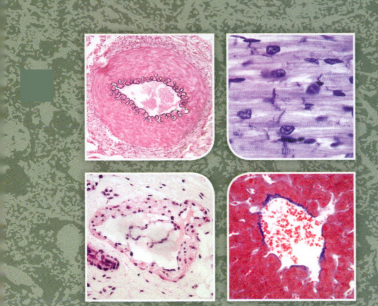

12

Cardiovascular System

Introduction to the Cardiovascular System

The cardiovascular system (Figure 12-1) consists of blood pumped by the heart through the blood vessels to all parts of the body. Its function is to carry materials from organs that exchange with the environment to and from cells buried deep in the body. Oxygen is picked up in the lungs and distributed throughout the body, whereas carbon dioxide is picked up from the cells and delivered to the lungs from which it is exhaled. Food absorbed by the digestive tract is distributed throughout the body, and wastes are picked up from cells and removed from the blood by the kidneys.

The postnatal human circulatory system consists of two closed-loop paths: the **pulmonary circuit** and the **systemic circuit**. Oxygen-poor blood is returned to the right atrium by the superior and inferior venae cavae. From there, it moves into the right ventricle and is pumped out into the pulmonary trunk where it is then sent to the lungs to pick up oxygen. It is returned to the left atrium by the pulmonary veins. This completes the pulmonary circuit. From the left atrium, the now oxygen-rich blood is sent into the left ventricle and is then pumped out through the aorta to be distributed by arteries to the capillaries of the entire body. Blood in the capillaries loses its oxygen to the surrounding tissues, picks up CO_2, and is sent through systemic veins and eventually the superior and inferior venae cavae back to the right atrium. This completes the systemic circuit.

A third path of blood flow is the **coronary circuit**, which begins with the coronary arteries (the first branches of the aorta). Blood is delivered to capillaries in the heart muscle and returned to the right atrium by the **coronary sinus**, located on the posterior of the heart.

12-1 Cardiovascular System
The cardiovascular system includes the heart, blood vessels, and blood, which is covered in Chapter 6.

Basic Blood Vessel Structure

Blood vessels are composed of as many as three layers, or tunics, that are modified according to the vessel's function. From innermost tunic to outermost these are the tunica (intima) interna, tunica media, and tunica (adventitia) externa. They are best demonstrated in arteries (Figures 12-2 and 12-3).

The **tunica (intima) interna** is a simple squamous endothelium supported by a thin layer of connective tissue. In arteries and the largest veins, an **internal elastic (lamina) membrane** is also present at the junction with the tunica media. The **tunica media** is composed of varying amounts of smooth muscle and elastic connective tissue oriented circularly around the vessel. In larger arteries, there may be an **external elastic (lamina) membrane** at the junction with the tunica externa. The **tunica (adventitia) externa** is composed of fibrous connective tissue that often blends with surrounding connective tissues, making the outer limit of the vessel difficult to see.

If the vessel's walls are thicker than the effective distance for diffusion of oxygen and nutrients, the wall may be penetrated with small blood vessels called **vasa vasorum**. They are especially common in larger veins due to the lower oxygen concentration in systemic venous blood.

▪▪ Types of Blood Vessels

Blood vessels are of three main types: arteries, veins, and capillaries. Each has a distinctive structure appropriate to its function. Arteries, veins, and nerves typically travel together to form a **neurovascular bundle** (Figure 12-4).

Arteries carry blood away from the heart at high pressure. As such, their walls are thicker than their corresponding vein. The two arteries that exit the heart are the aorta and pulmonary trunk. These branch into smaller and smaller arteries and eventually lead to the capillaries of the systemic circuit and pulmonary circuit, respectively. As arteries get smaller, the proportion of elastic tissue decreases and the smooth muscle increases (relative to the wall's thickness). When viewed under the microscope arteries typically have a circular lumen and distinct layers, with the tunica media being the thickest of the three (Figures 12-2 through 12-6).

Elastic arteries (Figure 12-5) are the largest and include the pulmonary trunk and aorta, and their major branches. The tunica media is dominated by elastic tissue in the form of **fenestrated membranes** (**lamellae**), which alternate with smooth muscle. Internal and external elastic membranes are present and prominent. It is this elasticity that allows the arteries closest to the heart to passively expand as blood is pumped into them (felt as a pulse if near the body's surface), and then recoil to propel the blood further along. The tunica externa is very thin and often has vasa vasorum.

Muscular arteries (Figure 12-6) are larger than 0.5 mm in diameter and include most of the named arteries. The internal elastic membrane is wavy in appearance, and the tunica media is composed of up to 40 layers of smooth muscle cells. An external elastic membrane may be present, and the tunica externa has collagen and elastic fibers and smooth muscle fibers oriented longitudinally along the vessel.

Arterioles (Figure 12-7) are the smallest arteries, with a diameter of 30 to 200 μm. The tunica media is composed of one to a few layers of smooth muscle. An internal elastic membrane is present in larger arterioles but is absent in smaller ones. The tunica externa is approximately the same size as the tunica media. The final arteriole before the capillary bed is called a **metarteriole**. Blood flow into the capillary bed is regulated by **precapillary sphincters**, made of circularly arranged smooth muscle fibers around the metarteriole and capillary junction. An **arteriovenous anastomosis** directly connects the arteriole and venule and allows blood to bypass the capillary bed when the sphincters are closed. (See page 132 for a description of how these work in the dermis to regulate body temperature.)

Capillaries (Figure 12-8) are the smallest blood vessels. They have a diameter of 4 to 10 μm and consist only of endothelium and basal lamina. Contractile **pericytes** may be present on capillaries (and some venules). They regulate blood flow.

Based on electron micrographs, three types of capillaries are recognized (Figures 12-2 and 12-9). **Continuous capillaries** have a complete endothelial lining. They are the most common and are found in muscle, nervous, and connective tissues, as well as the lungs. In **fenestrated capillaries**, membrane-covered pores 60 to 80 nm in diameter are present. These are found in endocrine glands, lamina propria of the small intestine, and kidneys (where there is no membrane covering the pores). **Sinusoidal capillaries** are larger than other capillaries and the surrounding cells determine their shape. Their discontinuous endothelium promotes exchange. They are found in bone marrow, the liver, spleen, and lymph nodes, as well as other places.

Veins carry blood toward the heart under low pressure, so their walls are thinner than the corresponding artery. Veins begin at the capillaries and end at the heart as either the inferior or superior vena cava or one of the pulmonary veins. Because they carry blood at low pressure and often against the pull of gravity, many veins are supplied with endothelial folds that form **valves**. When viewed under the microscope, veins often are collapsed and have an irregularly shaped lumen; the layers are indistinct and the thickest layer is the tunica externa (compare the artery and vein in Figure 12-4). In general, vessels of the pulmonary circuit have thinner walls than systemic vessels of the same size because they carry blood at lower pressure.

The smallest veins are called **venules** (Figure 12-7). Venules are structurally similar to capillaries, but are larger in diameter. As they emerge from the capillary bed, pericytes are present, but these are replaced with smooth muscle in the tunica media as the venules get larger. **High endothelial venules** are found in certain lymphatic organs and have a cuboidal endothelium. They play an important role in lymphocytes leaving the blood and entering lymphatic tissue.

Medium veins are less than 1 cm in diameter (Figure 12-10). Their tunica interna is composed of endothelium and connective tissue, but there is no internal elastic membrane. The tunica media consists of smooth muscle, and the tunica externa has collagen and elastic fibers, and smooth muscle. Valves formed by pockets of tunica interna are present in medium systemic veins that carry blood against gravity (Figure 12-11). If blood flows the wrong way, the pockets fill with blood and the lumen is closed.

Large veins (Figure 12-12) have a thicker tunica interna due to more connective tissue. The tunica media is generally absent, though smooth muscle cells are present in veins carrying blood against gravity. The tunica externa is the thickest layer and is composed of elastic and collagen fibers. Vasa vasorum are also present.

:: The Heart

The heart is a hollow, muscular organ. It consists of four chambers: the **right atrium** and **ventricle**, and the **left atrium** and **ventricle**. The superior vena cava brings blood from the head and upper limbs to the right atrium, whereas the inferior vena cava does the same for the lower limbs and abdomen. The pulmonary trunk emerges from the right ventricle and divides into pulmonary arteries that carry blood to each lung. The four pulmonary veins bring blood from the lungs to the left atrium and the aorta carries blood out of the left ventricle and distributes it body-wide through its numerous branches.

Valves in the heart ensure blood travels in the correct direction. Between each atrium and its ventricle is an **atrioventricular valve**. The **tricuspid valve** is between the right atrium and ventricle and consists of three flaps. The **bicuspid (mitral) valve** has two flaps and separates the left atrium and ventricle. At the start of the aorta and pulmonary trunk are the aortic and pulmonary **semilunar valves**, respectively. They are made of endothelial pockets similar in construction to the valves of veins. These valves prevent backflow into the ventricle during ventricular relaxation (diastole).

The heart wall consists of three layers. The **endocardium** is comparable to the tunica interna of blood vessels (Figure 12-13). It consists of endothelium plus a loose connective tissue. The endocardium folds inward and is reinforced with connective tissue to form the flaps of the bicuspid and tricuspid valves. A deeper connective tissue layer, called the **subendocardial** layer, is where **Purkinje fibers** are located (see below). The **myocardium** (Figure 12-14) is the middle and thickest layer of the heart wall. **Epicardium** is on the outer surface of the heart (Figure 12-15). It is also called **visceral pericardium** and is made up of a simple squamous mesothelium plus underlying fibrous connective tissue, which sometimes accumulates fat. It also is the layer in which the **coronary vessels** travel.

Cardiac muscle cells have an intrinsic contraction rate, but the **sinoatrial (SA) node** (also called the cardiac **pacemaker**), located at the junction of the superior vena cava and the right atrium, and made up of modified cardiac muscle cells, regulates that rate. The SA node and the following structures constitute the conduction system of the heart. The SA node's signal spreads over the atria, causing their contraction. It also reaches the **atrioventricular (AV) node** located in the myocardium at the level of the tricuspid valve near the entrance of the coronary sinus. When stimulated, the AV node sends its own signal via conducting fibers of the **bundle of His** (and its branches) down the interventricular septum to the heart's apex. From there, the signal spreads upward through the ventricular myocardium along specialized cardiac muscle fibers, called Purkinje fibers, which cause contraction (Figure 12-16). Purkinje fibers are located deep to the endocardium and are distinctive due to their large size, poorly defined striations (due to myofibrils being in the periphery), and pale cytoplasm. They are sometimes binucleate and have intercalated disks.

The **cardiac skeleton** is made up of dense connective tissue (Figure 12-13). It separates the atria from the ventricles and is also found at the bases of the pulmonary trunk and aorta. It is an attachment site for cardiac muscle and prevents transmission of impulses from the atria to the ventricles except via the bundle of His.

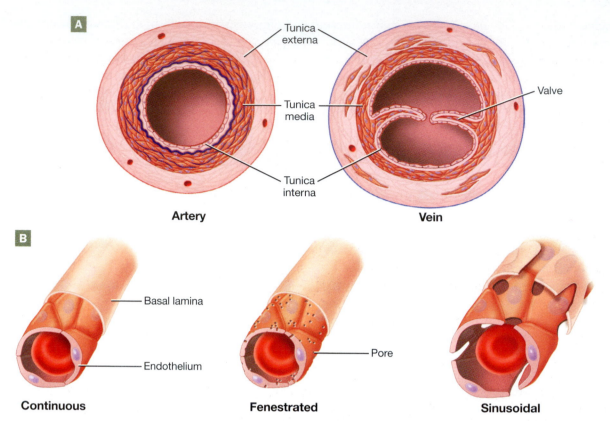

Artery   **Vein**

Tunica externa

Tunica media

Tunica interna

Valve

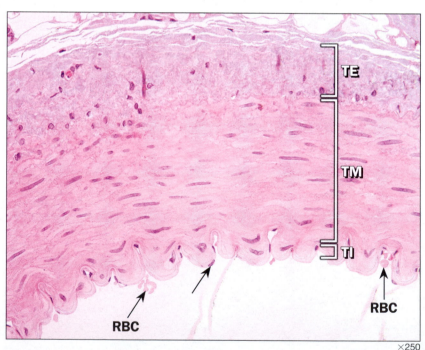

Basal lamina

Endothelium

Pore

Continuous   **Fenestrated**   **Sinusoidal**

12-2 **Comparison of Basic Artery, Capillary, and Vein Structure** ■ (**A**) The walls of arteries and veins are composed of three layers: a tunica (intima) interna next to the lumen, a middle tunica media, and an outer tunica (adventitia) externa. The endothelium lines all blood vessels and the heart. As a rule, the tunica media is the thickest layer in arteries, whereas the tunica externa is thickest in veins. The tissue composition of the outer two layers varies depending on the size of the vessel. Additionally, veins often have valves. Blood is carried in the lumen, the open region formed by the vessel's wall. (**B**) Capillaries consist only of endothelium and its basal lamina. Three capillary types have been identified based on the continuity of the endothelium: continuous, fenestrated with membrane-covered pores, and sinusoidal with gaps between cells.

TE

TM

TI

RBC

RBC

×250

12-3 **Blood Vessel Structure** ■ This artery illustrates the three layers found in blood vessel walls. The innermost layer, the tunica interna (TI), is composed of a simple squamous endothelium (arrow) and underlying connective tissue. Endothelium is the only layer found in all blood vessels (and the heart). Depending on the vessel, the tunica media (TM) is made of fibrous and/or elastic connective tissue and smooth muscle. In this artery it is mostly smooth muscle. The tunica media is absent in capillaries. The tunica externa (TE) is on the outside of vessels other than capillaries. Notice how it blends in with surrounding connective tissue. Also note the red blood cells (RBC) in the lumen. (×250)

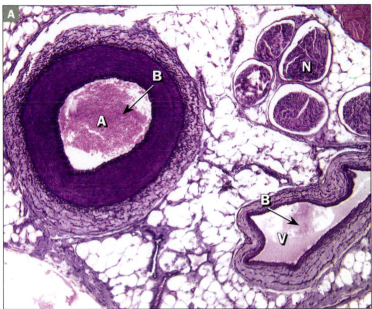

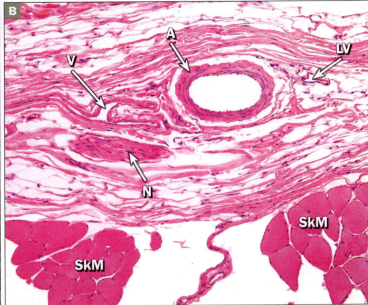

×60

×120

12-4 **Neurovascular Bundle** ◼ Typically, arteries (A), veins (V), and nerves (N) are found together in the body. Collectively, they are known as a neurovascular bundle. (**A**) Shown in this micrograph is a fairly large neurovascular bundle. Notice the round lumen and thicker wall layers in the artery. Corresponding layers in the walls of the artery and vein stain the same, as does the blood (B) in both. (×60) (**B**) This is a much smaller neurovascular bundle. The vein might be overlooked because it is so collapsed. The presence of an artery is a clue to look for a corresponding vein. Notice that the nerve, unlike the blood vessels, is cut in oblique section in this preparation. A small lymph vessel (LV), characterized by walls even thinner than veins, is also visible. Skeletal muscle (SkM) is at the bottom of the field. (×120) (**C**) In this much higher magnification, the neurovascular bundle stands out clearly because of the surrounding adipose tissue, as opposed to the fibrous connective tissue in (**B**). Notice all the branches of the nerve, as well as the small lymph vessel (LV). (×400)

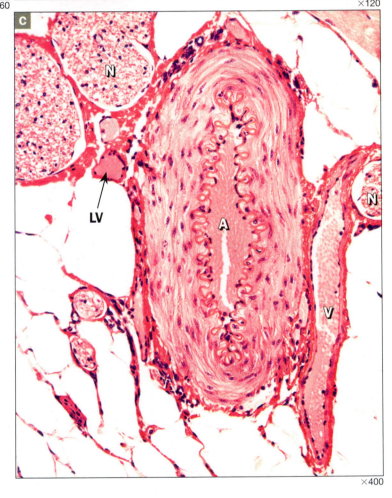

×400

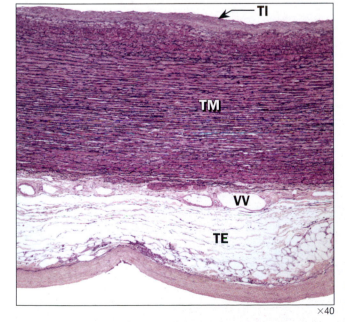

×40

12-5 **Aorta** ◼ In this specimen of the aorta, the fenestrated elastic lamellae are visible in the tunica media (TM) as black lines. They account for the elasticity of this large artery. The tunica interna (TI) and tunica externa (TE) are visible above and below the tunica media, respectively. Vasa vasorum (VV) are also visible. (×40)

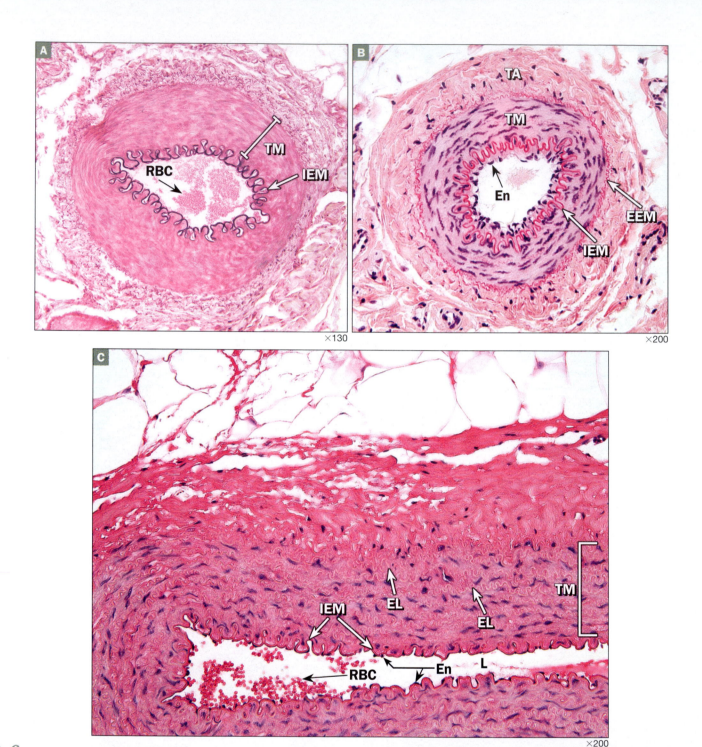

×130

×200

×200

12-6 **Muscular Arteries** ● Medium-sized arteries are also known as muscular arteries because of the abundance of smooth muscle fibers in the tunica media (TM). Notice in both specimens that the tunica media is the thickest layer, a feature typical of arteries in general. Red blood cells (RBC) are visible in both specimens. Because of their usually uniform size (between 7 and 8 µm in diameter), RBCs can be used to estimate magnification and sizes of other structures in the field. (**A**) Because it was stained to demonstrate elastic fibers, the internal elastic membrane (IEM) of this small muscular artery is obvious as a dark, squiggly line. (And, in turn, notice how little elastic tissue is present in the tunica media!) The endothelium (En) is hardly visible at this magnification. (×130) (**B**) This artery, stained for elastic fibers, shows an external elastic membrane (EEM), in addition to the internal elastic membrane. (×200) (**C**) The internal elastic membrane is still visible in this specimen, even though it was not stained for elastin. Once you see what elastic tissue looks like in this preparation, careful examination will reveal more elastic lamellae (EL) in the tunica media (TM). The endothelium is seen only as dark, flattened nuclei at the edge of the lumen (L), which is about all that is expected at this magnification. (×200)

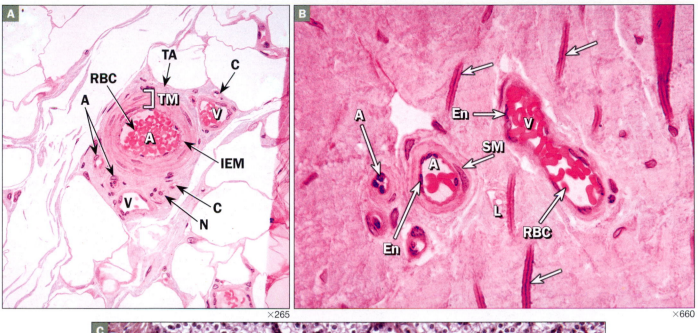

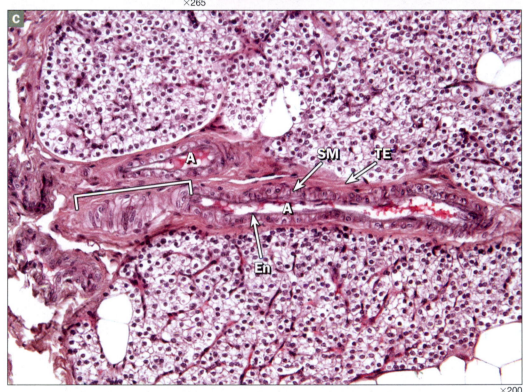

12-7 **Arteriole and Venule** ▪ (**A**) Arterioles (A) are less than 200 μm in diameter. In this specimen, the endothelial lining and internal elastic membrane (IEM) are visible and the tunica media (TM) is about three muscle cells thick. Notice that the tunica adventitia (TA) blends in with the surrounding connective tissue. Two smaller arterioles are also present, each with a single layer of smooth muscle. To the right and below the largest arteriole are two smaller venules (V). Note their thin walls. A couple of capillaries (C) and a small nerve (N) are also visible, as are red blood cells (RBC). (×265) (**B**) In this specimen, the nuclei of smooth muscle cells (SM) in the arterioles are larger and lighter than the endothelial cells' nuclei (En). Notice that the tunica media of the smallest arterioles consists of one layer of smooth muscle. The wall of the venule is extremely thin, but the lumen is relatively large. There is also a small lymphatic vessel (L) visible in the field. Structures marked by arrows are artifacts of preparation. (×660) (**C**) Two arterioles (A) are present in this micrograph of the parathyroid gland. The upper one was sectioned obliquely, but the lower one was sectioned longitudinally, which is somewhat of a rarity. Nuclei of the endothelium (En) are dark and flat. What looks like simple cuboidal epithelium is the single layer of circularly arranged smooth muscle cells (SM) of the tunica media. At the far left (bracket), the section only passes through tunica media and misses the arteriole's lumen. This dramatically demonstrates how smooth muscle cells of the tunica media wrap around the arteriole and can regulate blood flow through it by contracting or relaxing. The tunica externa (TE) stands out against the background tissue of the parathyroid gland. Red blood cells (RBC) are also present.

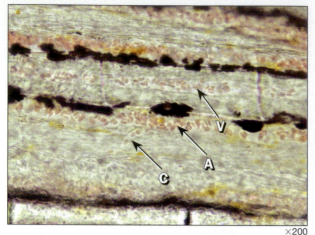

×200

12-8 Capillaries ▪

Capillaries are the smallest of blood vessels and are the site of material exchange between the blood and tissues. They can be recognized by the wall consisting only of endothelium and the red blood cells (RBC) lining up single file in the lumen. This micrograph is a wet mount of a living guppy's tail. A capillary (C) is shown branching off an arteriole (A), which was carrying blood from right to left. Because the guppy wasn't stained, the endothelial cells do not stand out. A venule (V) is also seen. Both the arteriole and venule were identified by their sizes and the direction of blood flow within the tail (arterioles carry blood toward the tail's tip; venules carry blood from the tail back to the body). This procedure was completed within minutes, and the female guppy "volunteer" happily swam away when returned to her bowl. As of this writing, she is in retirement and living with my grandchildren. Her name is "Herstology." She is a girl, after all. (×200)

×600

×400

12-9 Capillary Types ▪

Capillary walls consist only of endothelium and the lumen is the same size as (or even smaller than) RBCs, making their recognition mostly a matter of adequate magnification. There are three types of capillaries recognized based on structures visible with the electron microscope. Although they can't be differentiated using light micrographs, following are examples of each type (see Figure 12-2b). In each micrograph, an arrow indicates the capillaries. (A) This lung specimen provides examples of continuous capillaries, the most abundant of the three. The capillaries are found in the walls of air sacs called alveoli (Al) (see Chapter 15). (×600) (B) Glomerular capillaries in the kidneys (see Chapter 16) are an example of the fenestrated type. (×400) (C) This liver specimen provides an example of sinusoidal capillaries (see Chapter 14). Their endothelium (En), seen as the lighter layer lining the white spaces, is not complete, and the liver cells around each sinusoid determine its overall shape. Notice that these are larger than the other capillary types as evidenced by the number of RBCs that fit across the diameter. The large vessel in the center is a vein (V) that receives blood from the sinusoids. (×400)

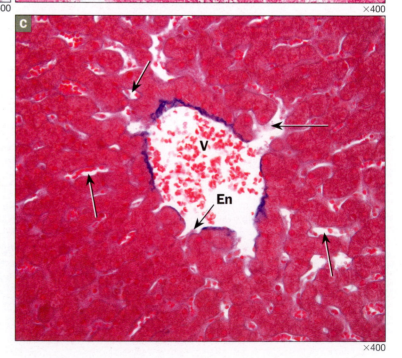

×400

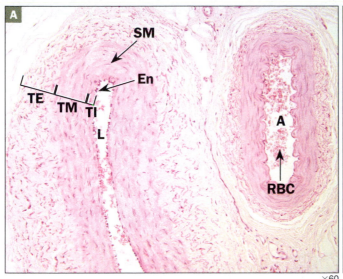

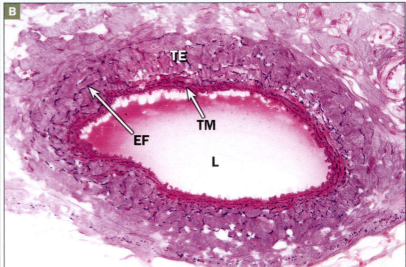

×60

×200

Key to symbols used

En	=	endothelium	**SM**	= smooth muscle
EF	=	elastic fibers	**TE**	= tunica externa
L	=	lumen	**TI**	= tunica interna
RBC	=	red blood cells	**TM**	= tunica media

12-10 **Veins** ▪ Veins are typically thin walled, and the tunica externa is the thickest layer. (**A**) The layers in this vein stain differently and are easily distinguished, although there is uncharacteristically little difference in the thicknesses of the tunica media and tunica externa. On a more subtle level, notice how the nuclei of the smooth muscle cells are uniformly distributed in the tunica media and are oriented in concentric circles around the lumen, and that the nuclei of the tunica externa (mostly fibroblasts) are scattered and have no particular orientation. The layers of this vein stain the same as the corresponding artery (A) in the field. (×60) (**B**) This specimen was prepared so that elastin was stained black. Notice that the few elastic fibers are primarily located in the tunica externa. (×200) (**C**) Staining of this specimen didn't differentiate well between the layers of this small vein, but endothelial cell nuclei are pretty obvious. The tunica media can be differentiated from the tunica externa based on the higher density of nuclei in the former. (Note: This is not a general rule, but it works for this specimen.) A tributary of this vein is visible in the lower right (arrow). (×260)

×260

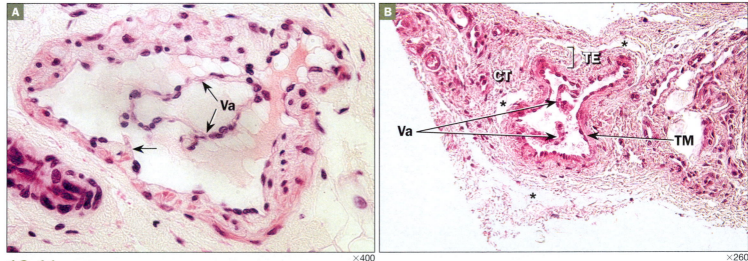

×400

×260

12-11 **Valves in Veins** ▪ Veins carrying blood against gravity often have pocket-shaped valves (Va) made of infoldings of tunica interna. (**A**) In this small vein, the more prominent valve has been sectioned in such a way that you are looking down into it. Only a piece of the other valve is visible on the opposite wall (arrow). (×400) (**B**) This is a more vertical section of two valves. Notice how the tunica externa (TE) is much thicker than the tunica (TM) and blends in with the surrounding connective tissue (CT). Spaces marked with asterisks (*) are artifacts of slide preparation. (×260)

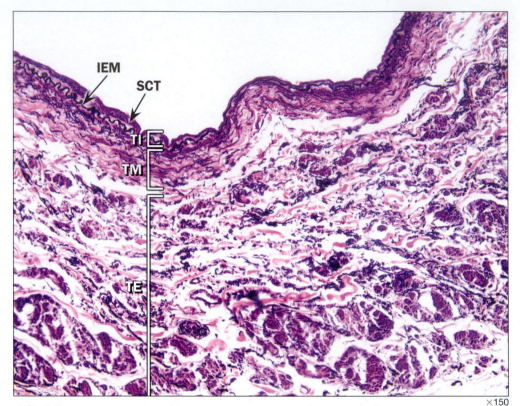

12-12 Vena Cava 🔴 Large veins have a relatively thick tunica interna (TI) because of a subendo-thelial connective tissue (SCT) layer. The tunica externa (TE) is by far the thickest layer. This specimen was stained for elastin and the internal elastic membrane (IEM), not seen in medium and small veins, is apparent. (×150)

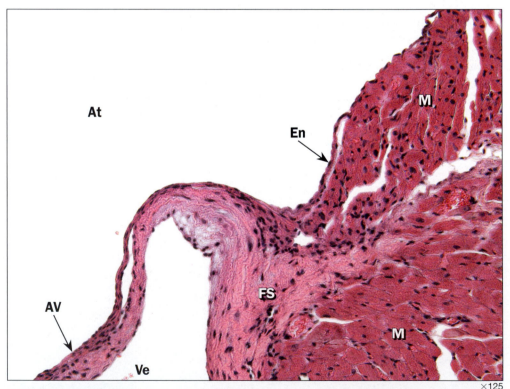

12-13 Endocardium 🔴 The inside of the heart is lined with endocardium composed of an endothelium (En) and loose connective tissue. Also shown is an atrioventricular valve (AV), which is composed of an interior of dense irregular connective tissue covered by endocardium. Atrioventricular valves separate the atrium (At) from the ventricle (Ve) on the same side of the heart and are anchored to the fibrous skeleton (FS). Myocardium (M) is also visible. (×125)

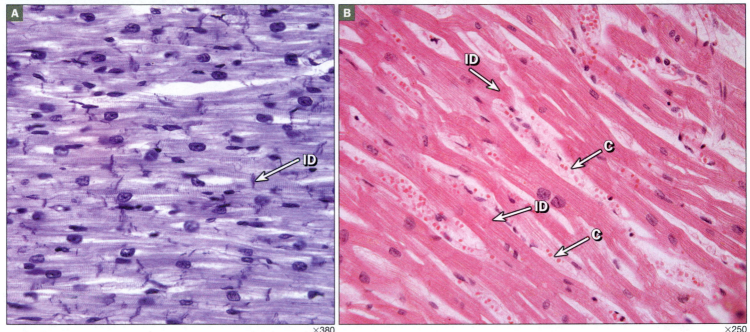

12-14 Myocardium ■ The thickest layer in the heart's wall is the myocardium, which is made up primarily of cardiac muscle. Shown here are two micrographs of cardiac muscle prepared with different stains. In (**A**) the striations and intercalated disks (ID) are easily seen. (×380) In (**B**) striations are difficult to see and the intercalated disks are faint, but the branching fibers are very obvious. Notice the numerous (continuous type) capillaries (C) between the fibers. (×250)

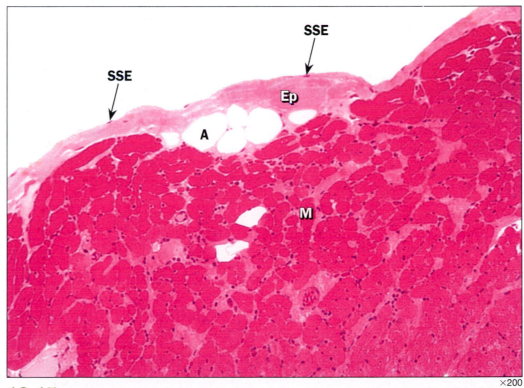

12-15 Epicardium ■ The outer surface of the heart is lined with serous membrane known as epicardium (Ep), or visceral pericardium. In this thin section, not many nuclei of the simple squamous epithelium (SSE) are visible, but the fairly substantial underlying connective tissue can be appreciated. Adipocytes (A), which can become quite numerous, and myocardium (M) are also shown. (×200)

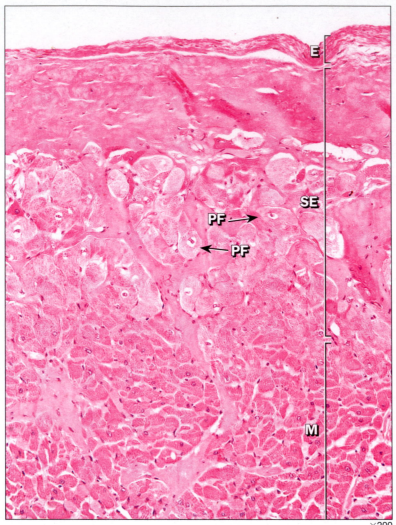

×200

12-16 **Purkinje Fibers** 🔲 Purkinje fibers (PF) are part of the heart's conduction system and are responsible for carrying the impulse from the apex upward across the ventricles. They are located in the subendocardial layer of connective tissue. Purkinje fibers are modified cardiac muscle cells, but are larger and lighter staining—compare their size to the cardiac muscle cells at the bottom of the field. Most are cut in cross section in this preparation. Other visible layers are the endothelium (E), subendothelial connective tissue (SE), and myocardium (M). (×200)

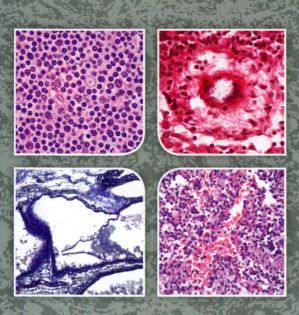

13

Lymphatic System

◼◼ Introduction to the Lymphatic System

A primary role of the lymphatic system (Figure 13-1) is that of immunity, of allowing the body to differentiate between "self" and "nonself." Nonself chemicals or cells are broadly referred to as antigens. (Immunologists define antigens more precisely than that, but this definition will serve our purposes.) The body's response to an antigen is either **humoral**, in which **antibodies** are secreted into tissue fluids (including serum), or **cellular**, in which the defense is provided directly by the immune cells. In either case, the response is specific for each antigen. (Other innate and nonspecific defenses, such as phagocytic cells and the protection from infection by epithelial barriers, are mentioned elsewhere.)

The lymphatic system is also involved in recovery and transport of tissue fluid as well as absorption of fats in the small intestine.

◼◼ Cells of the Immune System

There are several types of immune cells, but they are mostly difficult to differentiate with the light microscope and traditional staining techniques. Identification and differentiation of these cells primarily relies on **immunostaining**, in which the stain binds specifically to biochemicals (called **markers**) unique to each cell type. Differentiation may also be made based on function, which will be addressed superficially, but an exhaustive description of functions is beyond the scope of this book.

Lymphocytes (Figure 13-2) are produced in bone marrow and constitute approximately 20–25% of all leukocytes seen in the blood. They are typically about the size of erythrocytes, but larger lymphocytes are also seen. Lymphocytes are categorized into one of three functional groups: **B cells, T cells,** and **NK cells.** When functional, they are not found in the blood, but rather in lymphoid organs or as aggregations in **extravascular tissues**. It has been estimated that approximately 70% of blood lymphocytes are T cells.

B cells possess an antigenic marker (B-cell marker) in their cytoplasmic membrane that identifies them. They are produced in the bone marrow and also become **immunocompetent** (functional) there. When stimulated, the appropriate B cell multiplies and differentiates into **plasma cells** and **memory B cells**. Plasma cells actively secrete antibodies (humoral immunity), whereas memory cells remain dormant until subsequent contact with the same antigen. Plasma cells are enlarged

Thymus

Spleen

Lymph vessel

Lymph nodes

13-1 Lymphatic System ◼
The lymphatic system is made up of lymph vessels, lymph nodes, and lymphoid organs, such as the tonsils, spleen, and thymus. However, lymphatic tissue is found throughout the body, especially within the walls of organs that open to the external environment.

and ovoid and have nuclear chromatin resembling a clock face. A light region near the nucleus and visible with the light microscope is the site of the Golgi apparatus. Consistent with their function of antibody secretion (which are glycoproteins), the electron microscope also reveals abundant rough endoplasmic reticulum. Memory B cells are indistinguishable from other lymphocytes in routine histological preparations.

T cells are produced in the bone marrow but become immunocompetent in the thymus. They are identified by a T cell antigenic marker (such as CD4 or CD8) and are involved in cell-mediated responses. When stimulated, T cells proliferate and differentiate into one of several functional groups. **Helper T (T_H) cells** (also known as CD4+ cells) assist other T cells or B cells in their immune response. **Cytotoxic T (T_c) cells** (also known as CD8+ cells) are active in killing foreign cells or virally infected cells. **Memory T (T_M) cells** perform the same function as their B cell counterparts. These T cells are indistinguishable from other lymphocytes in routine histological preparations.

Natural killer (NK) cells are large lymphocytes that lack the T and B cell antigenic markers, and as such belong to the population of **null cells**. NK cells kill cells coated with antibodies in a process called **antibody-dependent cell-mediated cytotoxicity**. Thus, their response is to the antibody itself and is not specific to the antigen. They also have the ability to kill tumor and virally infected cells.

Another category of cells involved in the immune response are **antigen-presenting cells (APCs)**, which are involved in processing an antigen and "displaying" it to the appropriate immune cell to begin the immune response. **Macrophages** (Figure 4-7) and **dendritic (Langerhans) cells** (Figure 11-5c), which reside in the skin, are examples.

Organs of the Lymphatic System

Lymphatic tissue is found in encapsulated lymphoid organs such as lymph nodes, the thymus, and the spleen, and also as unencapsulated clusters in the walls of other organs such as those of the digestive and respiratory tracts.

Thymus

The **thymus** (Figure 13-3) is found in the mediastinum, the region of the thoracic cavity between the lungs. It is most highly developed at puberty, and although it remains active, it becomes largely replaced with adipose tissue as the individual ages. A dense connective tissue **capsule** covers the thymus, and connective tissue **trabeculae** or **septa** arising from it divide the organ's two lobes into incompletely separated **lobules**. The outer portion is the **cortex** and the inner part is the **medulla**.

The **thymic cortex** (Figure 13-4) stains darker and more basophilic than the medulla, and is occupied by numerous developing T lymphocytes (**thymocytes**) that have migrated from the bone marrow. They proliferate and, as they mature,

they move toward the medulla. They become immunocompetent at the periphery of the cortex. **Epithelioreticular cells** separate the cortex from blood vessels in the trabeculae and form part of the blood-thymus barrier that prevents antigens from contacting thymocytes prematurely. Other epithelioreticular cells perform other functions. Cortical macrophages remove thymocytes that are not developing properly.

Thymocytes that have passed the preliminary screening for proper development in the cortex migrate to the **thymic medulla** (Figure 13-5). The thymic medulla is eosinophilic and has fewer thymocytes and more abundant epithelioreticular cells than the cortex. **Thymic (Hassall's) corpuscles** are the most distinctive features of the medulla. They are concentrically arranged keratinized epithelioreticular cells, which are thought to produce chemicals (interleukins) necessary for T cell maturation. After further development, a second screening occurs and thymocytes that react with "self" are removed. A final stage of development commits thymocytes to either being cytotoxic T cells (T_C, or CD8+) or helper T cells (T_H, or CD4+). These enter blood or lymphatic vessels and spread throughout the body to populate other lymphatic organs.

Lymph Nodes and Lymph Vessels

Lymphatic vessels (Figure 13-6) return tissue fluid to the blood vascular system. The lymph vasculature begins as blind capillaries consisting of a simple squamous endothelium. The capillaries are tributaries to small lymph vessels, which continue to converge and get larger. Ultimately, lymph vessels empty into the right lymphatic duct and the thoracic duct, which drain lymph into the right and left subclavian veins, respectively. Lymphocytes occasionally may be seen in lymph vessels, but RBCs are not.

In addition to their pattern of convergence, lymph vessels also resemble veins in being thin walled (but thinner) and having valves. The tunics are indistinct in most lymph vessels, but the tunica media of the lymphatic ducts has longitudinal and circular layers of smooth muscle in it.

Lymph nodes (Figure 13-7 and 13-8) are lymph filters located periodically along the length of lymph vessels. B and T cells, as well as macrophages, populate them. Antigens in tissue fluid enter the lymph and are removed by these cells before they can get into the blood.

Lymph nodes are bean shaped and are covered with a dense connective tissue **capsule**. **Afferent lymph vessels** carry lymph to the node and enter along the node's convex surface. The indentation is the **hilus** and is the point of entry and exit for blood vessels as well as the exit of the **efferent lymph vessel** (Figure 13-9).

Internally, the node is divided by extensions of the capsule called **trabeculae** (Figure 13-10) and is supported by reticular connective tissue. Connecting the afferent vessels with the efferent vessel is a series of channels called sinuses, each named according to its location. The **subcapsular sinus** is on the periphery of the node, and the **cortical** and **medullary sinuses** are in the node's cortex and medulla, respectively. As lymph passes through the sinuses, it contacts macrophage pseudopods, which subsequently engulf antigens and other material. This antigen filtration is the first step in one mechanism of initiating an immune response by B cells. Antigens in lymph also can escape the sinuses and contact lymphocytes and dendritic cells directly, which also initiates an immune response.

Lymphocytes densely populate lymph nodes by entering through the artery, **high endothelial venules** (**HEVs**–see below), or the afferent vessels. While in the node, the framework of reticular fibers coursing through it provides them with support. Lymphocyte organization and location are associated with their function. The three regions are the cortex, paracortex (deep cortex or thymus-dependent cortex), and medullary cords.

In the cortex (Figure 13-11), lymphocytes are found in dense, spherical clusters called **lymph follicles** or **lymph nodules**. **Primary follicles** are uniform in appearance and are mostly composed of small, inactive B cells. **Secondary follicles** have a light-staining **germinal center** composed of proliferating B cells (and other cells) surrounded by a darker **mantle zone** populated by inactive B cells. The proliferating B cells develop into memory B cells, which may enter the blood and take up residence in other lymphatic tissues, and plasma cells, which migrate to the medullary cords to their complete development. A lighter **marginal zone** may be seen around the mantle zone.

T lymphocytes dominate the deepest portion of the cortex, called the **paracortex,** and are not organized into follicles. It has been estimated that approximately 60% of the lymphocytes populating a lymph node are T cells. High endothelial venules (HEV), so named because of their unusual cuboidal to columnar epithelial cells, are located in the paracortex.

In the medulla, lymphocytes are organized into elongated **cords** (Figure 13-12). Plasma cells from the cortex secrete antibodies into the lymph (which eventually enters the blood) and die after a few days.

Spleen

The spleen is a lymphoid organ that occupies the left upper quadrant of the abdominal cavity. It is responsible for immune responses to blood antigens as well as phagocytosis of worn out RBCs and other particulate matter. As such, it is a filter of blood.

The **capsule** (Figure 13-13) is composed of fibrous connective tissue and smooth muscle. Connective tissue **trabeculae** penetrate the spleen from the capsule, and reticular fibers form a framework in which the lymphocytes are suspended. Branches of the splenic artery and tributaries of the splenic veins may be found in trabeculae.

Spleen tissue is divided into regions referred to as **red pulp**, which comprises the majority of the spleen, and **white pulp**. Red pulp (Figure 13-14) is the blood vascular component and includes venous **sinuses** and the intervening **splenic cords** composed of macrophages, lymphocytes, plasma cells, RBCs, and other blood cells. The sinus walls are made up of elongated endothelial cells that are encircled by reticular fibers. Gaps up to 3 μm between endothelial cells are common and allow only flexible RBCs to pass into the sinus. Older, inflexible RBCs are removed by macrophages. Concurrently, hemoglobin is degraded and its iron is recycled. Another function of red pulp is acting as a reservoir of RBCs. **Myofibroblasts** in the trabeculae and capsule can contract and squeeze more RBCs into circulation, if needed.

White pulp (Figure 13-15) performs immunological functions and is composed of lymphocyte aggregates. T cells form **periarterial lymphatic sheaths** (**PALS**) around branches of the splenic artery called **central arteries. Splenic nodules,** with B cells in germinal centers and mantle zones, form as expansions of PALS and have an eccentric central artery. (They resemble lymphatic follicles, but can be differentiated from them by the central artery.) A lighter marginal zone of active macrophages is found at the periphery of splenic nodules and is the primary site of contact with blood antigens.

Other Unencapsulated Lymphatic Tissue

Lymphatic tissue is found scattered in various organs. In some cases, the lymphocytes are just dispersed in other connective tissues. In other cases they are organized into lymph follicles supported by a reticular framework.

Lymphocytes associated with mucous membranes are referred to as **mucosa associated lymphatic tissue** (**MALT**). Scattered lymphocytes are frequently seen in the lamina propria and epithelium of various organs. T cells are the primary occupants of this diffuse lymphatic tissue, but some B cells are also present (Figure 13-16). In other regions, the MALT is more organized, as described below.

Tonsils are probably the most well-known examples of MALT. They are small aggregations of unencapsulated lymphatic tissue located in the oropharynx and nasopharynx. They are drained by efferent lymph vessels, but lack afferent vessels. The two **palatine tonsils** (Figure 13-17) are located at the junction of the oral cavity and the oropharynx. They consist of lymph follicles, most with germinal centers. The stratified squamous epithelium of the oral mucosa covers them and penetrates downward as **tonsillar crypts.** Dendritic cells in the epithelium act as APCs. Connective tissue **trabeculae** are present and there is a deep connective tissue capsule, but the tonsils are not surrounded by it. The **pharyngeal tonsil** (Figure 13-18) is located in the nasopharynx. It is covered with PSCC and some stratified squamous epithelium. There are no crypts, but the mucosa is folded into epithelial invaginations. Like the palatine tonsils, it has a partial capsule. The **lingual tonsils** (Figure 13-19) are at the base of the dorsum of the tongue. They are covered with stratified squamous epithelium. Each has a single crypt and lacks even a partial capsule.

Gut associated lymphatic tissue (GALT) is composed of lymph follicles in the walls of digestive organs (Figure 13-20). They are most abundant in the **Peyer's patches** of the ileum (see page 174). GALT is drained by efferent lymph vessels, but has no afferent vessels. Instead, special epithelial cells called **M cells** overlie the follicles and transfer antigens to dendritic cells occupying pockets in their basal region. Dendritic cells in turn present antigens to T and B cells.

GALT is also abundant in the colon and the **vermiform appendix**, a tubular extension of the cecum.

Bronchus associated lymphatic tissue (BALT) is common at the branch points of the respiratory tree, where M cells replace the respiratory epithelium (Figure 13-21). B cells are the most abundant cells, but APCs and T cells are also present.

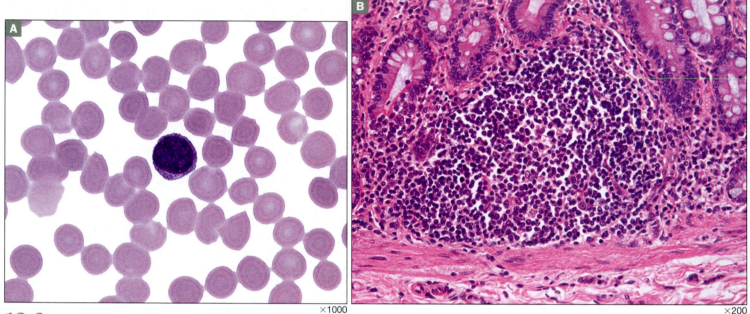

×1000   ×200

13-2 **Lymphocytes** ■ (A) Lymphocytes are the second most abundant leukocyte in blood. They are about the size of an RBC, or slightly larger, and their nucleus fills most of the cell, leaving only a thin ring of cytoplasm at the periphery. This accounts for the aggregations of lymphocytes you will see in subsequent micrographs in this and other chapters staining as dark spots. While they can't be differentiated with traditional staining methods, immunostaining has shown that approximately 70% of blood lymphocytes are T cells. (×1000) (B) Lymphocytes are found in blood, but they are usually functional outside the bloodstream. Shown here is a spherical aggregation of lymphocytes in the wall of the digestive tract. Most of the tiny purple spots are lymphocyte nuclei. (×200)

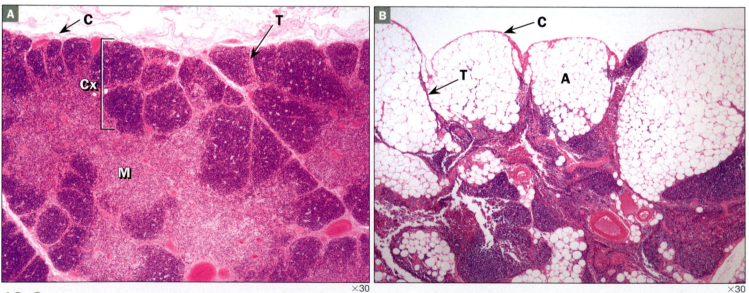

×30   ×30

13-3 **Thymus** ■ (A) The thymus is covered with a connective tissue capsule (C). Trabeculae (T) are projections of the capsule into the thymus that incompletely divide it into lobules. (Those lobules that appear to be completely surrounded by connective tissue have been cut in cross section.) The cortex (Cx) and medulla (M) are clearly seen. (×30) (B) After puberty, the thymus begins degenerating (a process called "involution") and the lymphatic tissue is largely replaced by adipose tissue (A). In this specimen, lobules are still evident because of the trabeculae. What lymphatic tissue remains continues to be active throughout a person's life. (×30)

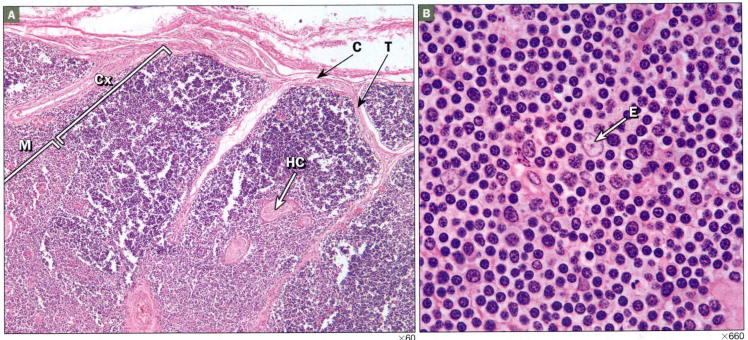

×60

×660

13-4 **Thymic Cortex** ■ The outer region of the thymus is called the cortex. (**A**) In this micrograph, the capsule (C) and trabeculae (T) are visible. The more basophilic cortex (Cx) stands out against the more eosinophilic medulla (M). Also visible in this preparation are medullary Hassall's corpuscles (HC). (×60) (**B**) Most of the cortical cells are thymocytes (developing T lymphocytes). Other cells of the cortex are macrophages and epithelioreticular cells (E—these are frequently difficult to see in normal preparations because of the numerous thymocytes). (×660)

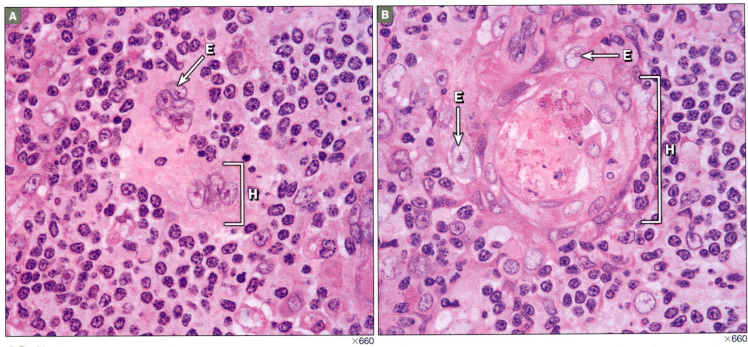

×660

×660

13-5 **Thymic Medulla** ■ The medulla is where T cell precursors differentiate and mature into functional T cells. Rounded and light-staining epithelioreticular cells (E) are more visible in the medulla than in the cortex. Keratinized clumps of epithelioreticular cells form Hassall's corpuscles (H), a distinctive feature of the thymus. (**A**) Epithelioreticular cells and an early Hassall's corpuscle are seen in this micrograph. (×660) (**B**) A more advanced Hassall's corpuscle is shown in this micrograph. Other epithelioreticular cells are also visible. (×660)

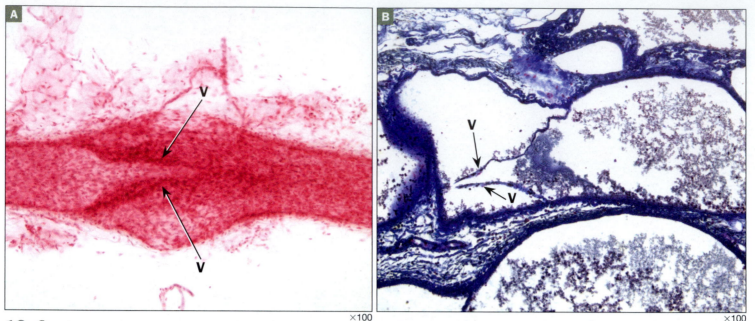

13-6 **Lymph Vessels** 🔲 Like veins, lymph vessels have valves, but they have thinner walls. (**A**) In this whole mount, the valve (V) and thin wall are apparent. Lymph would flow left to right. If it flowed from right to left, the pockets of the valve would fill and close the lumen. (×100) (**B**) This is an oblique section through a lymph vessel with valves. Lymph would flow right to left in this specimen. (×100)

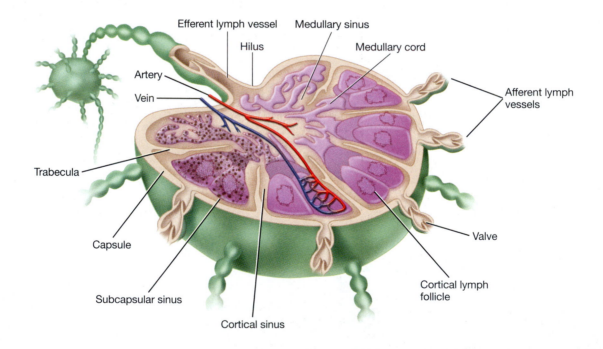

Efferent lymph vessel   Medullary sinus

Hilus   Medullary cord

Artery

Vein   Afferent lymph vessels

Trabecula

Capsule   Valve

Subcapsular sinus   Cortical lymph follicle

Cortical sinus

13-7 **General Structure of a Lymph Node** 🔲 Lymph nodes are located periodically along lymph vessels and are a primary means of lymphocytes contacting antigens and responding to them. Notice the orientation of valves in the afferent and efferent lymph vessels that ensures lymph flow in the correct direction.

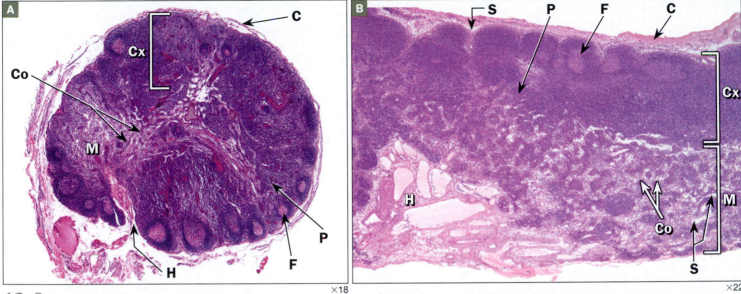

13-8 Lymph Node ◼ Each lymph node is covered by a connective tissue capsule (C). Lymphatic tissue comprising the cortex (Cx) is arranged in spherical follicles (F) or in irregular masses in the paracortex (P), whereas it is organized into cords (Co) in the medulla (M). Sinuses (S) run between masses of lymphatic tissue. Blood vessels and efferent lymph vessels connect at the hilus (H). Both micrographs are panoramic views of lymph nodes. (**A**) (×18) (**B**) (×22)

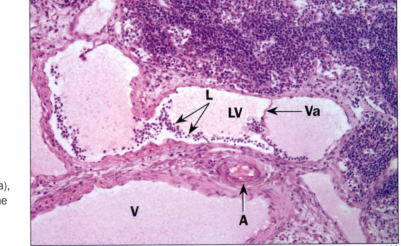

13-9 Efferent Lymph Vessels ◼ In this micrograph, an efferent lymph vessel (LV) emerging from the hilus is visible. Note the valve (Va), the lymphocytes (L), and the absence of RBCs in the lymph vessel. The hilus is also the point of entry and exit for blood vessels serving the node. In this section, an arteriole (A) and vein (V) are visible. (×120)

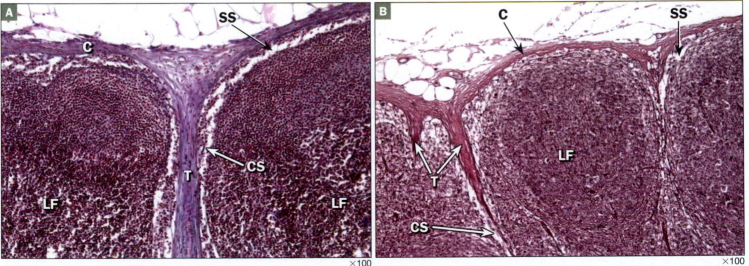

13-10 Lymph Node Trabeculae and Sinuses ◼ (**A** and **B**) The interior of the lymph node is penetrated by connective tissue trabeculae (T) arising from the capsule (C). The subcapsular sinus (SS) and cortical sinuses (CS) are visible in places, but are obscured in others by lymphocytes from the lymph follicles (LF). Reticular fibers (thin, black lines) are stained in (**B**). (Both **A** and **B** are ×100)

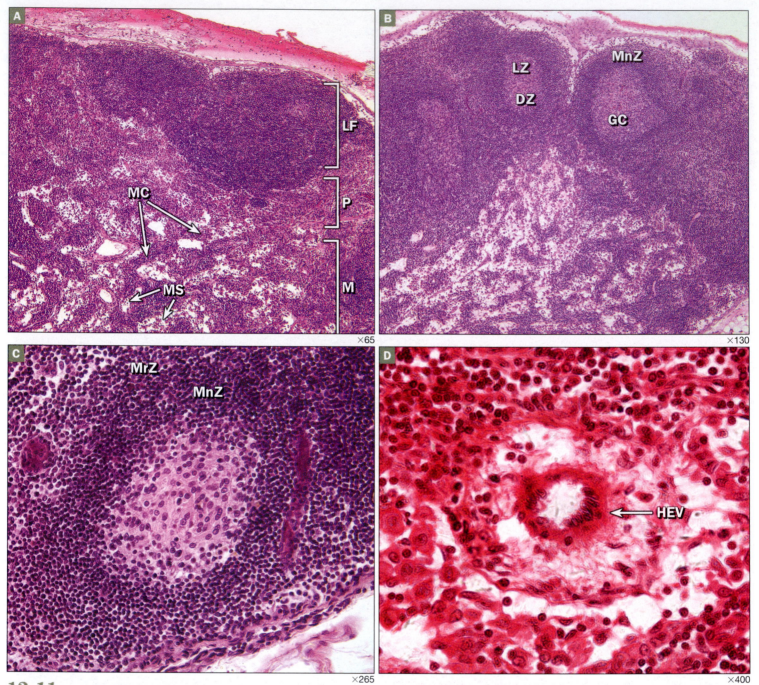

13-11 **Lymph Node Cortex and Paracortex** (**A**) The cortex of a lymph node is composed of spherical aggregations of B lymphocytes called lymph follicles (LF). Deep to the follicles is the paracortex (P), occupied mainly by T cells. The medulla (M), medullary cords (MC), and medullary sinuses (MS) are also visible in this micrograph. (×65) (**B**) Shown in this field are secondary follicles demonstrating the lighter germinal center (GC) and darker mantle zone (MnZ). Notice that the mantle zone is thicker on the side of the capsule and that the germinal center has a dark zone (DZ) toward the medulla and is lighter (LZ) toward the capsule. Secondary follicles have multiplying B cells in the germinal center. (×130) (**C**) This is a secondary follicle. In addition to the germinal center and mantle zone, the lighter marginal zone (MrZ) is visible. (×265) (**D**) High endothelial veins (HEV) return lymphocytes to lymphatic tissue as well as absorbing up to 30% of the lymph in a node into the blood. They are unusual in their cuboidal to columnar endothelial lining. (×400)

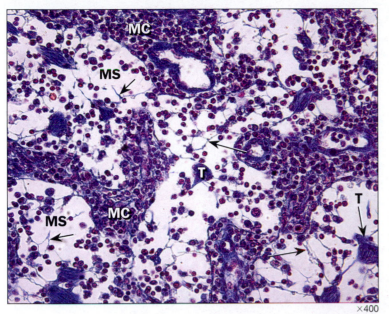

×400

13-12 **Lymph Node Medulla** ◼ The lymphocytes of the medulla (mostly plasma cells) are arranged into cords (MC) and are separated by medullary sinuses (MS). Plasma cells secrete antibodies into the lymph, which carries them to the blood vascular system to be distributed throughout the body. The reticular connective tissue framework is visible (arrows), as are trabeculae (T). (×400)

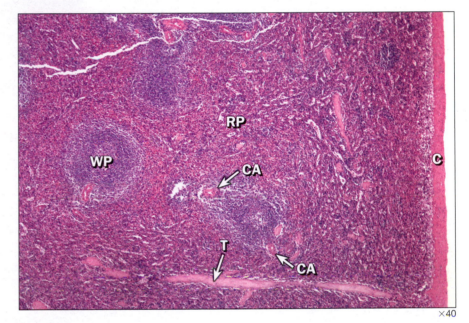

×40

13-13 **Spleen** ◼ This panoramic view of the spleen shows the connective tissue capsule (C) and trabeculae (T). Red pulp (RP), made up of blood sinuses, and white pulp (WP), made up of lymphocytes, are also visible. Central arteries (CA) that may not be "central" are visible in the white pulp. (×40)

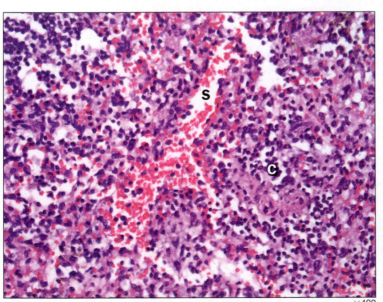

×400

13-14 **Splenic Red Pulp** ◼ The portion of splenic parenchyma composed of blood sinuses (S), cords (C) of lymphocytes, and macrophages is called red pulp because of its appearance in fresh specimens. Blood in central arteries is carried to open capillaries surrounded by macrophages and enters splenic cords, where it is screened by macrophages prior to entering the sinuses. In doing so, RBCs must pass through slits in the basement membrane of the sinuses, a task likely to break old, brittle RBCs. This contact with macrophages and difficult passage into the sinuses is the mechanism for removing antigens and RBCs from circulation. (×400)

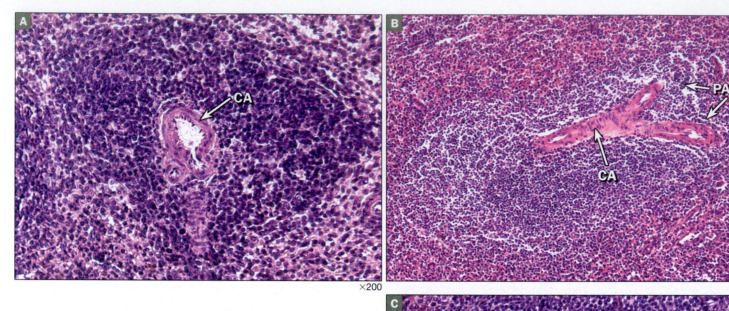

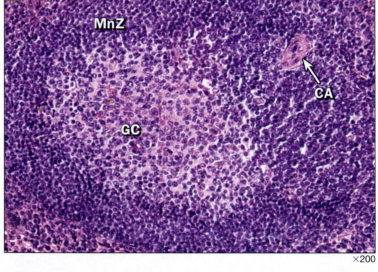

13-15 **Splenic White Pulp** 🔳 White pulp is found in two forms: periarterial lymphatic sheaths (PALS), and splenic nodules. **(A)** Shown is a single PALS, which is made up of T cells surrounding a central artery (CA). (×200) **(B)** In this specimen, the central artery has been cut obliquely and shows two branches, each of which is surrounded by PALS. (×100) **(C)** Upon exposure to antigen, PALS may form expanded regions of B cells called splenic nodules, which frequently have a germinal center (GC) and mantle zone (MnZ). Their expansion pushes the "central artery" to an eccentric position, as seen in this splenic nodule. (×200)

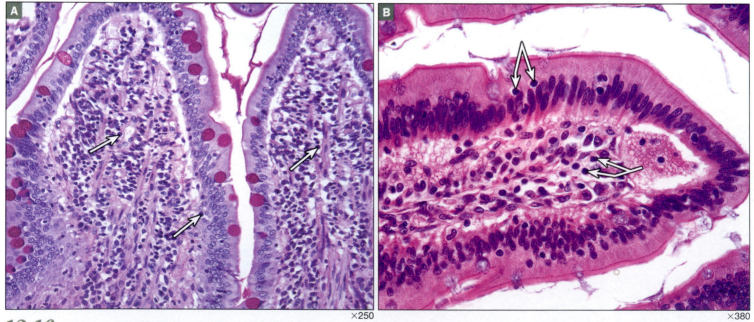

13-16 **Diffuse Lymphatic Tissue** 🔳 Lymphocytes (arrows) are often found scattered in the connective tissue layer of a mucous membrane. They are characterized by small, dark-staining nuclei. **(A)** The majority of cells occupying the lamina propria of this small intestine preparation are lymphocytes. (×250) **(B)** This is another small intestine specimen. Lymphocytes are present in the connective tissue, but are also seen in the epithelium. (×380)

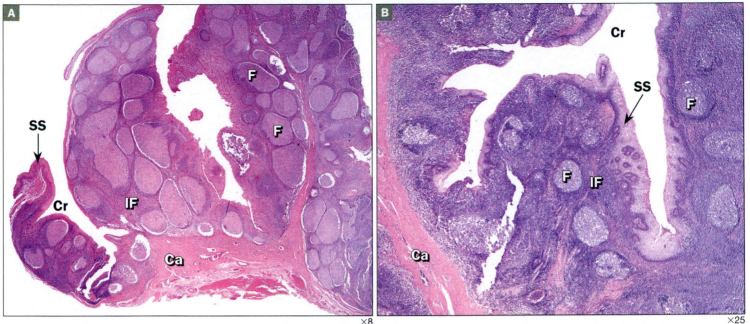

13-17 Palatine Tonsils ■ The palatine tonsils are covered by stratified squamous epithelium (SS) that projects down into tonsillar crypts (Cr). The bulk of the tonsil is composed of follicles with germinal centers (F), with interfollicular (IF) regions composed of T cells making up the remainder. A fibrous capsule (Ca) marks the lower margin of the tonsil. (**A**) ×8 (**B**) ×25.

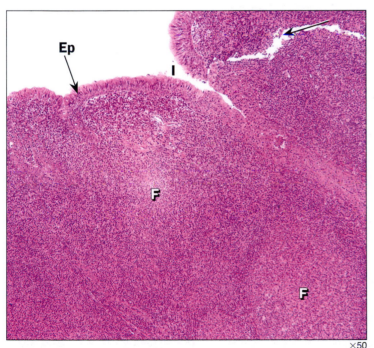

13-18 Pharyngeal Tonsil ■ The pharyngeal tonsil is similar in construction to the palatine tonsils, but has a thinner capsule, is covered with PSCC (Ep), and has shallower invaginations (I) than the crypts. Lymph follicles (F) are abundant. The white region indicated by the arrow is an artifact of preparation. (×50)

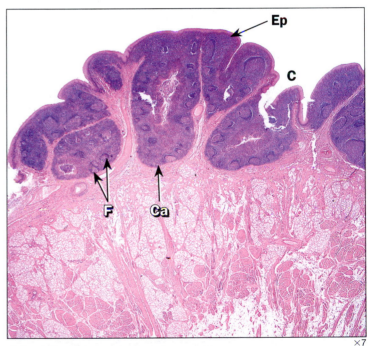

13-19 Lingual Tonsil ■ Each lingual tonsil has a single crypt (C), a thin capsule at its base (Ca), and is covered with stratified squamous epithelium (Ep). Follicles (F), some with germinal centers, are also present. (×7)

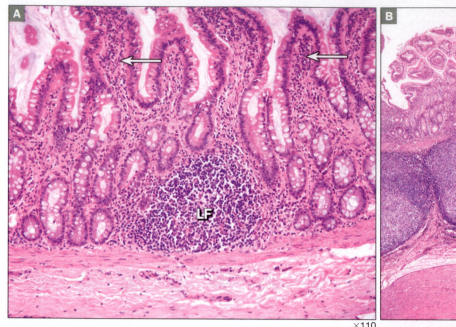

×110

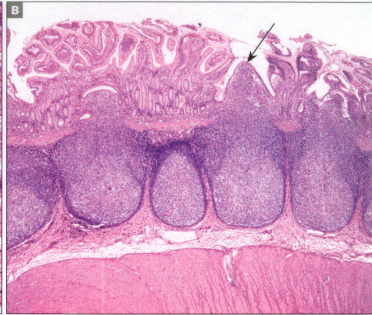

×25

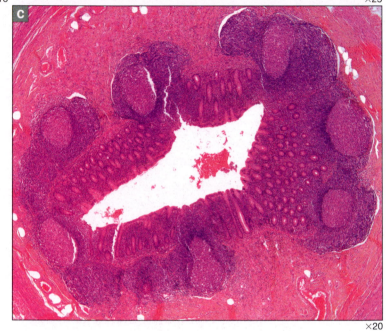

×20

13-20 **Gut Associated Lymphatic Tissue (GALT)** 🟥 Lymph follicles (LF) are present in the mucosa of many digestive organs. (**A**) Here is a single follicle in the small intestine's mucosa. Diffuse lymphatic tissue is also present (arrows). (×110) (**B**) Aggregates of lymph follicles in the ileum are known as Peyer's patches. They are found in the submucosa. The mucosa overlying them lacks villi (arrow), but the epithelium contains M cells that capture and transfer antigens to nearby dendritic cells for presentation to B and T cells. Also see Figure 14-29 (×25) (**C**) The vermiform appendix is found on the cecum of the large intestine. It has abundant lymphatic tissue in it, as this cross section illustrates. (×20)

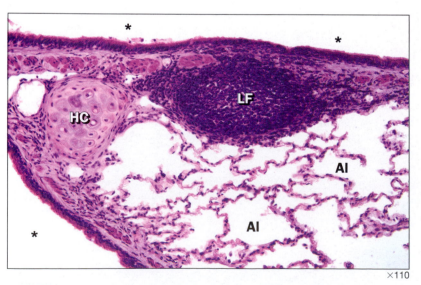

×110

13-21 **Bronchus Associated Lymphatic Tissue (BALT)** 🟥 Lymph follicles (LF) are also found associated with the respiratory tree, especially at branch points. Regions marked with asterisks (*) are the lumen of the bronchus. Also visible is a piece of hyaline cartilage (HC) and numerous alveoli (AI) of the lung. (×110)

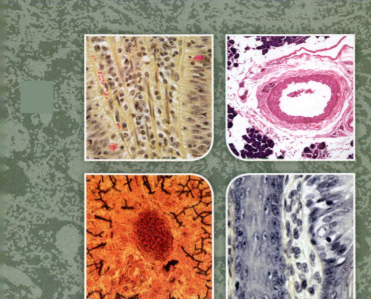

14

Digestive System

Introduction to the Digestive System

The digestive system (Figure 14-1) is involved in the ingestion, mechanical and chemical digestion, and absorption of food. It consists of the organs of the oral cavity (teeth and tongue), digestive tube (esophagus, stomach, small intestine, and large intestine) and accessory glands (salivary glands, liver, gallbladder, and pancreas).

Organs of the Oral Cavity

Mouth and Oral Cavity

The oral **mucosa** (mucous membrane) is composed of a stratified squamous epithelium with an underlying loose connective tissue layer called **lamina propria.** In many ways it resembles

Oral cavity
Pharynx
Esophagus
Liver
Gallbladder
Stomach
Small intestine
Large intestine

14-1 Digestive System ◼ The digestive organs are many and varied, ranging from those of the digestive tube (esophagus, stomach, small intestine, and large intestine), to accessory glands (salivary glands, pancreas, liver, and gallbladder), to those of the oral cavity (teeth and tongue), most of which are used in breaking down food to a size and form that can be absorbed into the blood by the small intestine for use by all body cells.

the cutaneous membrane (skin), with the lamina propria being equivalent in position and function to the skin's papillary layer. In some parts of the oral cavity there is a deeper and denser connective tissue layer (variously called **reticular layer** or **submucosa**). These connective tissue layers contain blood vessels, nerves, sensory receptors, and lymphatics—including lymph vessels, lymphatic nodules, and the palatine and lingual tonsils. There are three different types of oral mucosa: lining mucosa, masticatory mucosa, and specialized mucosa.

Most of the oral cavity (cheeks, soft palate, lips, floor of the mouth, alveolar surfaces, and inferior surface of the tongue) is covered with a **lining mucosa** composed of nonkeratinized stratified squamous epithelium and a lamina propria. Connective tissue papillae (comparable to dermal papillae, see Chapter 11, page 132) project into the base of the epithelium. With the exception of the inferior surface of the tongue, a denser connective tissue **submucosa** underlies the lamina propria. Small accessory salivary glands may be found in the submucosa. Skeletal muscles, such as the orbicularis oris surrounding the mouth, the buccinator in the cheeks, and muscles of the tongue and soft palate are deep to the submucosa. Figure 14-2 shows the mucosa of the lip.

Masticatory mucosa is found in regions where abrasion due to chewing is most severe, such as the **gingivae** (gums) and hard palate (Figure 14-3). The epithelium is keratinized (but sometimes the cells retain their nuclei and are referred to as **parakeratinized**) and the papillae are deeper and more abundant than in lining mucosa to resist the shearing forces associated with chewing. The lamina propria fibers, depending on location, may intertwine directly with the periosteum of the mandible or maxillae to provide firm anchorage.

The **specialized mucosa** of the tongue's dorsal surface will be discussed below.

Chemical digestion of starch begins in the oral cavity, but the main function is the mechanical digestion of food as it is broken up by the teeth and mixed with saliva to form a bolus.

Salivary Glands

Salivary glands (Figure 14-4) produce a secretion called **saliva**. Saliva is about 99% water, with mucin (mucus), the enzymes α-amylase and lysozyme, antibodies, and electrolytes comprising most of the remaining 1%. Lysozyme and antibodies are involved in microbial control; whereas α-amylase begins carbohydrate digestion. The high water content and mucin moisten food (and the oral mucosa), which aid taste bud stimulation and facilitate swallowing.

The secretory cells are arranged into acini of two types: **serous acini** and **mucous acini**. Serous acini produce a watery secretion containing enzymes and antibodies. They are typically basophilic and have a granular cytoplasm as a result of numerous protein-containing secretory vesicles. The cells of mucous acini generally appear pale with a smooth cytoplasm as a result of the mucinogen granules (mucin precursors) being extracted during specimen preparation. Nuclei are generally pushed toward the basement membrane. Their secretion is viscous due to the mucin in it. Occasionally, serous and mucous acini are found together, with the serous cells forming a cap over the mucous cells, a structure referred to as a **serous demilune**. Electron micrograph evidence shows that these are artifacts of traditional specimen fixation and that the serous and mucous cells are actually adjacent to one another.

Acini empty into ducts made of secretory cells called **intercalated ducts**, which lead to larger, **striated ducts**. Intercalated ducts are lined with a simple cuboidal epithelium with no particular identifying features other than their position between acini and striated ducts. They are longer in serous and mixed glands, and their cells modify the composition of the gland's saliva by secreting bicarbonate and absorbing chloride ions. They are comparatively short and difficult to identify in mucous glands.

Striated ducts are distinctive features of salivary glands. They are so named because radial striations (relative to the *duct* viewed in cross section) are visible in their simple columnar epithelial cells when viewed in routine preparations with the light microscope. Striations are the product of numerous infoldings of the basal plasma membrane that increase the surface area for membrane-bound ion pumps, which modify saliva by removing sodium ions and secreting bicarbonate and potassium ions. As a consequence of the folded membrane, nuclei tend to be located in the middle of the cell.

The main antibody of saliva is **secretory immunoglobin A (sIgA)**. It is produced by plasma cells (Chapter 13) occupying the connective tissue between acini. These antibodies bind to receptors in the basal membranes of acinar cells, which endocytose them and subsequently release them into the saliva via their apical membranes.

Each acinus is associated with a flattened, contractile **myoepithelial cell** with processes that wrap around the acinus. Upon contraction, myoepithelial cells assist in moving the secretion into the duct.

There are three main salivary glands. The largest are the **parotid glands** (Figure 14-5), located anterior to each ear; their ducts empty into the oral cavity near the second maxillary molar. A connective tissue **capsule** sends **septa** into the gland and divides it into **lobules**. Acini are the serous type and striated ducts are easily seen. Adipocytes become more abundant with age.

The **sublingual glands** (Figure 14-6) are located in the floor of the oral cavity. They are composed primarily of mucous acini, some with serous demilunes. Sublingual glands are small and their ducts are short, making them difficult to see. Adipocytes may be present, especially in adults, because they increase in number with age.

The **submandibular glands** (Figure 14-7) contain both serous and mucous acini, some with serous demilunes. The relatively long-striated ducts make them abundant in sectioned specimens.

Teeth

Humans typically have 20 **deciduous teeth** that are replaced by 32 **permanent teeth**. There are 16 permanent teeth in each adult dental arch and the pattern in the mandibular and maxillary arches is the same, with two incisors, one canine, two premolars, and three molars on each side (Figure 14-8), producing the dental formula 2.1.2.3. The deciduous dental formula is 2.1.0.2 with no premolars.

Each tooth (Figure 14-9) consists of a **crown**, which projects above the **gingivae**, or gums. The crown is covered with **enamel**, the hardest material in the body (95% calcium salts and 5% organic substances). Below the gumline, one or more **roots** project into **alveoli** (sockets) in the bone. The roots are covered with **cementum**, a bone-like material that lacks the Haversian systems and blood vessels of bone. The fibrous **periodontal ligament** (periodontal membrane) connects the cementum with the alveolar bone and acts as its periosteum. The **neck** of the tooth is a constriction at the junction of the crown and roots. Internally, the tooth consists of bone-like **dentin** (70% calcium salts) and a **pulp cavity** filled with vascular loose connective tissue containing nerves called **dental pulp**. The gingiva is a mucous membrane that covers the bone tissue of the maxilla and mandible up to the tooth's enamel. It has a keratinized stratified squamous epithelium.

Deciduous teeth develop from an invagination of thickened embryonic oral epithelium called the **dental lamina** in each jaw (Figure 14-10). The dental lamina dilates and forms an **enamel organ** for each tooth, then eventually degenerates. Deep to the enamel organ, mesenchyme begins to form the **dental papilla**. Concurrently, the enamel organ becomes cap-shaped as it grows around the papilla. It now comprises continuous layers of epithelium: the **inner** and **outer enamel epithelium**. Tall, columnar, enamel-producing **ameloblasts** begin to develop from the inner enamel epithelium, and dentin-producing **odontoblasts** form between the ameloblasts and the dental papilla. Further growth of the enamel organ results in a bell-shaped structure that determines the form of the particular tooth's crown. Connective tissue around the enamel organ differentiates into the **dental follicle,** the precursor of the periodontal ligament. It also forms the cementum of the root.

Odontoblasts secrete dentin between the odontoblast and ameloblast layers. As they do so, they migrate inward. A long, thin, cytoplasmic process of each odontoblast remains in the dentin as the odontoblastic process, visible in light micrographs as a **dentinal tubule.** Subsequently, ameloblasts deposit enamel next to the dentin. Thus, the odontoblast and ameloblast layers become separated by the dentin and enamel each has secreted. At about the time a tooth erupts through the gingival surface, ameloblasts die and no new enamel can be formed.

Tongue

The tongue (Figure 14-11a) is a muscular (skeletal) organ covered with mucous membrane consisting of a stratified squamous epithelium and lamina propria. It possesses general sensory receptors as well as chemoreceptors for taste called **taste buds.** In addition, it is responsible for mixing chewed food with saliva to form a bolus, and then assisting in swallowing. It is also involved in speech.

The bulk of the tongue is skeletal muscle arranged in horizontal, transverse, and longitudinal bands. These are responsible for producing the complex movements of the tongue. Filling in between the muscle and epithelial layers is a loose connective tissue lamina propria with occasional mucous and serous salivary glands.

The dorsal surface of the tongue is covered by **papillae** of four types. **Filiform papillae** (Figure 14-11b) are the most numerous and are conical in appearance. Their epithelium is keratinized and gives the tongue a whitish-gray coloration. Lacking taste buds, their primary function is to furnish a rough surface that assists in mixing food during mechanical digestion. **Fungiform papillae** (Figure 14-11c) are globular (mushroom shaped) with a nonkeratinized or slightly keratinized stratified squamous epithelium and vascular connective tissue within, which makes them appear reddish. They are most numerous at the tip of the tongue, but a few are scattered over its entire dorsal surface. Roughly a dozen **circumvallate (vallate) papillae** (Figure 14-11d) are located in a row in the region known as the **sulcus terminalis,** about two-thirds of the way back on the tongue. Each is surrounded by a **cleft** into which serous **von Ebner's glands** drain. Most taste buds are located in the mucosa of these papillae.

The epithelium of **foliate papillae** contains taste buds. The papillae are located along the lateral edges of the tongue, with their clefts running perpendicular to its long axis. They are more easily seen in children.

Taste buds (Figures 9-3 and 14-11) are light-staining, oval objects found in the epithelium of the oral cavity and all but filiform papillae of the tongue. At the surface is the **taste pore.**

Three cell types comprise a taste bud: **gustatory (taste, neuroepithelial) cells, support cells,** and **basal cells.** The first two are long and slender with microvilli that emerge from the taste pore at the taste bud's surface. Microvilli of gustatory cells receive chemical stimuli and are innervated by sensory neurons of facial (CN VII), glossopharyngeal (CN IX), or vagus (CN X) nerves. Basal cells are small stem cells that produce the other two types. For more information about the function of taste buds, see Chapter 9, page 108.

▪▪ Organs of the Digestive Tube

The digestive tube consists of the esophagus, stomach, small intestine, and large intestine. The wall is divided into four main layers that are modified from one organ to another, reflecting differences in function (Figure 14-12). From the lumen outward, these layers are the **mucosa, submucosa, muscularis externa,** and **serosa** or **adventitia.**

The mucosa is composed of either a stratified squamous epithelium or a simple columnar epithelium. Deep to it is a vascular loose connective tissue layer called the lamina propria. In addition to blood vessels, it contains nerves, macrophages, lymphocytes, and plasma cells, the latter of which produce antibodies (mostly sIgA) that are secreted into the lumen via the epithelial cells. In some organs, exocrine glands are also present. Together, the epithelium and lamina propria form the mucous membrane of the gut. Finally, one or two thin layers of smooth muscle (skeletal muscle in the proximal esophagus) form the **muscularis mucosae.**

Deep to the mucosa is the **submucosa,** a loose connective tissue that houses blood vessels, nerves, and lymphatics, as well as glands derived from the surface epithelium in some organs.

The **muscularis externa** is composed of smooth muscle in most organs, but skeletal muscle is seen in the proximal esophagus and anal canal. It is composed of an **inner circular layer** and an **outer longitudinal layer,** the coordinated contraction of which results in the propulsive movement called **peristalsis.** The stomach has an additional innermost oblique layer between the submucosa and circular muscle layer.

If the organ is in the peritoneal cavity, the outer surface is covered with a serous membrane called **visceral peritoneum,** and this constitutes the **serosa.** It is composed of a simple squamous mesothelium and a deeper fibrous connective tissue. In most parts of the gut, the serosal layer joins itself on one side of the organ and forms the double-layered **mesentery** that suspends the organ and carries blood vessels, nerves, and lymphatics to and from it. If the organ is outside the peritoneal cavity, it is covered with a fibrous **adventitia** that blends in with surrounding connective tissues.

Also present in the wall throughout the length of the digestive tube are components of the **enteric nervous system (ENS)** composed of sensory neurons, interneurons, motor neurons, and support cells. This extensive (and underappreciated) system is composed of neurons that equal or exceed the total number of neurons in the spinal cord! The ENS can work independently, but is also under control of the sympathetic and parasympathetic nervous systems to regulate gut motility, blood flow, and glandular secretion. As a rule, parasympathetic stimulation activates digestive activity, whereas sympathetic stimulation inhibits it. Although their fibers can be found throughout the wall, the ENS cell bodies are organized into ganglia named for their locations: the **submucosal plexus (of Meissner)** in the submucosa and the **myenteric plexus (of Auerbach)** between the longitudinal and circular layers of the muscularis externa (Figures 8-30 and 14-13). These are aggregations of parasympathetic postganglionic neuron cell bodies that supply the glands (submucosal plexus) and muscle (myenteric plexus).

Esophagus

The **esophagus** (Figure 14-14) is a muscular tube found in the mediastinum of the thoracic cavity leading from the laryngopharynx to the stomach. Peristaltic waves convey the bolus of food to the stomach. A physiological sphincter normally prevents food from being regurgitated from the stomach into the esophagus.

The relaxed esophageal mucosa is highly folded, but it flattens as the esophagus distends to accommodate a swallowed bolus. The epithelium is a nonkeratinized stratified squamous, and the lamina propria is thin. Near the distal end of the esophagus, mucus-secreting **esophageal-cardiac glands** occupy the lamina propria. The muscularis mucosae is thicker in the esophagus than in any other organ of the digestive tube.

The submucosa is composed of an elastic connective tissue (to accommodate swallowing) and contains compound tubular mucous **esophageal glands**.

Because swallowing is a voluntary action, the proximal one-third of the esophagus contains skeletal muscle in the muscularis externa and muscularis mucosae. By the distal one-third of the esophagus, the muscle layers are made exclusively of smooth muscle. The muscularis externa is thick and has well-defined layers.

All but the distal centimeter of the esophagus is located in the mediastinum and as such is covered by a fibrous adventitia. The terminal part of the esophagus, which has passed through the diaphragm to join the stomach, is covered with a serosa.

Stomach

The stomach (Figure 14-15) is divided into four regions. The esophagus enters at the **cardia**. Superior to the cardia is the **fundus**, and inferior to it is the main portion called the **body**, or **corpus**. The terminal portion that joins the small intestine is the **pyloris**.

Chemical digestion of carbohydrates, begun in the oral cavity, continues in the stomach. In addition, **gastric glands** produce **gastric juice,** which contains enzymes for protein and lipid digestion. Mechanical digestion continues as muscular contractions mix the stomach's contents to form semiliquid **chyme**.

An empty stomach has a larger diameter than the esophagus, but as it fills with food, it expands further. To accommodate this stretching imposed on the wall, the gastric mucosa is folded into **rugae** (Figures 14-15 and 14-16) that flatten as the stomach fills.

The mucosa changes abruptly as the esophagus joins the cardia (Figure 14-17). At the **esophageal-cardiac junction**, the stratified squamous becomes a simple columnar epithelium. The lamina propria becomes occupied by gastric (cardiac) glands (see below). All other layers are continuous across the junction.

The simple columnar epithelium is composed of tall, **surface mucous cells** with basal nuclei. They secrete viscous, insoluble, alkaline mucus that coats the mucosa and protects it from the enzymes and acid of gastric juice. Depressions into the mucosa called **gastric pits** (Figure 14-18) are also lined with surface epithelium. Pits are deepest in the pyloris, where they penetrate approximately halfway into the mucosa. Pits are shallowest in the fundus and body, with pits of intermediate depth in the cardia (Figure 14-19).

Leading from each gastric pit and extending through the lamina propria downward to the muscularis mucosae are branched, tubular **gastric glands** (Figures 14-18 and 14-19). In the cardia and pyloris, the glands (referred to as cardiac and pyloric glands, respectively) are coiled and secrete mucus. Glands of the fundus and body are the most abundant and are long, straight, and branched, but not abundantly so; a single bifurcation is common. Each gland is divided into three regions: the **isthmus**, a short segment that opens into the gastric pit; the **neck**; and the **body**, which is branched. Five cell types are identifiable in these glands with the light microscope and appropriate staining. These are: mucous neck cells, parietal cells, chief cells, stem cells, and enteroendocrine cells.

- **Mucous neck cells** are found in the gland's neck region and are cuboidal to irregular in shape with a spherical nucleus. Their water-soluble mucus is released only when the stomach is active.

- **Parietal cells** are large, eosinophilic cells that appear reddish with H&E stains. They secrete hydrochloric acid and intrinsic factor (necessary for absorption of vitamin B12). They are most abundant in the upper neck region, but may be found throughout the gland.

- **Chief (zymogenic) cells** are distributed throughout the gland, but are most abundant near the base. These cells are basophilic and their granular cytoplasm appears purplish with H&E stains. They secrete the precursor to the enzyme **pepsin** and a **lipase**.

- **Stem cells** are undifferentiated, low, columnar cells found in the isthmus and neck of gastric glands. After division, their daughter cells differentiate and migrate to the surface to replace worn out mucous cells, or migrate downward to replace secretory cells. They are not easily identified, but if you see a mitotic figure, it is likely in a stem cell.

- **Enteroendocrine cells** are small cells found throughout the gastrointestinal tract. They are pale staining with H&E and frequently don't reach the luminal surface. Their hormones, which typically have an effect on some aspect of digestion, are secreted into blood vessels of the lamina propria. For example, **gastrin** from **G cells** in the stomach stimulates gastric acid secretion. Immunochemical stains have replaced more traditional metallic stains (e.g., silver and chromium) and allow identification of specific hormones in enteroendocrine cells.

The stomach's submucosa is not remarkable, but the muscularis externa has an additional innermost oblique layer (Figure 14-20). At the pyloric-duodenal junction, the circular layer thickens to form the **pyloric sphincter** (Figure 14-21). The outer surface is covered with a serosa.

Small Intestine

The **small intestine** (Figure 14-22) is approximately 3 meters in length. It begins at the duodenum (25 cm long), which is retroperitoneal,[1] continues as the jejunum (1 m long), and ends with the ileum (2 m long). Each segment has characteristic features (see below). The small intestine is anchored to the dorsal body wall by a fan-shaped mesentery that supplies blood vessels, nerves, and lymphatics.

Chemical digestion of chyme continues in the small intestine as it is mixed with enzymes in pancreatic juice and secretions of the intestinal mucosa. It is also the primary site of nutrient absorption into the blood. Consistent with its absorptive function, the mucosa is modified to increase surface area (to an amazing 600 m^2!). On a gross level, **plicae circulares** (Figure 14-23) are permanent mucosal folds that are visible to the naked eye. Extending from the mucosal surface are the fingerlike **villi**, which are just barely visible to the naked eye and give the internal surface an appearance of velvet. Lastly, most epithelial cells have microscopic **microvilli** extending from their surface, visible with the light microscope as a **striated border**.

Villi are a distinctive feature of the small intestine (Figure 14-24). They are mucosal projections that extend into the intestinal lumen to increase surface area for absorption. Between villi are **intervillous spaces. Intestinal glands** (**crypts of Lieberkühn**) are depressions into the mucosa between the bases of villi. The lumen within a crypt is small compared to the intervillous spaces, making differentiation between gastric pits and intervillous spaces (which is problematic for novice

histologists) easier. Crypts contain stems cells capable of producing all epithelial cell types discussed below (Figure 14-25).

The intestinal mucosa is lined by a simple columnar epithelium with a striated border. Two major cell types are present. **Enterocytes** are "typical" columnar cells with a striated border. They have enzymes in their apical membranes that catalyze the final stages of chemical digestion that produce molecules small enough for absorption. In addition, they produce an **enterokinase** that converts inactive precursors of pancreatic enzymes (called proenzymes) to their active form. Thus, enterocytes participate in chemical digestion in addition to absorption. Goblet cells (Chapter 3) comprise the other major cell type and produce lubricating mucus. When viewed with the microscope, they may appear "empty" as a result of slide preparation removing the mucin. Enterocytes diminish and goblet cells increase in abundance from duodenum to ileum.

Other cells of the intestinal mucosa include enteroendocrine cells, which have many of the same functions as those found in the stomach, **Paneth cells**, and **M cells**. Paneth cells are located deep in the crypts, especially in the ileum, and produce a variety of antimicrobial chemicals, including the antibacterial enzyme **lysozyme**. They possess eosinophilic granules in their apices and thus are easily recognizable in routine specimen preparations. **M cells** are specialized epithelial cells that have **microfolds** (hence, "M" cell) in place of microvilli. They are located in epithelium overlying lymphatic nodules (especially Peyer's patches–see below) and assist in the immune response of MALT (Chapter 13) by endocytosing and transporting cellular and molecular antigens to lymphocytes and macrophages occupying pockets in their lateral and basal margins.

The lamina propria within each villus has a capillary bed, a lymphatic lacteal (capillary), an abundance of scattered lymphocytes, and vertically oriented smooth muscle cells that may assist in lymph movement through the lacteal.

Each segment of the small intestine has distinctive features (Figure 14-26). Duodenal villi tend to be shorter and broader than in other segments of the small intestine, but this qualitative feature is difficult to determine in histological sections. Of greater utility for identification of the duodenum is the presence of **Brünner's (duodenal) glands** in the submucosa (Figure 14-27). They are compound tubular glands that produce a mucoid alkaline secretion that counteracts the acidity of the chyme entering from the stomach. The secretory cells have a typical mucus-secreting cell appearance. That is, they are pale staining with a flattened nucleus near the base. The duct empties into the base of an intestinal crypt.

Other than long, thin villi, the jejunum has no microscopic features that differentiate it from the duodenum and ileum (Figure 14-28). In most instances, it must be identified by the absence of Brünner's glands and Peyer's patches.

---

[1] "Retroperitoneal" literally means "behind the peritoneal cavity." The parietal peritoneum forms a sac (the peritoneal cavity) within the abdominal cavity. Some organs, such as the duodenum, are located outside of the peritoneal sac, between it and the body wall, making them retroperitoneal.

The ileum (Figures 13-20b and 14-29) is characterized by **Peyer's patches**, aggregations of several dozen lymph follicles in the submucosa on the side of the intestine opposite the mesentery. Whereas isolated lymph follicles are visible in all parts of the small intestine, only the ileum has them in this great a quantity. Ileal villi are shorter and less abundant than those in the jejunum.

The small intestine's muscularis externa is smooth muscle and the circular and longitudinal layers are well defined. A serosa lines the outer surface, except for the posterior of the duodenum, which is retroperitoneal.

Large Intestine

The **large intestine** (Figure 14-30) is divided into a **cecum, ascending colon, transverse colon, descending colon,** and **rectum**. Its primary function is to absorb water from the undigested, unabsorbed material entering from the small intestine. The large intestine begins at the **ileocecal junction** and the ileocecal valve prevents backflow of material into the small intestine.

Nonpermanent folds of the colon's mucosa may be present, but there are no villi (Figure 14-31). The epithelium is a simple columnar with abundant goblet cells. Straight **crypts of Lieberkühn** extend down to the muscularis mucosae. These are involved in absorption of water and production of new cells by mitosis. Lymphatic follicles and diffuse lymphatic tissue may be seen in the lamina propria.

The muscularis mucosae is usually prominent. The inner circular layer of the muscularis externa is unremarkable, but the outer longitudinal layer is modified to form three bands called **taenia (or teniae) coli muscles** (Figure 14-32). The surface is covered with serosa, except for parts of the ascending and descending colon, which are retroperitoneal.

The **vermiform appendix** (Figure 13-20c and 14-33) is a short, narrow, tubular structure arising from the cecum. Its mucosa resembles the rest of the large intestine, but there is an abundance of lymphocytes in the lamina propria and the submucosa, and the longitudinal muscle layer is uniform in thickness.

The **rectum** is the straight, terminal portion of the large intestine. Its mucosa resembles the rest of the large intestine, but the crypts are shallower and goblet cells are more abundant. At the **rectoanal junction** (Figure 14-34), the simple columnar epithelium abruptly changes back to a stratified squamous. Thickening of the circular muscularis externa forms the **internal anal sphincter**. A ring of skeletal muscle outside the muscularis externa forms the **external anal sphincter**.

▪▪ Glands of the Digestive Tract

The liver, pancreas, and gallbladder are derived as outgrowths of the embryonic digestive tube and they retain their connection with the gut's lumen in the postnatal individual via bile ducts, pancreatic duct(s), and the cystic duct, respectively.

Liver

The **liver** is located inferior to the diaphragm in the upper right abdominal quadrant and is the largest internal organ of the body. It is divided into four lobes, which are further divided into microscopic **lobules** (Figures 14-35 through 14-37). Traditionally, lobules have been considered the structural and functional units of the liver, but other interpretations also have merit. This being a histology book and not a physiology book, the traditional view of the classic hepatic lobule will be emphasized.

The **hepatic artery** and the **hepatic portal vein** provide two sources of blood to the liver. The former supplies oxygen-rich blood, whereas the latter brings nutrient-rich blood from the digestive organs to be processed by **hepatocytes**, the cells of the liver.

The liver performs a variety of functions, including detoxification of chemicals, phagocytosis of worn-out RBCs, synthesis of plasma proteins and plasma lipoproteins, glucose metabolism (starch storage and gluconeogenesis), storage of certain vitamins, and production of bile.

All liver functions are performed by the hepatocytes, and most of them require close contact with the blood. As such, the hepatocytes are arranged in **plates,** or **cords,** of cells separated by large capillaries called **sinusoids** (see Chapter 12). The cords are usually a single cell thick, and the sinusoids are lined with endothelial cells and phagocytic **Kupffer cells** (derived from monocytes). Blood from branches of the hepatic artery and hepatic portal vein enters the sinusoids at several points along the periphery of the lobule. As the mixture of arterial and venous blood flows by the hepatocytes, they remove and deposit whatever nutrients are appropriate. The blood is drained from the lobule by a **central vein** and ultimately leaves the liver through one of the hepatic veins,[2] which empty into the inferior vena cava.

Small intercellular channels called **bile canaliculi** (Figure 14-38) carry bile produced by the hepatocytes. The canaliculi only exist as small, sealed spaces between cells; they are not tubes apart from the cells. Bile flows through the canaliculi toward the periphery of the lobule and empties into a **bile duct**. Bile ducts converge and ultimately lead to hepatic ducts that emerge from the liver.

---

[2] Be careful not to confuse the hepatic portal vein (which delivers blood to the liver) and the hepatic veins (which drain it).

The system of bile ducts and the branches of the hepatic artery and hepatic portal vein travel together within the liver and constitute a **hepatic (portal) triad** (Figure 14-39), a poorly chosen term because efferent lymph vessels are also present! Materials within each triad's vessels flow in opposite directions: Blood is coming into the liver and bile and lymph are leaving.

It is this differential flow of blood and bile that has led to newer functional interpretations of liver lobules beyond the classic one.[3] The bile duct of a hepatic triad is at the center of a **portal lobule** (rather than the central vein) with three central veins at the corners of a triangular region incorporating parts of three classic lobules (Figure 14-40a). Bile produced by hepatocytes in this triangular region flows into the same bile duct, thus forming a structural and functional unit. An **acinar lobule**, or **portal acinus** (Figure 14-40b), emphasizes blood flow into adjacent classic lobules. At its center is the shared side with portal triads at each end. At the apices of the acinar lobule are the two central veins. Together, they form a diamond-shaped region of hepatocytes supplied by blood from branches of the hepatic portal vein and hepatic artery in each triad.

Gallbladder

The **gallbladder** (Figure 14-41) is a small, blind sac found inferior to the liver. It receives bile from the **common hepatic duct** via the **cystic duct**. Once in the gallbladder, bile is concentrated and stored until it is needed.

The mucosa is folded into **rugae** and is lined by a simple columnar epithelium with microvilli that concentrates bile by absorbing water and electrolytes. The lamina propria is rich in lymphocytes and plasma cells. There is no muscularis mucosae or submucosa, so the lamina propria rests directly on the muscularis externa, which is made of indistinct smooth muscle layers. Most of the gallbladder's surface is covered by a serosa.

Fats in the duodenum stimulate enteroendocrine cells to produce the hormone **cholecystokinin (CCK)**, which, among other actions, causes the gallbladder to contract and eject concentrated bile out through the cystic duct, into the common bile duct, and ultimately into the duodenum. Bile is alkaline and assists in neutralizing the acidic chyme entering the duodenum from the stomach. In addition, it contains **lecithin** and **bile salts (bile acids)** that emulsify fats and promote fat digestion. Other compounds, such as cholesterol and bilirubin, are also present.

Pancreas

The pancreas is a retroperitoneal organ covered by a thin, fibrous **capsule** that sends septa into the gland to divide it into lobules (Figures 14-42 and 14-43). It has both endocrine (Chapter 10) and exocrine components. It is the latter that we are concerned with here.

The exocrine component is devoted to producing **pancreatic juice**, which is composed of proenzymes produced by **secretory acini**, and a watery, alkaline secretion produced by **intercalated ducts**. Unlike bile, pancreatic juice is not concentrated. Once activated by duodenal enterocytes, the proenzymes are responsible for the bulk of chemical digestion, being capable of digesting molecules within the four biochemical families (protein, lipid, carbohydrate, and nucleic acid). Acidic contents in the duodenum stimulate enteroendocrine cells to release CCK and **secretin**, which stimulate the acinar cells and duct cells, respectively, to release their secretions.

Secretory acini cells are roughly triangular and have a granular cytoplasm typical of zymogenic (enzyme secreting) cells. That is, they have a basophilic cytoplasm because of the extensive rough endoplasmic reticulum. They also have eosinophilic granules at their apex. There are no myoepithelial cells associated with the acini.

Each acinus empties its secretion into a short intercalated duct. An unusual aspect of these ducts is that they begin *within* the acinus as squamous, pale-staining **centroacinar cells**. Intercalated ducts empty into **intralobar ducts**, which in turn empty into **interlobar ducts** located within the gland's septa. Eventually, pancreatic juice is delivered to the duodenum by the main and accessory (if present) pancreatic duct(s). The main pancreatic duct (usually) joins the common bile duct (Figure 14-44) in the wall of the duodenum at the **hepatopancreatic ampulla (of Vater)**. Together they empty into the duodenum at the **major duodenal papilla**. The **minor duodenal papilla** is in the more proximal duodenum and contains the opening of the accessory duct, if present.

Once in the duodenum, intestinal enterokinases convert **trypsinogen** to **trypsin**, which in addition to digesting proteins in food, converts other pancreatic proenzymes to their active form. The alkalinity of pancreatic juice works with bile to bring the acidic chyme entering from the stomach to near neutral pH.

---

[3] Note that these interpretations do not change the structure of the classic nodule, but rather are simply different ways of viewing how they function.

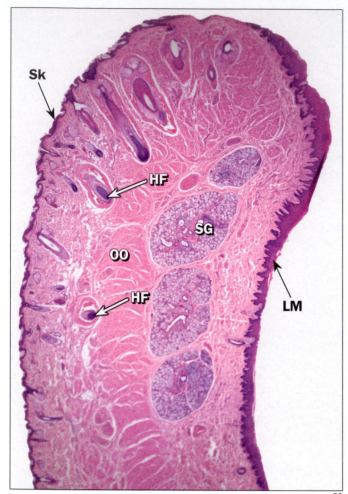

×60

14-2 **Lip** Shown is a vertical section of the lip, with skin (Sk) on the left and nonkeratinized stratified squamous epithelium of the lining mucosa (LM) on the right. Accessory salivary glands (SG) are present in the submucosa. The skeletal muscle orbicularis oris (OO—the "kissing muscle") and hair follicles (HF) are also visible. (×60)

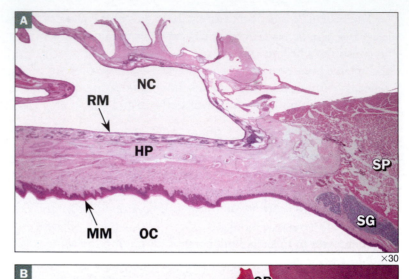

×30

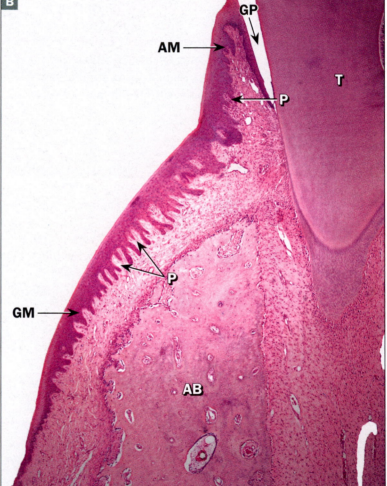

×40

14-3 **Masticatory Mucosa of the Oral Cavity** In both micrographs, epithelium of the masticatory mucosa is keratinized (though difficult to see at these magnifications). (**A**) Shown is a parasagittal section of the hard palate (HP) separating the nasal cavity (NC) from the oral cavity (OC). Masticatory mucosa (MM) is found on its inferior surface, whereas respiratory mucosa (RM) is on its superior surface. A portion of the soft palate (SP) is visible at the right and contains accessory salivary glands (SG) in the submucosa. (×30) (**B**) Shown is the mucosa associated with a tooth (T). The masticatory gingival mucosa (GM), gingival pocket (GP), alveolar bone (AB), and lining alveolar mucosa (AM) are visible. Notice the relatively numerous and deep papillae (P) of the lamina propria of the masticatory mucosa and the sparse, shallow papillae of the lining mucosa. (×40)

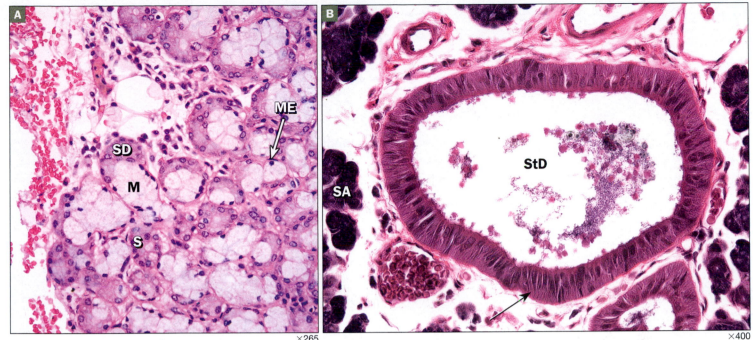

×265

×400

14-4 **Basic Components of a Salivary Gland** 🔴 (**A**) This section of the sublingual gland shows several acini composed of secretory mucous (M) and serous (S) cells. Mucous cells tend to be light staining with the nuclei pushed toward the basement membrane. They secrete mucus. Serous cells tend to be darker staining (basophilic) and granular, an appearance typical of enzyme-secreting cells. On occasion, serous demilunes (SD) form over a mucous acinus, but these apparently are artifacts of slide preparation. Myoepithelial cells (ME) wrap around the acini and assist in moving the secretion out the ducts. (×265) (**B**) Striated ducts (StD) are lined with a simple columnar epithelium and are unique to salivary glands. Their nuclei are toward the apical edge and the basal cytoplasm is vertically striated (arrow). Purple serous acini (SA) are visible at the periphery of the field. This specimen is from the parotid gland. (×400)

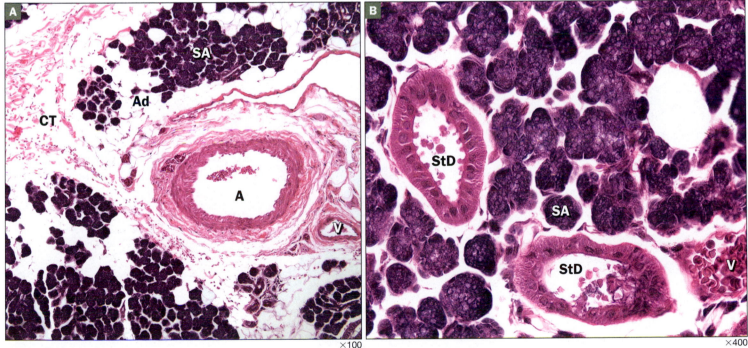

×100

×400

14-5 **Parotid Gland** (**A**) The parotid gland is divided by connective tissue (CT) septa into lobules of dark-staining serous acini (SA). Also visible are adipocytes (Ad), and an artery (A) and vein (V). (×100) (**B**) This higher magnification shows two striated ducts (StD), numerous serous acini (SA), and a venule (V). (×400)

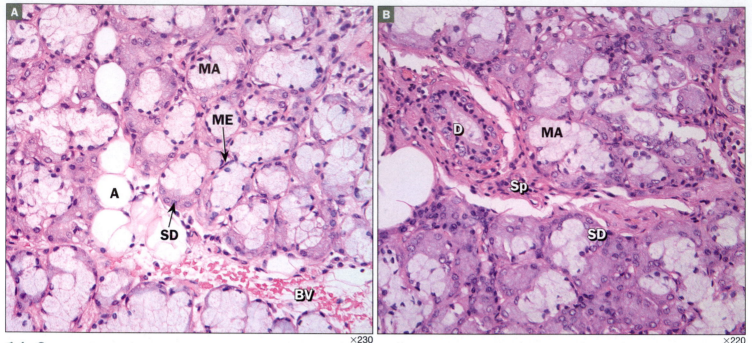

14-6 **Sublingual Gland** ■ The sublingual gland consists mostly of mucous acini (MA), some with serous demilunes (SD). **(A)** In addition to the acini, myoepithelial cells (ME) and adipocytes (A) are visible in this specimen, as is a blood vessel (BV). (×230) **(B)** A duct (D) is seen in a connective tissue septum (Sp) in this specimen. (×220)

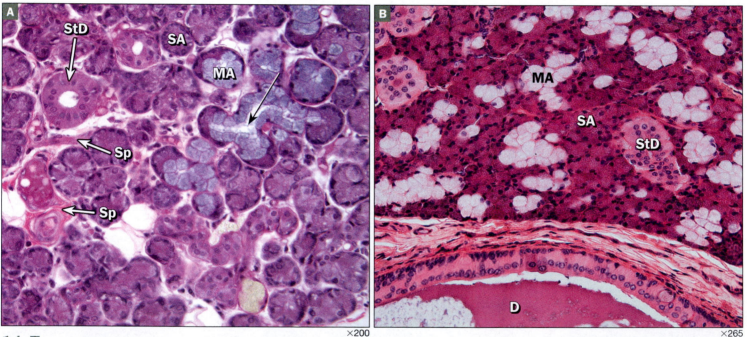

14-7 **Submandibular Gland** ■ The submandibular gland is a tubuloacinar gland, with the serous acini (SA) outnumbering the mucous acini (MA). The mucous cells are often in a tubular arrangement. Striated ducts (StD) and connective tissue septa (Sp) are also present. **(A)** In this specimen, the tubular arrangement of mucous cells is clearly seen (arrow). (×200) **(B)** A major duct (D) is visible in this specimen at the bottom of the field. It is lined with a stratified columnar epithelium. (×265)

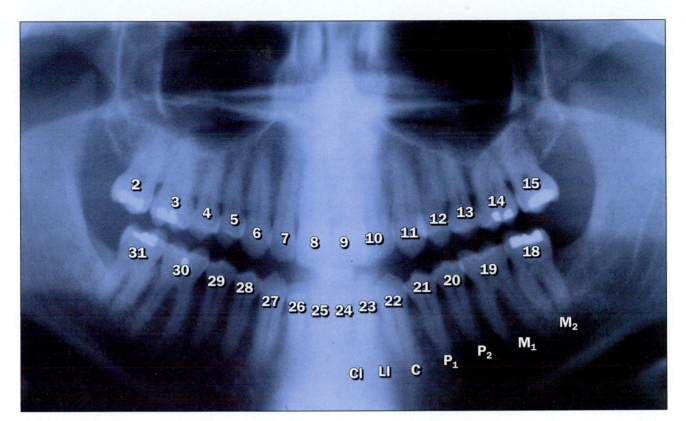

14-8 **The Adult Dentition** ◼ Shown is a radiograph of maxillary (upper) and mandibular (lower) dental arches. Starting from the center of each arch are the central (CI) and lateral incisors (LI), the canine (C), the first (P_1) and second premolars (P_2), and the first (M_1), second (M_2), and third molars. Note: the third molars of each dental arch are the wisdom teeth and they have been removed from this patient. Teeth are also identified by Arabic numerals in most parts of North America using the American (Universal) system. Teeth are numbered beginning with the right third maxillary molar (#1) and continuing to the left third maxillary molar (#16). That is, from the posterior of the right upper quadrant to the posterior of the left upper quadrant. Numbering resumes with the left lower quadrant, starting with the left third mandibular molar (#17) and continuing around to the right lower mandibular quadrant, ending with the third mandibular molar (#32). The missing wisdom teeth correspond to numbers 1, 16, 17, and 32.

(Courtesy of Paul C. Howard, D.M.D.)

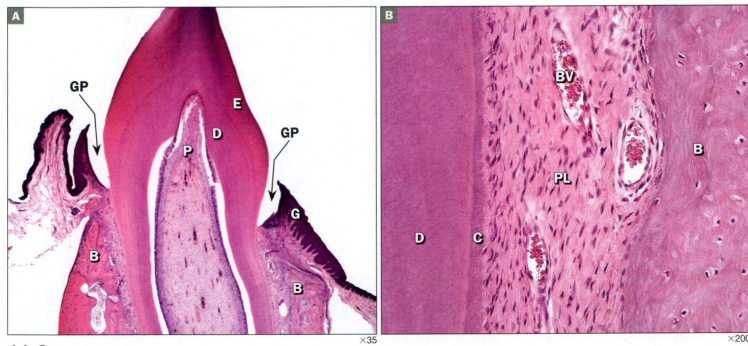

14-9 **Tooth** ◼ (**A**) In this section of a tooth, dentin (D), enamel (E), pulp (P), gingivae (G), gingival pocket (GP), and alveolar bone (B) are visible. (×35) (**B**) Each tooth is anchored to its alveolus by a periodontal ligament (PL), which is made of vascular connective tissue. Its collagen fibers are anchored in the cementum (C) surrounding dentin (D), and penetrate the bone (B) as Sharpey's fibers. Note the numerous blood vessels (BV). (×200)

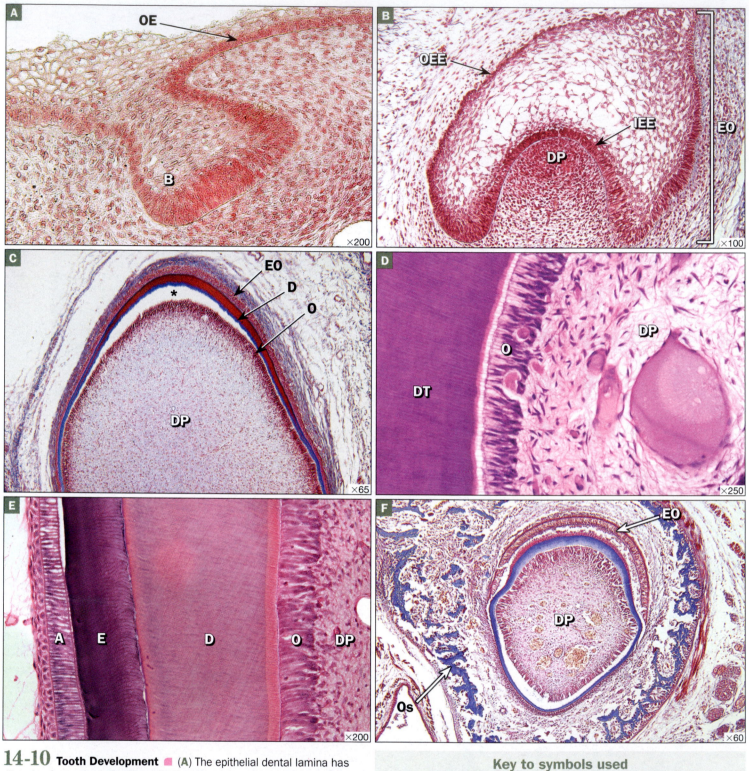

14-10 Tooth Development 🔲 (**A**) The epithelial dental lamina has dilated to form a bud, the first evidence of an enamel organ in an embryo. (×200) (**B**) The cap stage is characterized by the formation of a connective tissue invagination called the dental papilla, that becomes surrounded by the developing enamel organ. Eventually, this will become dental pulp. Inner and outer enamel epithelium have formed as a result. The inner enamel epithelium will become enamel-secreting ameloblasts. (×100) (**C**) In this much later stage, the enamel organ is fully formed. (×65) (**D**) This micrograph shows dentin formation, with odontoblasts and dentinal tubules. (×250) (**E**) This micrograph shows how the ameloblasts secrete enamel inward and odontoblasts secrete dentin inward so that both layers are in contact with one another. It also explains why ameloblasts and odontoblasts move farther apart as the tooth develops. (×200) (**F**) This is a cross section of a developing tooth. Notice that the connective tissue has begun to produce membrane bone (Os) of the jaw, or more accurately, the alveolus. (×60)

Key to symbols used

A = ameloblasts		**IEE** =	inner enamel epithelium
B = bud			
D = dentin		**O** =	odontoblasts
DP = dental papilla		**OE** =	oral epithelium
DT = dentinal tubules		**OEE** =	outer enamel epithelium
E = enamel			
EO = enamel organ		**Os** =	ossification
		* =	artifactual space

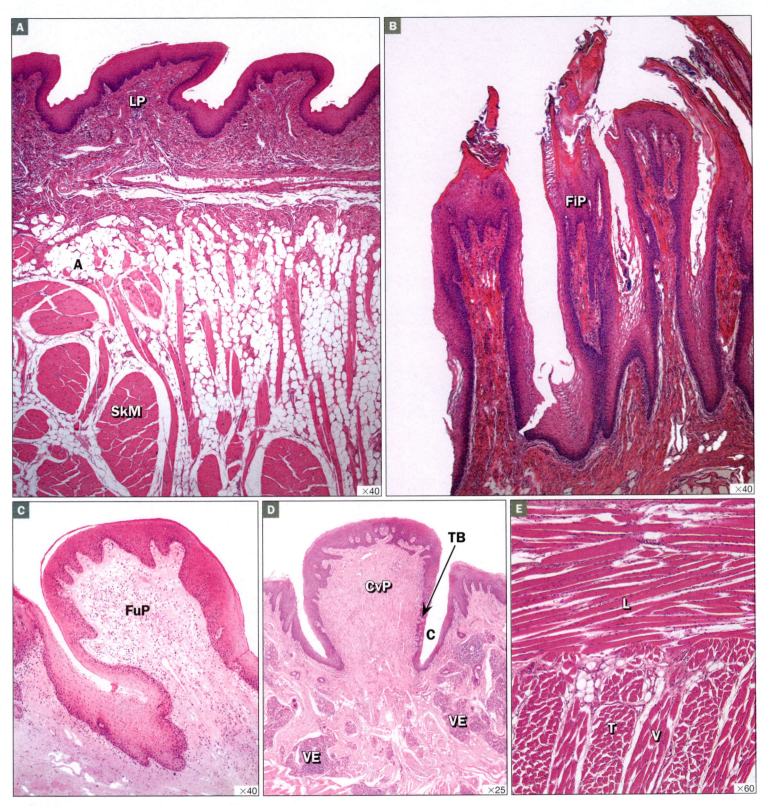

14-11 **Tongue** ■ (**A**) Lingual papillae (LP) are visible on the dorsal surface of this specimen, as are skeletal muscle fibers (SkM) and adipose tissue (A). (×40) (**B**) Elongated filiform papillae (FiP) are the most numerous of papillae and are covered with a keratinized stratified squamous epithelium. They have no taste buds, but their keratinized surface assists in mechanical digestion of food. (×40) (**C**) Mushroom-shaped fungiform papillae (FuP) are interspersed between filiform papillae. In life, they often can be seen without magnification due to their reddish color, a consequence of extensive vasculature in their lamina propria. Fungiform papillae are lined with a lightly keratinized stratified squamous epithelium and, although taste buds are present in their epithelium, this section doesn't show any. (×40) (**D**) Humans have about a dozen or so circumvallate papillae (CvP), which have the highest density of taste buds (TB) in their epithelium. For taste bud details, see Figures 9-3A and 9-3B. Each papilla is surrounded by a gutter-like cleft (C), into which drain serous von Ebner's glands (VE). (×25) (**E**) Skeletal muscle in the tongue is arranged into vertical (V), longitudinal (L), and transverse (T) bands, all of which are seen in this specimen. These multiple orientations allow the tongue to produce complex movements. (×60)

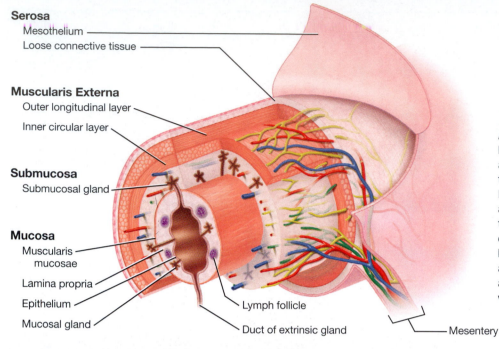

Serosa
- Mesothelium
- Loose connective tissue

Muscularis Externa
- Outer longitudinal layer
- Inner circular layer

Submucosa
- Submucosal gland

Mucosa
- Muscularis mucosae
- Lamina propria
- Epithelium
- Mucosal gland
- Lymph follicle
- Duct of extrinsic gland
- Mesentery

14-12 Basic Plan of the Digestive Tube 🔲
All parts of the digestive tube are built on this basic plan, with modifications in each organ appropriate to their different functions. Notice the alternation of muscle with connective tissue: lamina propria, muscularis mucosae, submucosa, and muscularis externa. In general, the connective tissue layers will stain the same, as will the muscular layers. This should help you in getting your bearings as you examine the following micrographs and your own slides. In this art, standard colors are used for arteries (red), veins (blue), lymph vessels (green), and nerves (yellow).

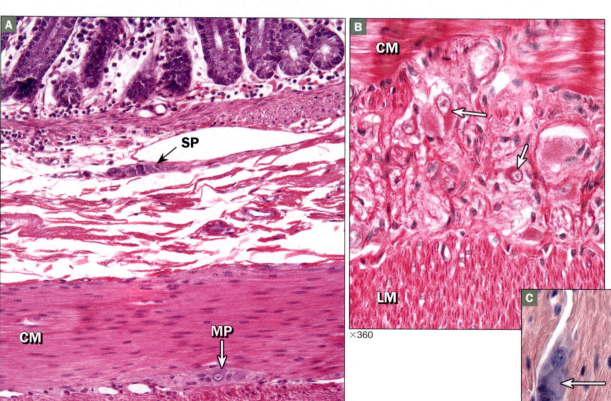

14-13 Autonomic Plexuses of the Gut 🔲 (A) Autonomic neuron cell bodies controlling gut activity are found in two locations of the gut: Submucosa (Meissner's) plexuses (SP) are found in the submucosa, and myenteric (Auerbach's) plexuses (MP) are positioned between the circular (CM) and longitudinal muscle (LM) layers of the muscularis externa. The former controls glandular secretion and the latter controls muscular contraction. (×180) (B) Myenteric plexuses are fairly easy to find because they stand out prominently against the smooth muscle tissue. In the higher magnification, you can see some multipolar neurons (arrows). (×360) (C) Submucosal plexuses are more difficult to find because they are smaller and their locations are not as restricted. Try searching specimens that don't have other dominating structures (e.g., Brünner's glands) in the submucosa and look for cells with large, circular nuclei and nucleoli. This specimen is from the jejunum and was stained so the neurons (gray) and the connective tissue (tan) are different colors. (×360)

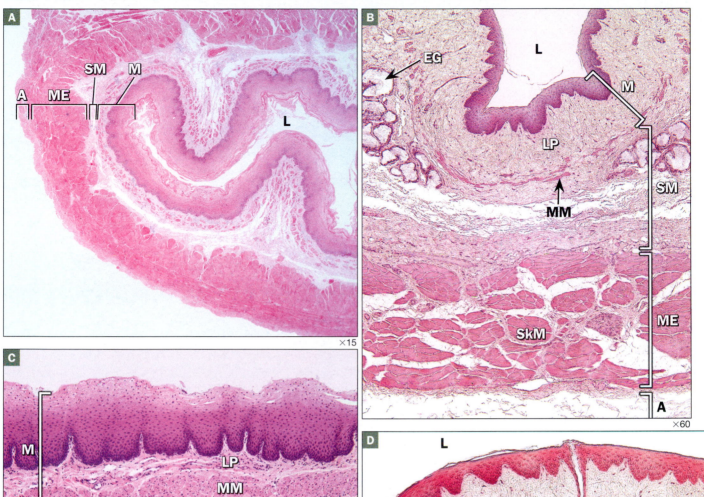

×15

×60

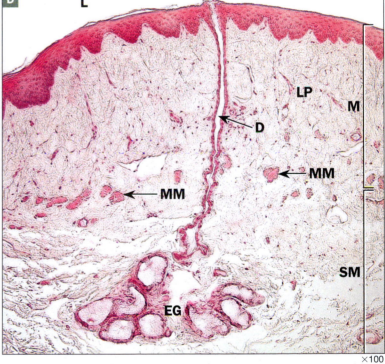

×65

×100

14-14 **Esophagus** (**A**) In this panoramic view, one can observe the collapsed lumen of the esophagus when empty. (×15) (**B**) This specimen is from the upper third of the esophagus as evidenced by skeletal muscle in the muscularis externa. Also note the esophageal glands in the submucosa and the incomplete muscularis mucosae. (×60) (**C**) Note the thick, nonkeratinized stratified squamous epithelium and the thick, but still incomplete, muscularis mucosae. The skeletal muscle in the muscularis externa tells us that the specimen is from the upper third of the esophagus. (×65) (**D**) Esophageal glands secrete lubricating mucus for the inner lining of the esophagus. Note the duct of one gland passing to the surface. (×100)

Key to symbols used

A	=	adventitia	**M** =	mucosa
D	=	duct	**ME** =	muscularis externa
EG	=	esophageal gland	**MM** =	muscularis mucosae
L	=	lumen	**SkM** =	skeletal muscle
LP	=	lamina propria	**SM** =	submucosa

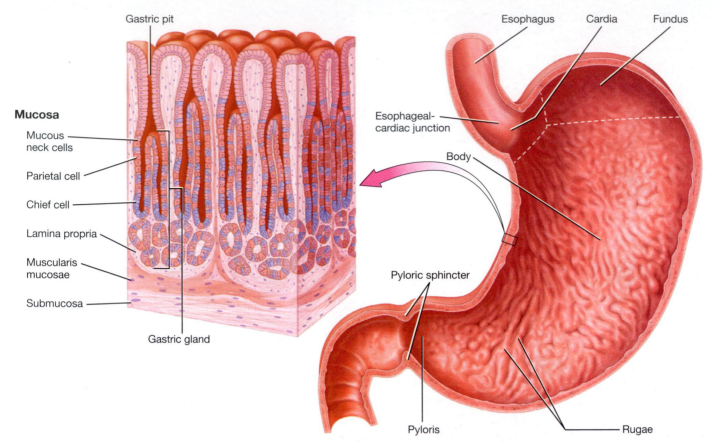

Mucosa

- Mucous neck cells
- Parietal cell
- Chief cell
- Lamina propria
- Muscularis mucosae
- Submucosa

Gastric pit

Gastric gland

Esophagus   Cardia   Fundus

Esophageal-cardiac junction

Body

Pyloric sphincter

Pyloris

Rugae

14-15 Stomach Gross Anatomy and Mucosal Structures ■ Refer to this figure as you look at specimens from the various stomach regions. The detail illustrates the basic microscopic structures of the gastric mucosa.

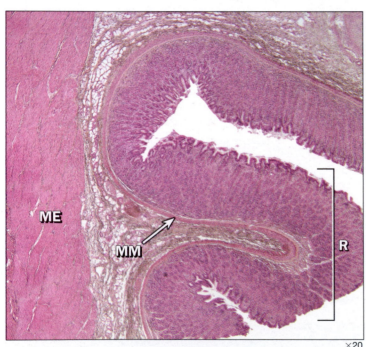

×20

14-16 Gastric Rugae ■ The stomach's mucosa presents nonpermanent longitudinal folds called rugae. These flatten as the stomach fills with food. One ruga (R) is shown in this micrograph. Notice that the muscularis mucosa (MM) is folded, indicating the whole mucosa is folded, but the muscularis externa (ME) is not. (×20)

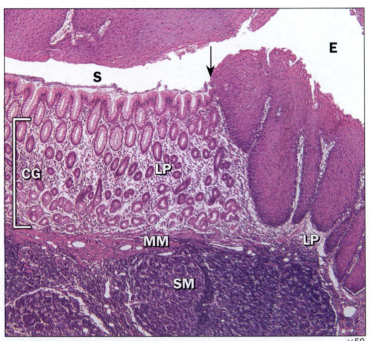

×50

14-17 Esophageal-Cardiac Junction ■ The stratified squamous epithelium stops abruptly (arrow) and becomes a simple columnar epithelium where the esophagus (E) joins the cardiac stomach (S). (Note: In this micrograph, food would be traveling from the right to the left.) All other layers are continuous between the two organs. Visible are the lamina propria (LP), muscularis mucosae (MM), and submucosa (SM). The ovals in the lamina propria are mucus-secreting cardiac glands (CG). (×50)

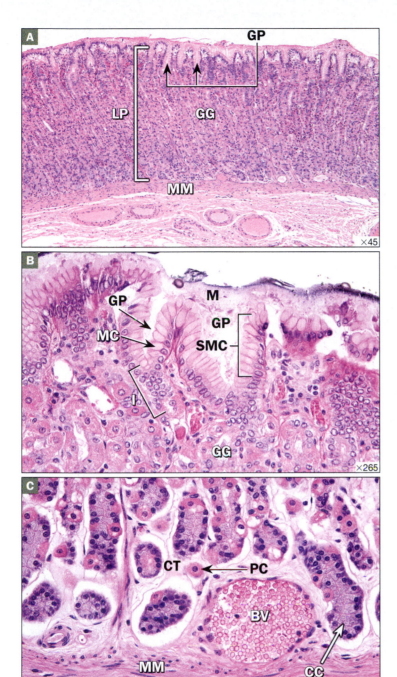

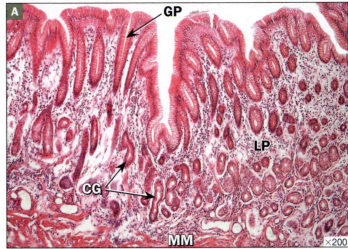

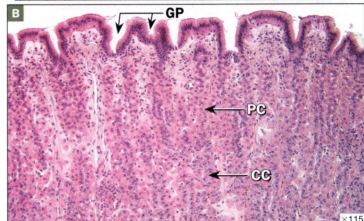

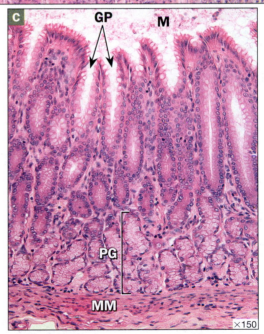

14-18 Gastric Mucosa 🔲 The stomach's mucosa is lined with a simple columnar epithelium. Depressions called gastric pits (GP) lead to gastric glands (GG), which extend to the muscularis mucosae (MM) and occupy most of the lamina propria (LP). (**A**) This micrograph shows the entire thickness of the gastric mucosa. (×45) (**B**) Shown here are two gastric pits (GP) and the beginnings of gastric glands (GG). Surface mucous cells (SMC) extend into the pits and possess a distinctive "mucous cup" (MC) at their apices. Connecting each pit to the deeper glands is a constricted region called the isthmus (I). The isthmus is populated by stem cells that give rise to new surface and gland cells. The most superficial part of a gastric gland is the neck, which contains (among other secretory cells) mucous neck cells, but these are often difficult to identify among all the other gland cells. Note the mucus (M) coating the surface. (×265) (**C**) This micrograph shows that gastric glands extend down to the muscularis mucosae. Enzyme-secreting chief cells (CC) and HCl-secreting parietal cells (PC) are indicated. Also present are enteroendocrine cells, but these are difficult to identify in standard light microscope preparations. Note the blood vessel (BV) and how little connective tissue (CT) of the lamina propria there is between glands. (×265)

14-19 Stomach Regions 🔲 The mucosa of each part of the stomach has a characteristic appearance. (**A**) In the cardiac stomach the gastric pits (GP) are deep and the coiled cardiac glands (CG) mostly secrete mucus. Most of the dark dots in the lamina propria (LP) are lymphocytes or plasma cells nuclei. The muscularis mucosae (MM) is barely visible at the bottom. (×200) (**B**) The body and fundus of the stomach have shallow pits and typical gastric glands with chief (CC) and parietal cells (PC). (×115) (**C**) Deep pits extending down about half the mucosa's thickness characterize the pyloric region. The pyloric glands (PG) secrete mucus (M). (×150)

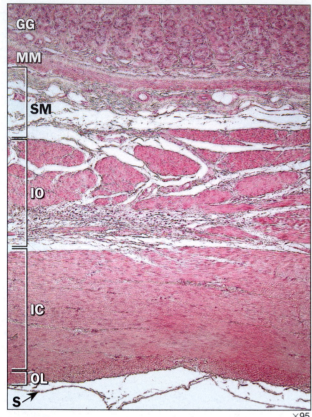

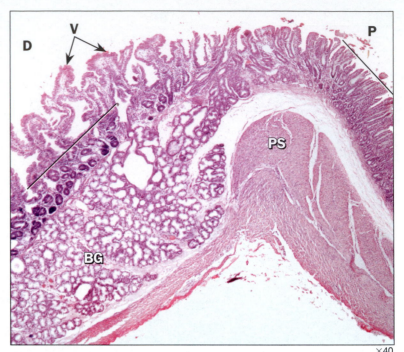

14-20 Gastric Muscularis Externa ■ Befitting an organ whose shape is not a simple tube, but rather one whose embryonic origin involves dilation, rotation, and bending, the muscularis externa is also not simply made of an inner circular (IC) and an outer longitudinal (OL) layer. It possesses an innermost oblique (IO) muscle layer of fibers. Also visible in this micrograph are the submucosa (SM), muscularis mucosae (MM), gastric glands (GG) in the lamina propria, and serosa (S). (×95)

×40

14-21 Stomach-Duodenal Junction ■ The most obvious change in the mucosa where the pyloris (P) joins the duodenum (D) is the presence of villi (V) in the latter. It takes some getting used to, but remember that the stomach has depressions into the mucosa—the gastric pits, whereas the small intestine has depressions into the mucosa—crypts of Lieberkühn, and projections out of it—villi. Lines are drawn to show the surface of each organ. Note the submucosal (Brünner's) glands (BG) in the duodenum and the thickened inner circular muscle layer of the pyloris—the pyloric sphincter (PS). (×40)

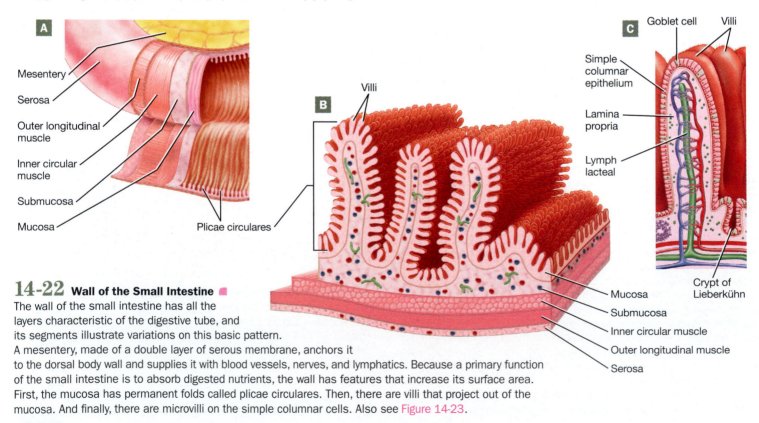

14-22 Wall of the Small Intestine ■
The wall of the small intestine has all the layers characteristic of the digestive tube, and its segments illustrate variations on this basic pattern.
A mesentery, made of a double layer of serous membrane, anchors it to the dorsal body wall and supplies it with blood vessels, nerves, and lymphatics. Because a primary function of the small intestine is to absorb digested nutrients, the wall has features that increase its surface area. First, the mucosa has permanent folds called plicae circulares. Then, there are villi that project out of the mucosa. And finally, there are microvilli on the simple columnar cells. Also see Figure 14-23.

14-23 Increasing Surface Area in the Small Intestine ◼ The mucosa of the small intestine has several modifications to increase surface area for absorption. (**A**) Plicae circulares (PC) are permanent mucosal folds. As with rugae, note that the muscularis mucosae (MM) is folded, but the muscularis externa (ME) is not. The submucosa (SM) just fills in the space between the two muscle layers. Note the well-defined inner circular (IC) and outer longitudinal (OL) layers of the muscularis externa (ME) and the serosa (S) with adipocytes. (×30) (**B**) Villi (V) extend from the mucosal surface. In this micrograph, the villi are projecting from the surface of a plica. Note that the muscularis mucosae does not follow the contours of the villi. Also notice that the inner circular (IC) layer of the muscularis externa has been cut in cross section, meaning this is a longitudinal section of the intestine. (×30) (**C**) Shown here are the adjacent sides of two villi. The simple columnar epithelium (enterocytes) covering villi is modified with microvilli, which in light micrographs is seen as a striated border (SB). Also note the goblet cells (GC) and lymphocytes (L). (×660)

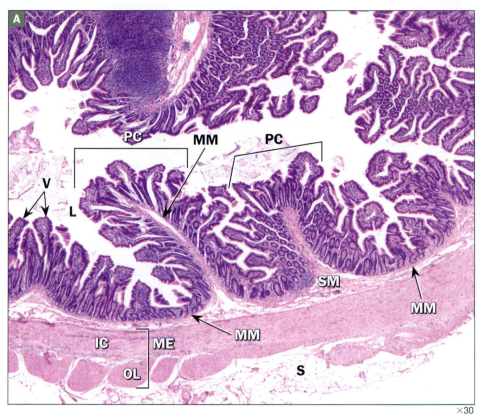

×30

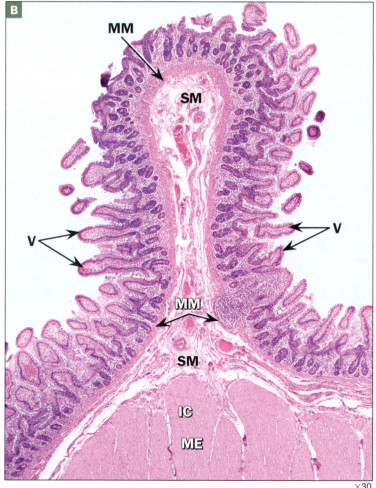

×30

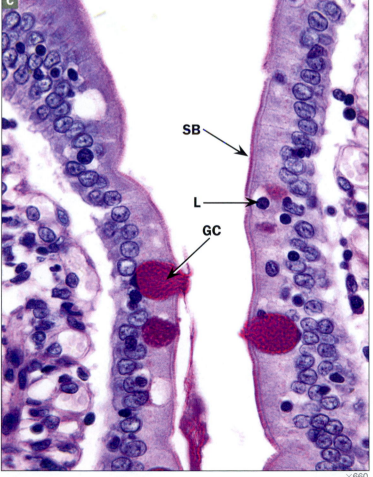

×660

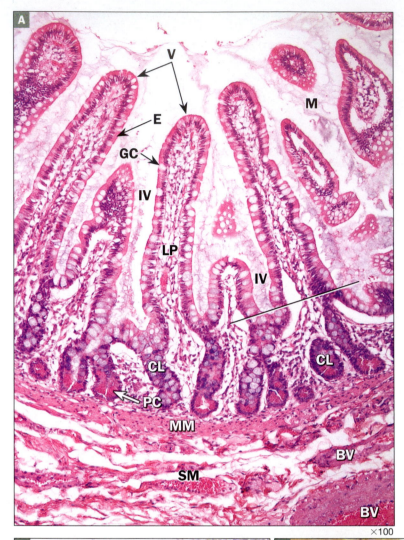

14-24 **Intestinal Mucosa-Villi** ■ The intestinal mucosa has villi (V) projecting from it and crypts of Lieberkühn (CL) projecting into it. The intervillous spaces (IV) are much larger than the space within the crypts, providing a clue as to where the intestinal surface actually is. Simple columnar enterocytes (E), goblet cells (GC), and Paneth cells (PC) are present in the epithelium. (**A**) The level of the intestinal surface is indicated with a line at the right of the field. Villi project up from the surface and crypts project below the surface. Note the dark nuclei of lymphocytes in the lamina propria (LP), the muscularis mucosae (MM), the submucosa (SM), blood vessels (BV), and the mucus (M) coating the surface. (×100) (**B**) This specimen has had its blood vessels injected with a red dye. Note the capillaries in the lamina propria of the villi. (×140) (**C**) This micrograph shows smooth muscle fibers (MF) and a capillary (C) in the lamina propria (LP) of a villus. A striated border (SB) and goblet cells (GC) are also visible. Many of the nuclei in the lamina propria are lymphocytes and plasma cells. (×480)

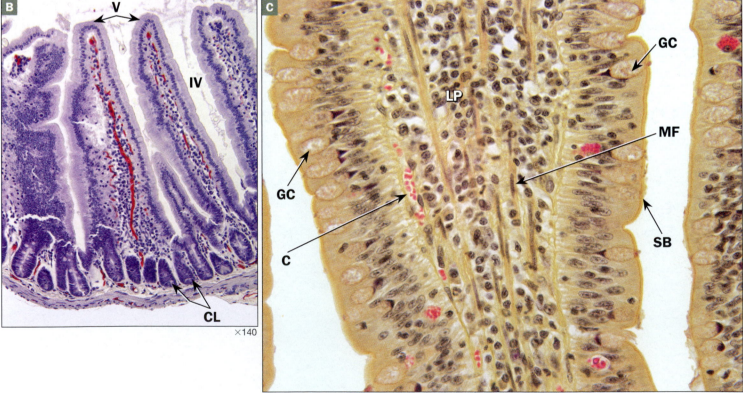

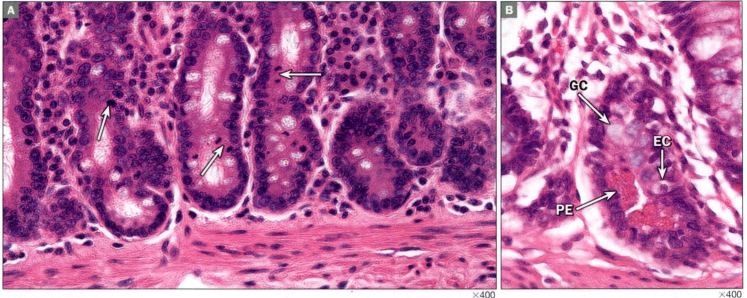

14-25 Intestinal Mucosa—Cells of the Intestinal Crypts ▪ **(A)** The intestinal crypts contain stem cells that divide and replace worn-out enterocytes, goblet cells, and others. Look for cells undergoing mitosis (arrows). (×400) **(B)** Also in the crypts are Paneth cells (PE) whose apical granules stain bright red in standard H&E preparations. They secrete antimicrobial chemicals, such as lysozyme, and are especially abundant in the ileum. The pale-staining, elongated cell is probably an enteroendocrine cell (EC). What appear to be secretory granules are between the nucleus and the basement membrane (unlike Paneth cells). Also visible are goblet cells (GC). (×400)

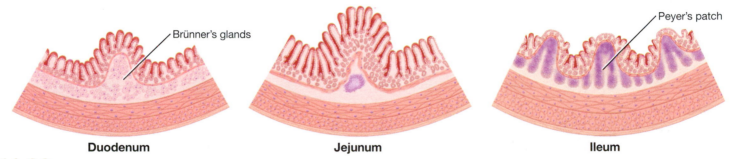

14-26 Histology of the Small Intestine Segments ▪ All three segments of the small intestine are variations on the basic digestive tube plan. The duodenum has mucous-secreting Brünner's (duodenal) glands in the submucosa and shorter, broader villi. The ileum has aggregations of lymphatic follicles in the submucosa called Peyer's patches. Its villi are short and less dense than the other two segments. The jejunum has long, thin villi and lacks Brünner's glands and Peyer's patches.

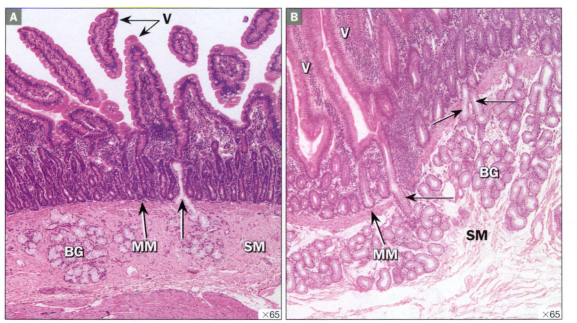

14-27 Duodenum ▪
The duodenum is identifiable by mucus-secreting Brünner's glands (BG) in the submucosa (SM) and short, broad villi (V). **(A)** In this micrograph, the Brünner's glands are not very dense. One duct is seen emptying into a crypt (arrow). Because they are in the submucosa, Brünner's glands are deep to the muscularis mucosae (MM). (×65) **(B)** The Brünner's glands are much denser in this specimen. Three ducts are seen emptying into the crypts (arrows). (×65)

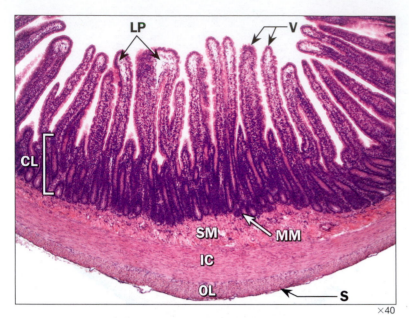

14-28 Jejunum ▰ Other than the villi being longer than other segments of the small intestine, the jejunum has no diagnostic features, and so must be provisionally identified based on the absence of Brünner's glands and Peyer's patches. (×40)

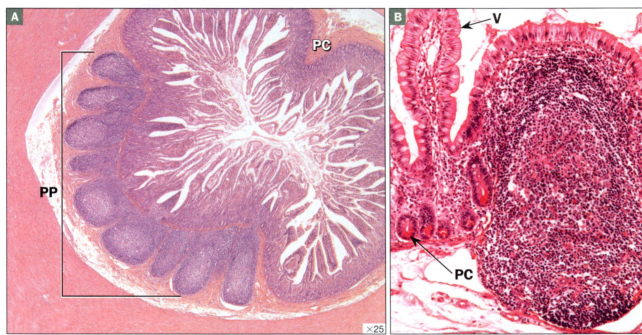

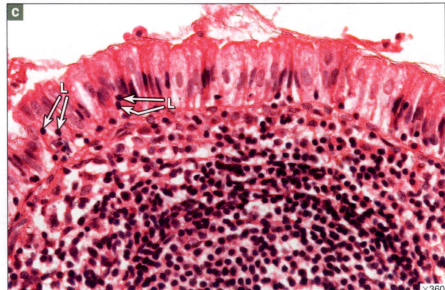

14-29 Ileum ▰ **(A)** The ileum has distinctive aggregations of lymphatic follicles called Peyer's patches (PP) in the submucosa and sometimes extending into the lamina propria. Note the plica circularis (PC). Also see Figure 13-20b. (×25) **(B)** Shown is a single lymph nodule in the ileum, and as is customary, it has no villi (V) covering it. Paneth cells (PC) are visible in the crypts of Lieberkühn. (×100) **(C)** M cells are found in the epithelium over the nodule. These cells capture antigens from the lumen and transport them to immune cells, such as dendritic cells, macrophages, and lymphocytes (L). Although the M cells cannot be identified with certainty in a standard light microscope preparation, the presence of intraepithelial lymphocytes is a good indication they are nearby. Electron micrographs reveal that they lack microvilli found in enterocytes. (×360)

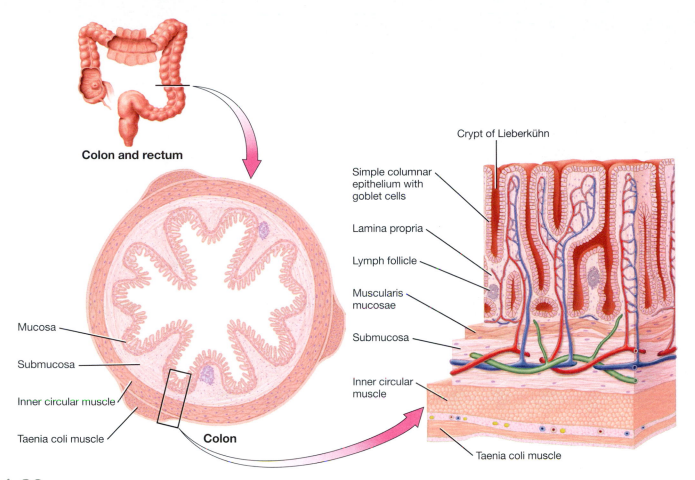

Colon and rectum

Crypt of Lieberkühn

Simple columnar epithelium with goblet cells

Lamina propria

Lymph follicle

Muscularis mucosae

Submucosa

Inner circular muscle

Taenia coli muscle

Mucosa

Submucosa

Inner circular muscle

Taenia coli muscle

Colon

14-30 **Large Intestine Mucosa** ■ The large intestine starts where the jejunum enters at the cecum. From there, it ascends the right side of the abdominal cavity as the ascending colon, crosses to the left as the transverse colon, and descends on the left side as the descending colon. It ends as the straight rectum. Note that the colon's longitudinal muscle is limited to three bands called taeniae coli muscles. Its mucosa has straight intestinal crypts with numerous goblet cells.

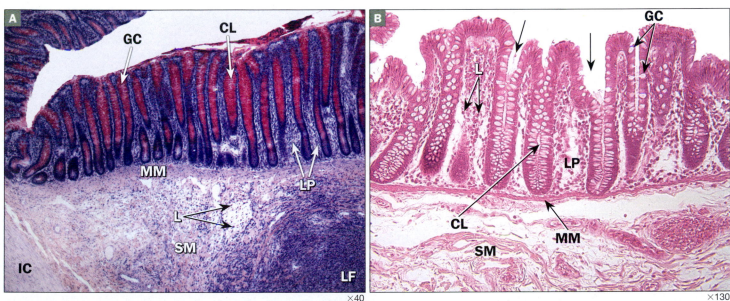

14-31 **Colon Mucosa** ■ (A) The colon's mucosa is characterized by long, straight crypts of Lieberkühn (CL) that penetrate the lamina propria (LP) to the muscularis mucosae (MM). The submucosa (SM) is also visible. Note the abundant goblet cells (GC) in the epithelium, which are stained red, and the lymphocytes (L) and lymph follicle (LF) in the lamina propria. The inner circular layer (IC) of the muscularis externa is visible in the lower left. (×40) (B) This is another micrograph of the colon. It is included because it might be confused with stomach, with the gaps near the surface (arrows) being mistaken for gastric pits and the crypts being mistaken for gastric glands. But, notice crypts are nowhere near as dense in the lamina propria as gastric glands. One might also confuse this with small intestine, with the gaps at the surface being mistaken for intervillous spaces, but that would make the villi exceptionally short. (×130)

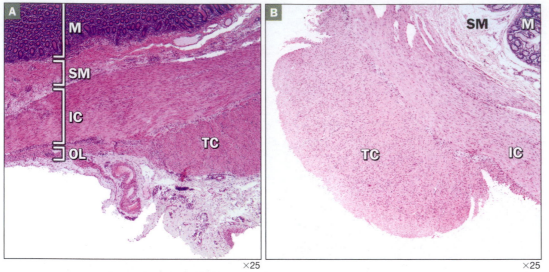

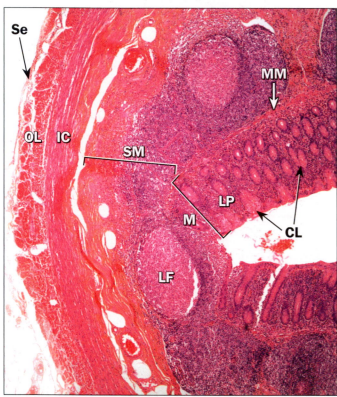

14-32 **Taenia Coli Muscles** ▪ The longitudinal layer of the muscularis externa in the colon is thicker in three strips called taenia (teniae) coli muscles (TC). As evidenced by these micrographs, the taeniae coli are not exceptionally thick for the outer longitudinal muscle layer (OL). It is the thin regions between them that make them prominent. Also visible are the mucosa (M), submucosa (SM), and inner circular (IC) layer of muscle. Both micrographs are ×25.

14-33 **Vermiform Appendix** ▪ Extending from the cecum is the small, tubular vermiform appendix. Structurally, it resembles the rest of the colon, with crypts (CL) in the mucosa (M), but the lamina propria (LP) and submucosa (SM) have a considerably higher density of lymphoid tissue. In this preparation, the muscularis mucosae is hardly discernable, but the inner circular (IC) and outer longitudinal (OL) layers of the muscularis externa and serosa (Se) are clear. (×40)

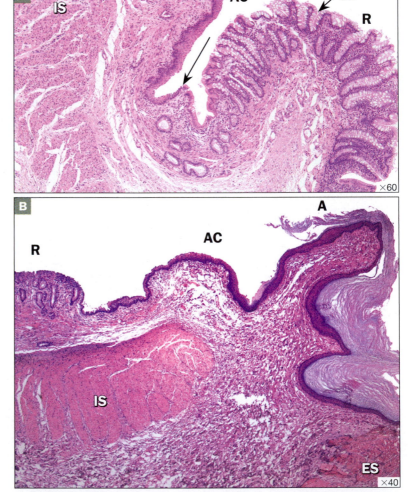

14-34 **Rectoanal Junction** ▪ Compared to the colon, the rectum has shorter crypts (CL) with more goblet cells. (**A**) For orientation, the anus would be at the top of the field, but is not in the micrograph. At the rectoanal junction (arrow), the simple columnar epithelium abruptly changes to a nonkeratinized stratified squamous epithelium in the anal canal (AC). The internal anal sphincter (IS) is a thickening of the inner circular muscle layer. (×60) (**B**) This longitudinal section shows the transition from rectum (R), to anal canal (AC), to anus (A) (with the keratinized stratified squamous epithelium). Also visible are the internal anal sphincter (IS), which is smooth muscle, and the external anal sphincter (ES), which is skeletal muscle. (×40)

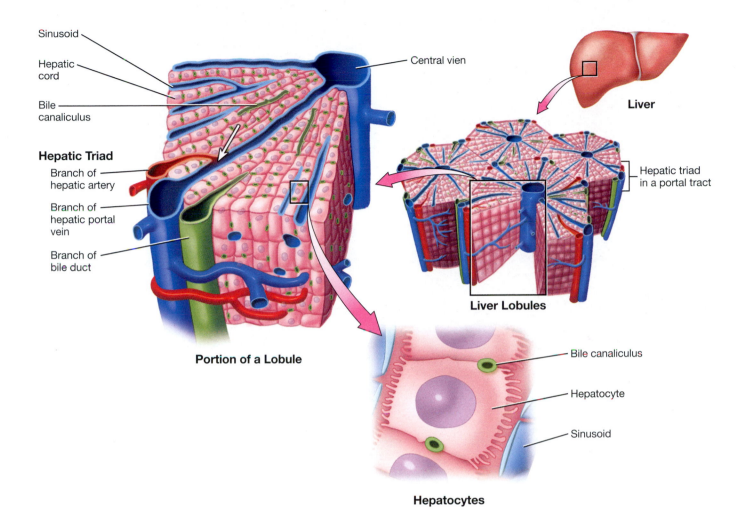

Sinusoid

Hepatic cord

Bile canaliculus

Hepatic Triad

Branch of hepatic artery

Branch of hepatic portal vein

Branch of bile duct

Portion of a Lobule

Central vien

Liver

Hepatic triad in a portal tract

Liver Lobules

Bile canaliculus

Hepatocyte

Sinusoid

Hepatocytes

14-35 **Liver Microanatomy** ■ Connective tissue divides the liver parenchyma into lobules, which are not very distinct in humans, but are the structural and functional unit of the liver (at least in the classical view—see Figure 14-40 for alternative interpretations). Each lobule is roughly hexagonal with a central vein in the middle. Radiating outward like spokes on a wheel are cords of hepatocytes, between which are blood sinusoids lined with endothelium. Branches of the hepatic artery, hepatic portal vein, and bile duct are found in the connective tissue around the lobule and are often close to its corners. These have traditionally been called a hepatic or portal triad (see pages 174–175). Unfortunately, this is a misnomer, because it ignores the presence of one or more lymphatic vessels in the grouping. Nevertheless, the terms *hepatic* and *portal triad* remain in use and emphasize the fact that the two blood supplies to the liver and the biliary duct system draining it travel and branch along the same paths. Just don't forget there are lymphatic vessels right there with them. The connective tissue region containing these vessels is called a portal tract. Blood from the hepatic artery and hepatic portal vein mixes in the sinusoids (arrow) and flows to the central vein. Bile flows to the lobule's periphery through canaliculi. Note that each bile canaliculus is formed by a space between hepatocytes, whose membranes are tightly joined to seal it.

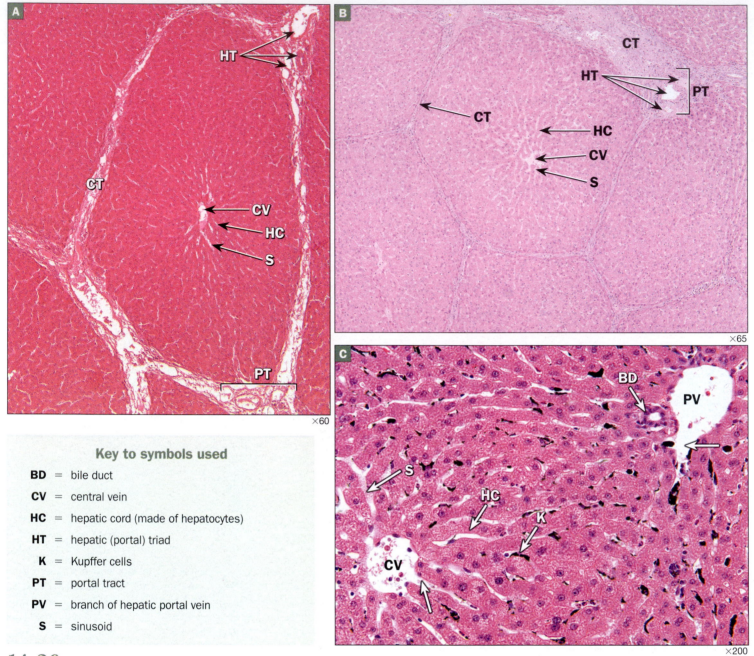

Key to symbols used

BD = bile duct

CV = central vein

HC = hepatic cord (made of hepatocytes)

HT = hepatic (portal) triad

K = Kupffer cells

PT = portal tract

PV = branch of hepatic portal vein

S = sinusoid

14-36 **Classic Liver Lobules** ■ (A) and (B) Shown are lobules from pig livers, where they are surrounded by connective tissue (CT). Magnifications are (A) ×60 and (B) ×65. (C) This is a section from a human liver and the lobules are not outlined by connective tissue. Only a portion of one lobule is shown. The portal vein can be differentiated from the central vein because of the bile duct next to the former. Note the continuity of each with sinusoids (arrows). The black splotches are phagocytic Kupffer cells (see Figure 14-37d). (×200)

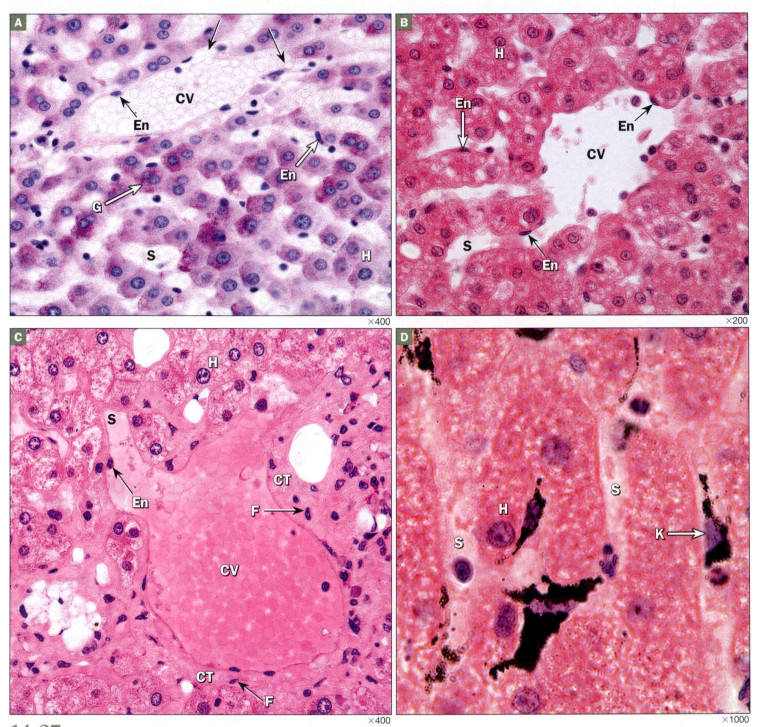

14-37 **Cells of the Liver Lobule** 🔲 Hepatocytes (H) are arranged into cords that are separated by the sinusoids (S), which carry blood to the central vein (CV). Sinusoids and the central vein are lined with flat endothelial cells (En), but the central vein has an additional layer of fibrous connective tissue (CT) in which fibroblasts (F) may be seen. Also in the sinusoids are phagocytic Kupffer cells (K). (**A**) In this preparation, a PAS + H stain was used to show glycogen (reddish-purple cytoplasmic patches—G) in the hepatocytes. Note the continuity of the sinusoid with the central vein (arrows). (×400) (**B**) In this section, the hepatocytes have a frothy appearance because glycogen and lipid were lost during preparation. (×200) (**C**) This is a thin section through the central vein. The hepatocytes have a frothy appearance because glycogen and lipid were lost during preparation. Fibroblasts can be distinguished from endothelial cells because of their deeper location. (×400) (**D**) In this specimen (and in Figure 14-36c) Kupffer cells are black because they phagocytosed carbon particles prior to specimen preparation. Along with the endothelial cells, Kupffer cells form the sinusoids' wall. Notice their irregular shape and how they project into the sinusoid lumen. (×1000)

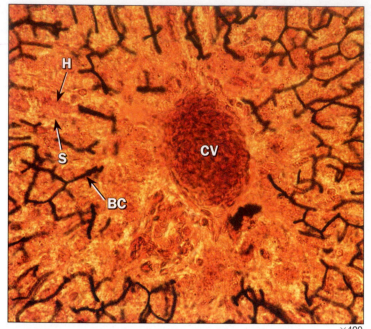

14-38 Bile Canaliculi ■ Bile production is among the many functions performed by hepatocytes. Bile canaliculi (BC) are tiny channels formed between hepatocytes that lead to a branch of the bile duct in the hepatic triad. These bile canaliculi have been injected with a black dye to make them more visible. Notice that they are only found between (or "over" in this section) hepatocytes (H, darker orange), not in the sinusoids (S, lighter orange). Normally, blood and bile don't mix. A central vein (CV) is also seen in this field. (×400)

×400

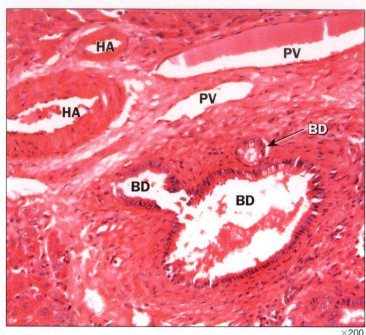

14-39 Hepatic (Portal) Triad ■ Branches of the hepatic artery (HA), hepatic portal vein (PV), and bile duct (BD) travel together throughout the liver and form a hepatic triad. Notice that the triad components are not unusual in appearance. That is, the artery is smaller and has a thicker wall than the vein, and the bile duct is lined with a simple cuboidal to columnar epithelium. This specimen was sectioned just above a branch point, so each component is represented more than once. (×200)

×200

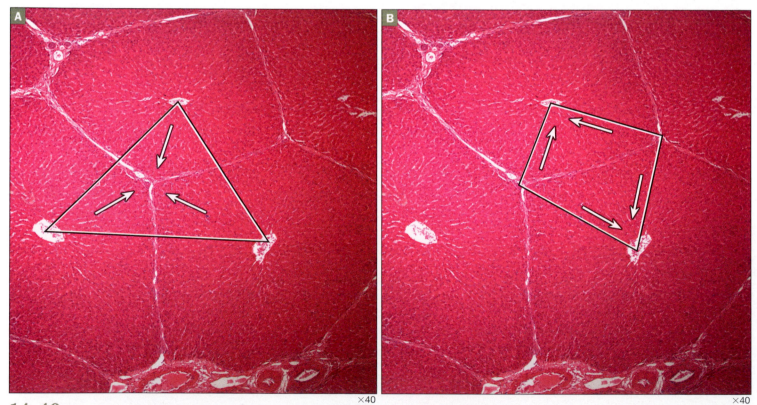

×40   ×40

14-40 Other Interpretations of Liver Lobules ■ **(A)** A portal lobule is drawn over this liver section. The portal lobule emphasizes bile drainage, with a bile duct at its center. **(B)** An acinar lobule (or portal acinus) emphasizes blood flow from the blood vessels in the portal triads toward the central veins of two adjacent classic lobules. Both micrographs are ×40.

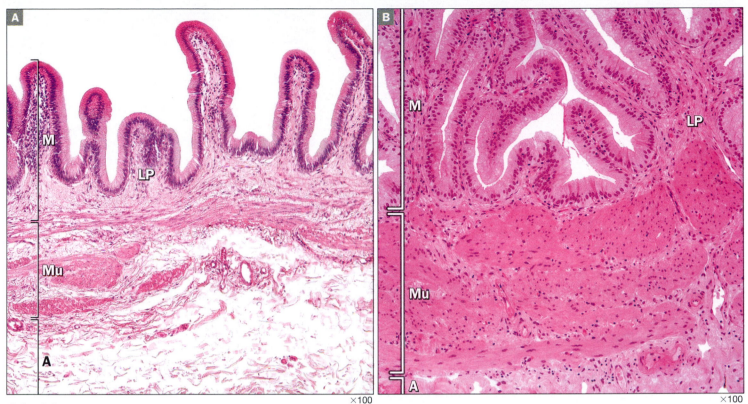

14-41 **Gallbladder** ■ The mucosa (M) of the gallbladder is folded longitudinally and is lined with a tall simple columnar epithelium with microvilli overlying a loose connective tissue lamina propria (LP). There is no muscularis mucosae or submucosa. Deep to it is the muscularis (Mu), which is made up of smooth muscle arranged into indistinct longitudinal, circular, and oblique layers. A thick adventitia (A) or serosa covers the outer surface. (**A**) This is a primate gallbladder. (×100) (**B**) This is a thin section of human gallbladder. (×100)

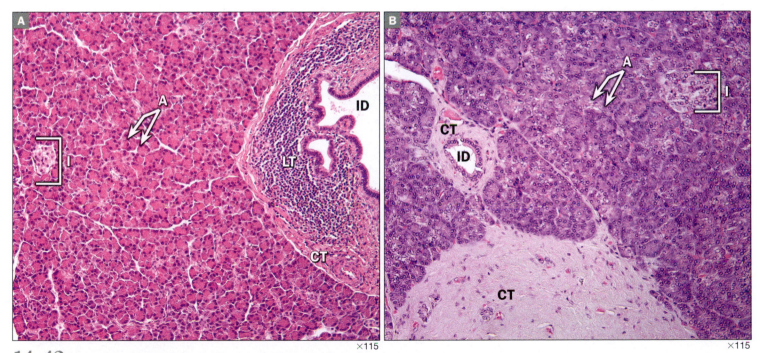

14-42 **Pancreas** ■ The pancreas has an endocrine component and an exocrine component. The endocrine islets of Langerhans (I) secrete the hormones insulin and glucagon. The exocrine pancreatic acini (A) secrete pancreatic juice, an alkaline fluid rich in enzyme precursors that will become active in the duodenum. Interlobar ducts (ID) are also present and are recognizable by the connective tissue (CT) covering. (**A**) Note the lymphatic tissue (LT) in the interlobar duct at the right. (×115) (**B**) The light-staining region at the bottom is the connective tissue of a large interlobar duct. Compare its appearance to that of the smaller interlobar duct above. (×115) Also see Figure 10-11.

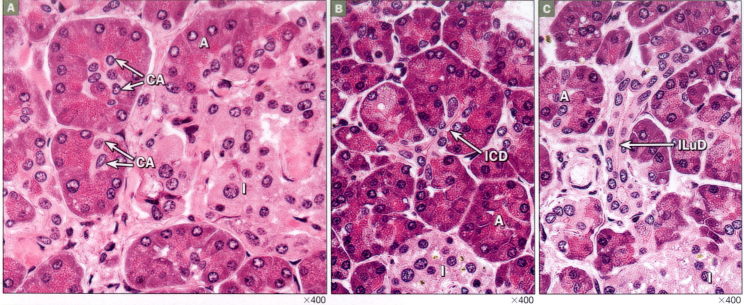

14-43 **Pancreas Detail** ■ This series of micrographs illustrates pancreatic acini (A), islets of Langerhans (I), and the duct system that delivers pancreatic juice from the acini to the duodenum. The acini are made up of enzyme-secreting serous cells and are basophilic and granular in appearance. The ducts begin with centroacinar cells (CA) that are found within the acini. These are the beginnings of intercalated ducts (ICD), that are made of squamous cells. Intercalated ducts drain into intralobular ducts (ILuD) that are composed of cuboidal epithelium and are found within pancreatic lobes. (Also see Figures 10-11 and 14-42 for an intralobular duct.) Intralobular ducts drain into interlobar ducts (ILoD) that are found in connective tissue (CT) between lobes and drain into the main or accessory pancreatic ducts, which empty into the duodenum. All specimens are thin sections and are ×400.

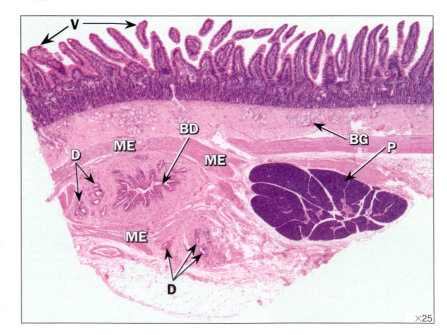

14-44 **Bile/Pancreatic Duct** ■ The common bile duct and the main pancreatic duct join within the duodenal wall and empty into the duodenum via the ampulla of Vater. Thus, pancreatic juice and bile are mixed. It is not clear whether the large duct (BD) shown is before or after the union of the common bile duct and the main pancreatic duct, but it is within the duodenal wall; note the disruption of the muscularis externa (ME). The other smaller ducts (D) complicate interpretation. Also visible in this micrograph are the pancreas (P) (note the lobes), villi (V), and Brünner's glands (BG). (×25)

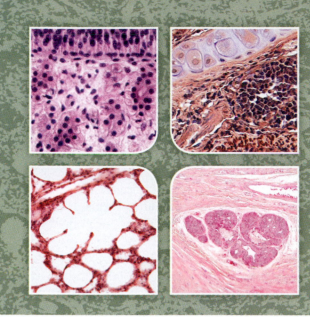

15

Respiratory System

Introduction to the Respiratory System

The respiratory system (Figure 15-1) is responsible for gas exchange between the environment and lung capillaries. Anatomically, it is divided into the **upper respiratory tract** including the nasal cavity, pharynx, and larynx, and the **lower respiratory tract** composed of the trachea, bronchial tree, and lungs. Besides conducting air, other important functions of the upper respiratory tract include warming and moistening the air to prepare it for gas exchange, filtering it to prevent infection and blockage of smaller airways, olfaction, and vocalization.

Functionally, the respiratory system is divided into a **conducting portion**, responsible for transmitting air to the lungs, and a **respiratory portion**, in which respiratory gas exchange occurs. The actual sites of gas exchange are called **alveoli**, microscopic sacs composed of a simple squamous epithelium and capillary-rich elastic connective tissue.

The abundant alveoli occupy the majority of lung volume, so a discussion of lung histology is primarily a discussion of alveolar anatomy. However, on a gross level, each lung is divided into lobes (three in the right lung, two in the left), which in turn are divided into segments (ten in the right lung, eight in the left). The lung's surface is covered with serous membrane called **visceral pleura** (Figure 15-2).

Nasal Cavity

The **nasal cavity** is formed from a framework of bone and cartilage with a vascular mucous membrane covering. The nasal septum divides it into right and left cavities. Just inside the **external naris** on each side is the **vestibule**, which is lined with stratified squamous epithelium and thick hairs, called **vibrissae**. These act as a coarse filter.

Most of the nasal cavity is lined by **respiratory epithelium**, a **pseudostratified ciliated columnar epithelium (PSCC)** with **goblet cells** (Figures 9-2 and 15-3). Deep to the epithelium is a very vascular **lamina propria** that also contains serous and mucous glands. Secreted mucus maintains a moist environment that humidifies the air. It also traps inhaled particles and microorganisms, which the cilia sweep to the pharynx where they are swallowed. The blood vessels of the lamina propria are responsible for providing heat to warm the air.

Olfactory epithelium (Figures 9-2 and 15-3) covers portions of the upper nasal cavity and superior conchae. It differs from typical respiratory epithelium in its thickness and lack of mucous cells. Bipolar neurons act as **olfactory receptors**, which are chemoreceptors. Taller **sustentacular (support) cells** and shorter **basal cells** are also present. Although they are difficult to differentiate in standard H&E preparations, high-percentage "guesses" can be made based on these

15-1 Respiratory System

The respiratory system consists of the lungs and the passageways that carry air into and out of them. The passageways, including the nasal cavity, pharynx, trachea, and bronchial tree, warm, filter, and moisten the air before it contacts the delicate respiratory membranes within the lungs.

Nasal cavity

Pharynx

Larynx

Trachea

Lung

Bronchus

characteristics: Sustentacular cell nuclei tend to stain dark and are located high in the epithelium (that is, near the cells' apices), whereas the nuclei of olfactory cells are located in the middle levels of the epithelium (and the centers of the cells) and frequently exhibit clearly distinct regions of hetero- and euchromatin. Basal cells are located near the basement membrane. Sustentacular cells play a role analogous to glial cells in nervous tissue by furnishing physical and metabolic support to the receptor cells. Basal cells are stem cells that divide to replace olfactory cells and sustentacular cells. **Bowman's glands** in the lamina propria produce a watery secretion that dissolves chemicals and makes them more able to bind to the receptors.

Larynx

The **larynx** is positioned between the pharynx and the trachea. It is made of a cartilagenous (mostly hyaline) framework lined with mucous membrane consisting of PSCC and a lamina propria. On its anterior and superior aspect is the **epiglottis** (Figure 15-4), which is made of a leaf-shaped elastic cartilage covered with stratified squamous epithelium over most of its surface, though the inferior laryngeal surface is covered with PSCC. It closes the opening to the larynx to prevent food from "going down the wrong pipe" when swallowing.

Within the larynx are two pairs of mucosal folds, each lined with stratified squamous epithelium (Figure 15-5). The **vestibular (ventricular, false) vocal folds,** which are not involved in sound production, are the superior pair. They form a protective cover for the **true vocal folds** (Figure 15-5), which produce sound as they vibrate as air passes by them. The space between the two vocal folds is called the **rima glottidis (glottis),** and the pockets formed between the true and false cords on each side are the laryngeal **ventricles.**

Within each true vocal fold is a **vocal ligament** and the **vocalis muscle,** which run from the thyroid cartilage to one arytenoid cartilage. Contraction of the vocalis and other muscles increase and decrease tension on the vocal folds by rotating the arytenoid cartilages to alter the pitch of the sound produced. Pitch is also affected by the length and thickness of the vocal ligaments. Sound is further modified by most parts of the throat, nasal cavity and its sinuses, and oral cavity, including teeth, tongue, hard palate, and lips.

Trachea

The **trachea** (Figure 15-6) is a tubular organ anterior to the esophagus. It begins at the junction with the larynx and continues to its bifurcation into the two **primary bronchi.** C-shaped hyaline cartilage rings, with their "open" portion oriented posteriorly toward the esophagus, provide support to keep the airway open. Fibroelastic connective tissue fills in between the cartilages to provide flexibility.

Histologically, the trachea is composed of a **mucosa,** a **submucosa,** a cartilagenous/fibromuscular layer, and an adventitia, and its structure establishes the basic plan for the rest of the respiratory tree (Figure 15-7). The mucosa is composed of a typical respiratory epithelium—a tall PSCC with goblet cells—and a loose connective tissue lamina propria. The epithelium also contains enteroendocrine cells that produce a variety of hormones, and small basal stem cells. Abundant lymphatic tissue, fibroblasts, and macrophages are interspersed among the collagenous and elastic fibers of the lamina propria. The transition into the submucosa is not an abrupt one, because its fibrous connective tissue is only slightly denser than that of the lamina propria. It ends where its fibers blend with the perichondrium, or in the absence of cartilage, where it blends with the adventitia. Exocrine **seromucous glands** are found in the submucosa and produce a glycoprotein-rich secretion. Glands are most abundant in the posterior wall where the cartilage ring is open. The smooth muscle fibers of the **trachealis muscle** (Figure 15-8) run transversely between the ends of the C-shaped cartilage rings. It can regulate, to some degree, the tracheal diameter and stabilize it. The adventitia is a loose connective tissue that blends in with the surrounding connective tissues.

Bronchial Tree

The trachea branches into two **primary bronchi,** each of which goes to a lung. Once in the lung, primary bronchi divide to form **secondary (lobar) bronchi.** (From the secondary bronchi on, all branches are intrapulmonary.) There are three secondary bronchi supplying the three lobes of the right lung and two supplying the two lobes of the left lung. Secondary bronchi divide to form **tertiary (segmental) bronchi,** each of which supplies a distinct lung segment. Further branching produces, in order, **bronchioles, terminal bronchioles, respiratory bronchioles, alveolar ducts,** and **alveolar sacs.**

The general trends seen in the bronchial tree are as follows:

- The diameter of the tubes decreases;
- The epithelium as a whole gets shorter and the cells get flatter, going from a tall PSCC in the trachea to a simple squamous in the alveoli;
- There is a decrease in the size of the cartilage, going from C-shaped rings in the trachea, to more platelike in the bronchi, to absent in the bronchioles;
- There is an increase (relative to the size of the tube) in the amount of smooth muscle and elastic tissue; and
- The number of glands and goblet cells decreases.

The bronchi (Figure 15-9) resemble the trachea, but the cartilage is platelike, with the plates being found on all sides (that is, there is no open side as with the C-shaped rings). Elastic fibers are more numerous and the smooth muscle becomes organized into a complete circular layer. Seromucous glands, scattered lymphocytes, and lymph nodules are also present in the thinner lamina propria and submucosa, especially at branch points of the airways. The epithelium is PSCC that gets progressively shorter.

Bronchioles (Figures 15-10 and 15-11) are about 1 mm in diameter or less, but they are easily identified because cartilage is absent from their walls. The epithelium is generally a simple ciliated columnar in larger bronchioles that transitions into a simple ciliated cuboidal, and then to a simple nonciliated cuboidal in the smallest bronchioles. Goblet cells are only seen in the largest of bronchioles. **Clara cells** constitute the majority of epithelial cells and are identified by their dome-shaped surface, cytoplasmic secretory granules, and lack of cilia. They are mitotically active and produce a variety of chemicals, including a surfactant (that reduces surface tension in the alveoli); lysozyme, an enzyme that digests mucus; and many others. Glands are absent from the lamina propria, but lymphoid tissue is often seen. Elastic fibers and spiral layers of smooth muscle occupy a majority of the wall.

The conducting portion of the bronchial tree ends with the **terminal bronchioles.** These are less than 0.5 mm in diameter. The epithelium is a simple ciliated cuboidal with nonciliated Clara cells. Elastic fibers and only a couple of muscle layers are present.

Terminal bronchioles divide to produce **respiratory bronchioles,** which represent the beginning of the respiratory portion of the bronchial tree (Figures 15-10 and 15-12). Histologically, these resemble terminal bronchioles but are identifiable by the presence of alveoli in their walls. In the distal portion of respiratory bronchioles, cuboidal epithelial cells no longer possess cilia. Notice that cilia extend farther down the respiratory tree than mucous glands and goblet cells.

As one progresses through the respiratory bronchioles, the alveoli become more and more numerous. Eventually, the wall is exclusively alveoli and the bronchiole has become an **alveolar duct** (Figures 15-10 and 15-13). A smooth muscle cell is positioned around the opening of each alveolus, giving the appearance of knobs at the entrance of the alveolus to the alveolar duct. At the end of the alveolar duct are a few clusters of alveoli called **alveolar sacs,** which share a common opening into the duct.

Alveoli

The diameter of an alveolus is about 200 μm, and between the two lungs there are about 300 million of them with a total surface area of approximately 150 m². The extensive surface area and the thin alveolar wall make them efficient in gas exchange with the blood. They also account for the spongy consistency of the lungs on a gross level.

There are three cell types found associated with alveoli (Figure 15-14). These are the type I pneumocytes, type II pneumocytes, and alveolar macrophages (dust cells). The majority of alveolar surface (> 90%) is covered by the simple squamous **type I pneumocytes,** although they comprise less than half of the alveolar cells. They are thin, even by squamous standards, having a thickness of as little as 80 nm. Their nuclei are infrequently seen in sectioned specimens because of the cells' extensive cytoplasm.

Type II pneumocytes (great alveolar cells) are cuboidal with a rounded apical surface and a central nucleus. They secrete surfactant that reduces surface tension and prevents the alveoli from collapsing during expiration.

Alveolar macrophages are often seen in the alveolar wall or lumen. They are derived from blood monocytes and phagocytose small particles that have slipped past the other defenses.

The **interalveolar septum** is composed of the epithelium of two alveoli separated by connective tissue containing numerous capillaries supported by elastic and collagen fibers. Tiny openings called **alveolar pores** join adjacent alveoli through the septum and allow pressure equalization within the various lung compartments. The actual **blood-air barrier** is composed of the type I pneumocytes and capillary endothelium, plus their fused basal laminae. Oxygen and carbon dioxide must diffuse through these layers during gas exchange between the air and blood.

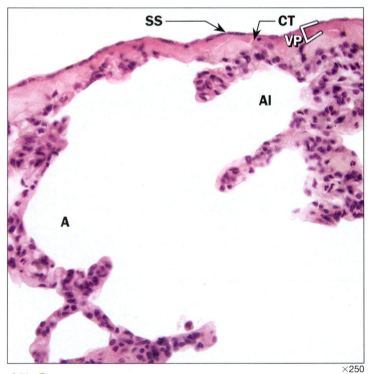

×250

15-2 Visceral Pleura ■ The outer surface of the lungs is covered with a serous membrane known as visceral pleura (VP). It consists of a simple squamous mesothelium (SS) and underlying connective tissue (CT). Pulmonary alveoli (AI) are seen deep to the pleura. (×250)

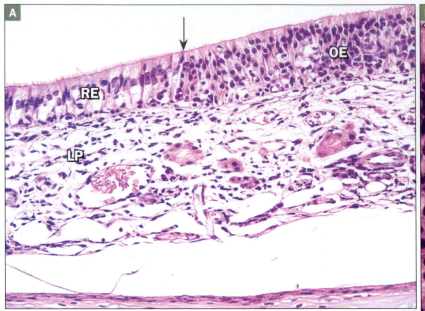

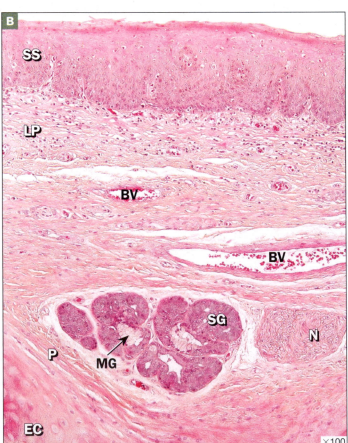

15-3 Nasal Epithelium ▪ **(A)** Respiratory epithelium (RE) is a PSCC with goblet cells. It lines most of the nasal cavity as well as the trachea and bronchi. In the superior portion of the nasal cavity, the typical respiratory epithelium is replaced by olfactory epithelium (OE), identifiable by its thickness and lack of goblet cells. An arrow marks the junction of the two epithelia. The vascular lamina propria (LP) is deep to the epithelium. (×230) **(B)** Cells within olfactory epithelium can be identified with reasonable certainty. Darker-staining nuclei located high in the epithelium are typical of sustentacular cells (SC). Olfactory cell nuclei (OC) are located in the middle and their nuclei generally exhibit regions of hetero- and euchromatin. Short basal cells (BC) are located near the basement membrane. Also seen in this section are Bowman's glands (BG), olfactory nerves (ON), and the layer of olfactory hairs (OH) and mucus. Also see Figure 9-2. (×340)

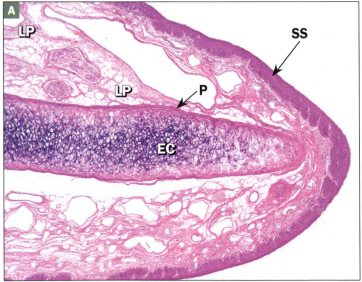

15-4 Epiglottis ▪ **(A)** The epiglottis projects over the larynx and prevents food from going down it during swallowing. (This is accomplished primarily by the larynx being elevated to the epiglottis by muscles during swallowing. Feel for yourself!) The superior and anterior portion is lined with nonkeratinized stratified squamous epithelium (SS), as shown here. Internally, there is a leaf-shaped piece of elastic cartilage (EC) surrounded by a perichondrium (P), which blends with the lamina propria (LP). (×20) **(B)** Visible are the stratified squamous epithelium (SS), lamina propria (LP), blood vessels (BV), mixed mucous (MG) and serous glands (SG), a nerve (N), and elastic cartilage (EC) with its perichondrium (P). (×100)

15-5 Larynx ■ **(A)** The larynx is made up of a framework of cartilage lined with mucous membrane. Fibroelastic connective tissue (FCT) and skeletal muscles (SkM) are also present. In this frontal section of a cat larynx, the thyroid (TC) and cricoid (CC) hyaline cartilages are seen, as is the elastic cartilage of the epiglottis (E). The hyoid bone (HB) has yet to ossify and is still hyaline cartilage. On the left, the vestibular (ventricular, or false vocal) fold (VeF), true vocal fold (VoF), ventricle (Vn), laryngeal tonsil (LT), and vocalis muscle (VM) are also seen. The space between the true vocal folds is the glottis (G). The space above the glottis that connects with the laryngopharynx is the vestibule (Ve) and that below it is the infraglottic cavity (IC), which leads to the trachea. (×8) **(B)** This is a higher magnification of a single true vocal fold from the right side of a similar specimen as in **(A)**, with the ventricle and glottis labeled for perspective. The stratified squamous epithelium (SS), vocalis muscle, vocal ligament (VL), and vocal cord (VC) are shown. Note that the vocalis is skeletal muscle. (×30)

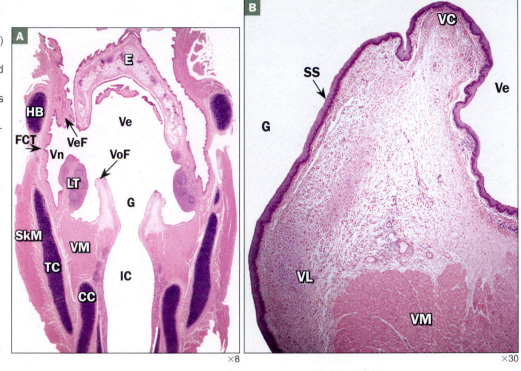

×8

×30

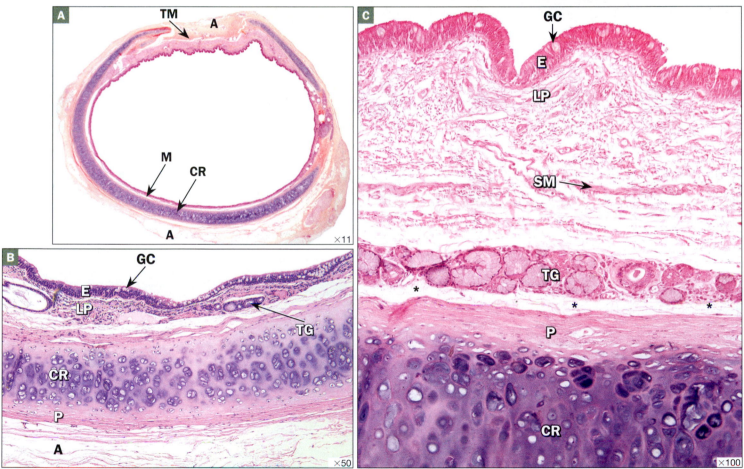

×11

×50

×100

15-6 Trachea ■ The tracheal mucosa (M) is a PSCC epithelium (E) with a loose connective tissue lamina propria (LP) that gradually blends into the submucosa (SM). Tracheal glands (TG) may be present in the submucosa. C-shaped cartilagenous rings (CR) made of hyaline cartilage and covered by a perichondrium (P) provide structural support and are found in the fibrous adventitia (A). The rings are positioned with their open side toward the esophagus. The trachealis muscle (TM) joins their ends. Outside the hyaline cartilage and trachealis muscle is a fibrous adventitia (A). **(A)** The entire trachea is shown in this micrograph. The esophagus would be at the top. (×11) **(B)** In this micrograph, the light-staining goblet cells (GC) in the PSCC are just barely visible. (×50) **(C)** Mixed seromucous tracheal glands are seen in the submucosa. The space indicated by the asterisks is a preparation artifact. (×100)

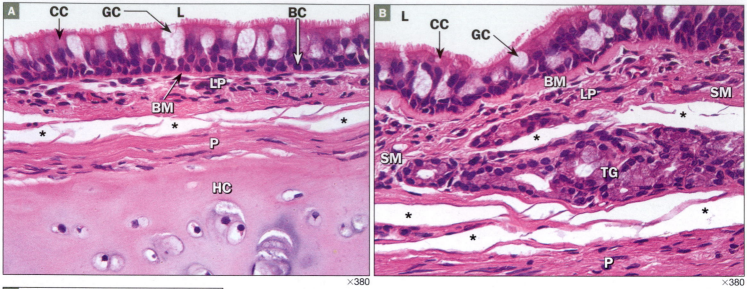

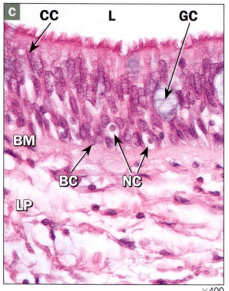

15-7 **Tracheal Mucosa** 🔲 The tracheal epithelium is a PSCC with tall ciliated cells (CC), goblet cells (GC), basal stem cells (BC), and neuroendocrine cells (NC). In these micrographs, also note the prominent basement membrane (BM), the lamina propria (LP), submucosa (SM), lumen, (L), and glands (TG). Asterisks (*) denote artifactual tears in the specimens. (**A**) In this specimen, there is very little lamina propria and submucosa separating the epithelium from the perichondrium (P) of the hyaline cartilage (HC). (×380) (**B**) This specimen has a tracheal gland in the submucosa. (×380) (**C**) In addition to the usual epithelial cells, probable neuroendocrine cells are visible in this preparation. They are located basally, have a clear cytoplasm, and are fewer in number than basal stem cells. These are provisionally identified here; usually, special staining techniques are required for positive identification. (×400)

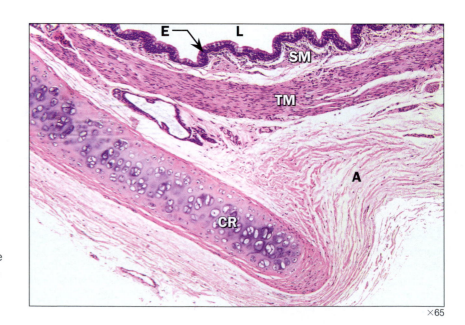

15-8 **Trachealis Muscle** 🔲 The trachealis muscle (TM) is smooth muscle located at the posterior of the trachea. The adventitia (A), hyaline cartilage ring (CR), PSCC (E), lumen (L), and submucosa (SM) are also visible. (×65)

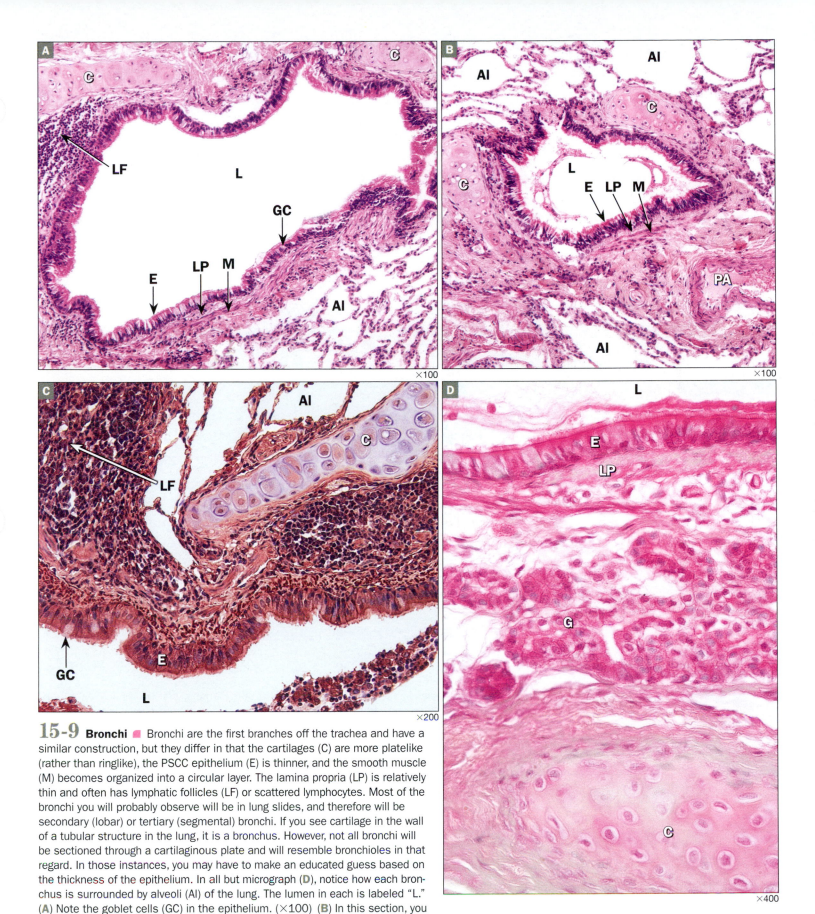

15-9 **Bronchi** ■ Bronchi are the first branches off the trachea and have a similar construction, but they differ in that the cartilages (C) are more platelike (rather than ringlike), the PSCC epithelium (E) is thinner, and the smooth muscle (M) becomes organized into a circular layer. The lamina propria (LP) is relatively thin and often has lymphatic follicles (LF) or scattered lymphocytes. Most of the bronchi you will probably observe will be in lung slides, and therefore will be secondary (lobar) or tertiary (segmental) bronchi. If you see cartilage in the wall of a tubular structure in the lung, it is a bronchus. However, not all bronchi will be sectioned through a cartilaginous plate and will resemble bronchioles in that regard. In those instances, you may have to make an educated guess based on the thickness of the epithelium. In all but micrograph (D), notice how each bronchus is surrounded by alveoli (AI) of the lung. The lumen in each is labeled "L." (A) Note the goblet cells (GC) in the epithelium. (×100) (B) In this section, you can see a branch of the pulmonary artery (PA), which typically accompanies the respiratory tree as it branches. (×100) (C) Note the goblet cells (GC) in the epithelium. (×200) (D) Here you see the layering of the bronchial wall, including submucosal glands (G). (×400)

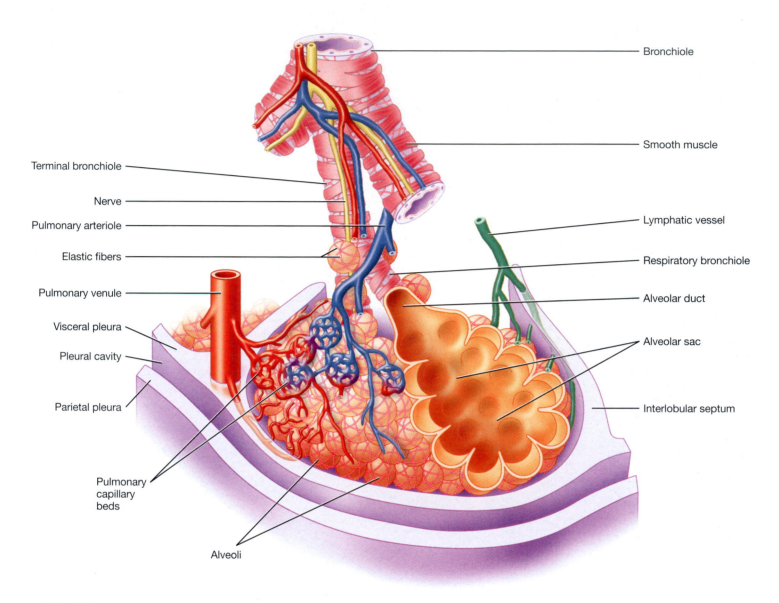

Bronchiole

Smooth muscle

Terminal bronchiole

Nerve

Pulmonary arteriole

Elastic fibers

Lymphatic vessel

Respiratory bronchiole

Pulmonary venule

Alveolar duct

Visceral pleura

Pleural cavity

Alveolar sac

Parietal pleura

Interlobular septum

Pulmonary
capillary
beds

Alveoli

15-10 **Respiratory Tree** ■ The final few branches of the respiratory tree are shown in this illustration. Terminal bronchioles represent the end of the conducting portion of the respiratory tree. Note the absence of hyaline cartilage. Beyond these, all components belong to the respiratory portion because they have alveoli and are involved in gas exchange.

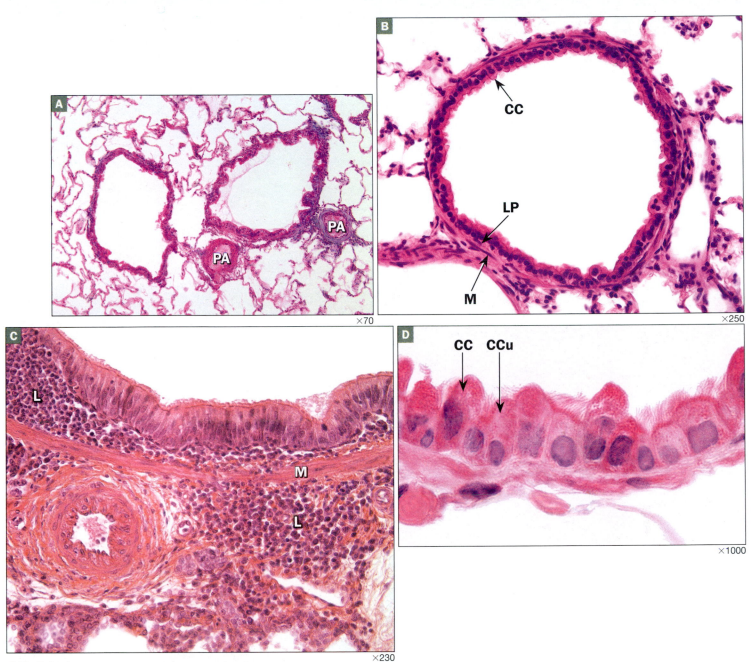

15-11 **Bronchioles** ◼ Bronchioles are only found within the lung and maintain the general appearance of the bronchi, only smaller. The absence of cartilage and, in many instances, goblet cells, distinguishes them from bronchi. The epithelium ranges from low PSCC to simple ciliated or nonciliated columnar. Smooth muscle and elastic fibers are present. (**A**) The mucosa of these bronchioles is folded, a result of the smooth muscle in the wall and the absence of cartilage. Notice the lung tissue around the bronchioles and the two branches of the pulmonary artery (PA). (×70) (**B**) This bronchiole is lined with a simple ciliated columnar epithelium with Clara cells (CC), which actually comprise the majority of cells. The remainder of the wall is a thin lamina propria (LP) and only one or two layers of smooth muscle cells (M). Notice the absence of goblet cells. (×250) (**C**) Lymphatic tissue (L) and smooth muscle (M) are seen in this bronchiole. Based on the PSCC epithelium, it can be concluded that this bronchiole is larger than the specimen in (**B**) even though only a portion of it is shown. (×230) (**D**) This is a thin section of a bronchiole showing simple ciliated cuboidal (CCu) epithelium and Clara cells (CC). Note the granular cytoplasm of the Clara cells typical of secretory cells. (×1000)

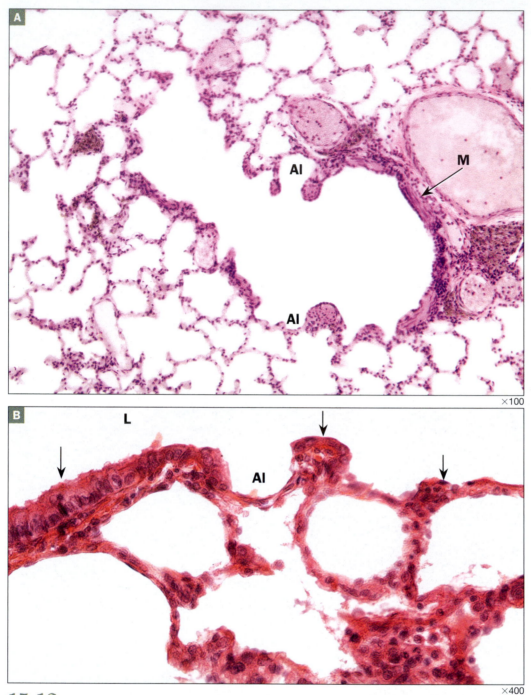

15-12 **Respiratory Bronchioles** ■ Respiratory bronchioles resemble terminal bronchioles in structure except for the alveoli (Al) in their walls. Clara cells are abundant in the simple cuboidal epithelium. Only a few of the epithelial cells are ciliated. A thin layer of smooth muscle (M) is also visible in (**A**). (**A**) Not every slide will provide longitudinal sections of respiratory bronchioles, as this one does. Patience and persistence will pay off. When you see slightly thicker regions in lung tissue, examine it carefully. It is probably a portion of a bronchiole. If it is a respiratory bronchiole, it will have thin pouches—alveoli—in it. (×100) (**B**) Only one wall of a respiratory bronchiole is shown here, with its lumen (L) at the top. Notice how its epithelium gets shorter from left to right (arrows) as it gets closer to an alveolar duct (not shown). (×400)

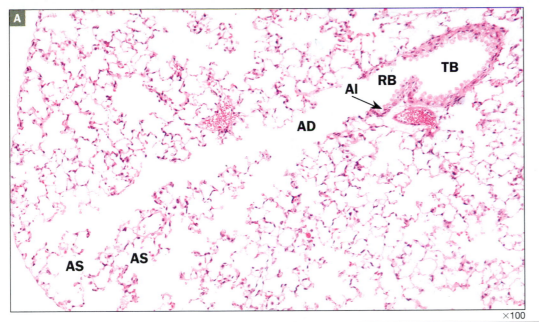

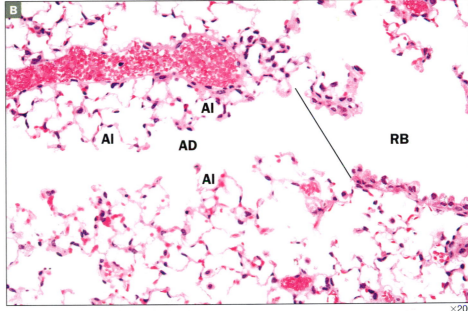

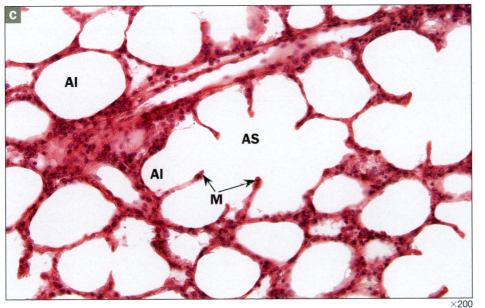

15-13 Alveolar Ducts and Alveolar Sacs

Arising from each respiratory bronchiole (RB) is an alveolar duct (AD) whose wall is made exclusively of alveoli (AI). Alveolar sacs (AS), which are clusters of alveoli that open to a common space, also branch off alveolar ducts. (**A**) This micrograph shows the airway from terminal bronchiole (TB), to respiratory bronchiole (RB), to alveolar duct (AD), to alveolar sacs (AS) cut in longitudinal section. (×100) (**B**) In this higher magnification, you can see the difference in wall thickness between respiratory bronchiole and alveolar duct. A line shows the approximate location of the transition between the two. (×200) (**C**) Most specimens are not going to show these passageways in longitudinal section. Here you see an alveolar sac cut in transverse section. Notice how the alveoli open into a common space. Smooth muscle fibers (M) produce the thickened wall at the opening of each alveolus. (×200)

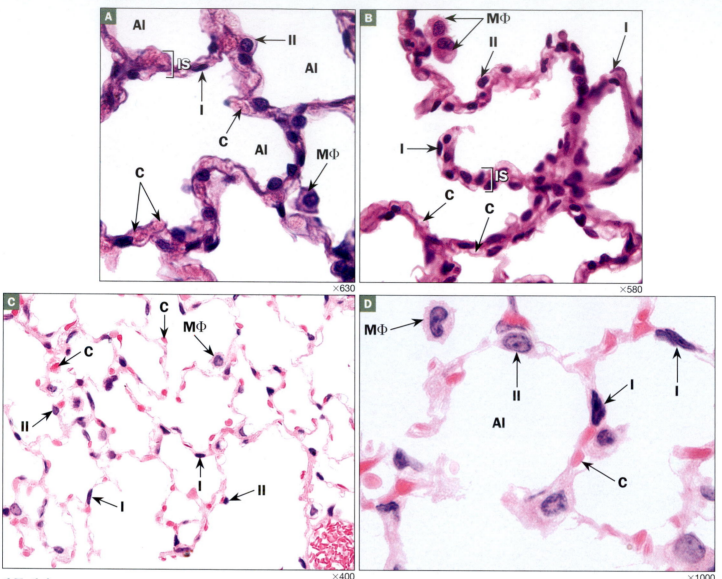

15-14 **Alveoli** (**A** and **B**) Each alveolus (Al) is mostly lined by a simple squamous epithelium that is difficult to see clearly in standard preparations such as these. More easily seen are the interalveolar septa (IS) formed from the epithelia of neighboring alveoli, plus the small amount of connective tissue with elastic and reticular fibers and capillaries (C) between them. The cells present are the simple squamous type I pneumocytes (I) and the cuboidal type II pneumocytes. The former participate in the blood-air barrier, whereas the latter produce surfactant. Alveolar macrophages (MΦ) may be seen in interalveolar septa and free in the alveolar spaces. Fine focusing through the specimen will help in identifying the cells present. Micrograph (**A**) is ×630 and (**B**) is ×580. (**C** and **D**) In these thin sections of lung, the cell types are more easily seen. Most of what you see of type I pneumocytes are their nuclei, because their cytoplasm is spread quite thin in forming blood-air barrier. Macrophages are also present. Micrograph (**C**) is ×400 and (**D**) is ×1000.

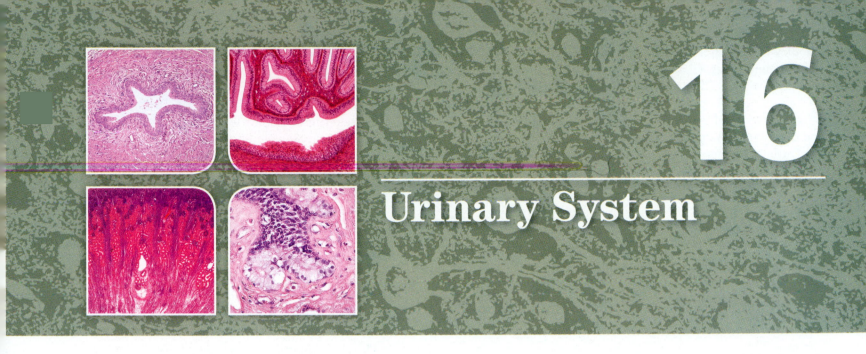

16

Urinary System

Introduction to the Urinary System

The organs of the urinary system (Figure 16-1) are the two kidneys and ureters, the urinary bladder, and the urethra. Its function is to maintain fluid and electrolyte homeostasis by filtering blood to remove wastes and excess ions, and conserve water and ions that are in short supply. It also is involved in maintaining blood pressure by adjusting blood volume.

Kidneys

Gross Anatomy

The kidneys (Figure 16-2) are paired organs that occupy the retroperitoneal region just inferior to the diaphragm on the dorsal body wall. They are kidney bean shaped (!) and the

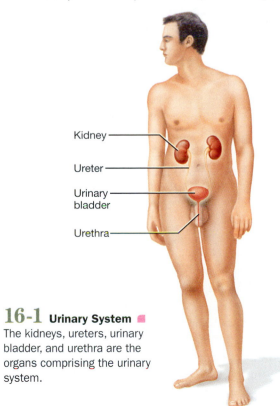

16-1 Urinary System ▪
The kidneys, ureters, urinary bladder, and urethra are the organs comprising the urinary system.

Kidney

Ureter

Urinary bladder

Urethra

indentation, called a **hilus**, faces medially. Renal blood vessels, lymphatics, and the ureter enter at the hilus. The **renal pelvis** is a dilation of the ureter's proximal end. It branches to form **major** and **minor calyces** that connect with the apices of the pyramids (see below). A dense, **fibrous capsule** covers the kidney's surface.

Internally, the kidney presents a **renal cortex** and **renal medulla**. In section, the medulla appears as 6 to 12 triangular and striated regions called **renal pyramids**, which accurately describes their three-dimensional shape. The apex of each pyramid projects into a minor calyx as a **renal papilla** and has approximately 20 openings called **papillary ducts (of Bellini)**. This forms the **area cribrosa**. The base of each pyramid is adjacent to the cortex. The cortex has a granular appearance and occupies the outer portion of the kidney, forming the **cortical arch**. Thin extensions of medullary tissue into the cortical arch are called **medullary rays**. **Cortical columns** are found between the pyramids.

Uriniferous Tubules

Uriniferous tubules constitute the functional units of the kidneys. Each tubule is composed of a **nephron** and a short **collecting tubule**, which empties into a collecting duct shared by many nephrons. Collecting ducts converge to form the ducts of Bellini.

There are approximately 1 million to 1.3 million nephrons in each kidney. Each nephron consists of a **renal corpuscle** (Bowman's capsule and glomerulus—see page 212), proximal convoluted tubule, loop of Henle, and distal convoluted tubule (Figure 16-3). **Cortical nephrons** are located in the cortex, with their loops of Henle barely penetrating the medulla. **Juxtamedullary nephrons** are located near the junction of the cortex and medulla. They have long loops of Henle that penetrate deep into the medulla.

The oval renal corpuscles (Figure 16-4) are the site of blood filtration. They are located in the cortex and are quite complex in structure. Each is composed of a capillary tuft called a **glomerulus**, which is surrounded by a **Bowman's capsule**. The glomerular capillaries are fenestrated capillaries (Figure 12-2) with openings up to 100 nm in diameter. A three-layered **basal lamina** is deep to the endothelial cells and contributes to the filtration barrier.

During development, the glomerulus pushes into the dilated and spherical Bowman's capsule at the proximal end of the nephron, not unlike a fist pushing into a deflated playground ball and collapsing it upon itself. This establishes the **vascular pole** of the renal corpuscle. The outer layer of Bowman's capsule, the **parietal layer**, is a simple squamous epithelium. The inner layer, which is in contact with the glomerular capillaries, is called the **visceral layer** and is composed of cells called **podocytes** (Figure 16-5). Podocyte processes, called **pedicels**, wrap around the glomerular capillaries, but leave small gaps about 25 nm wide called **filtration slits**.

Blood enters the glomerulus through the **afferent arteriole** and leaves through the **efferent arteriole**, both of which penetrate the renal corpuscle at its vascular pole (Figures 16-3 and 16-6). The afferent arteriole is larger than the efferent arteriole, resulting in resistance to blood flow. The pressure produced by this size difference forces fluid and smaller molecules from the blood through the filtration slits and basal lamina, and into the interior of Bowman's capsule, **Bowman's space**. The fluid is called **glomerular ultrafiltrate**. In healthy kidneys, blood cells and large molecules are absent from the ultrafiltrate.

Intraglomerular mesangial cells are associated with the glomerulus and are phagocytic in function. Their primary role is to remove molecules trapped on the basal lamina that would impede filtration if they weren't removed. They are also contractile and adjust blood flow through the glomerulus. **Extraglomerular mesangial cells** are located at the vascular pole.

Emerging from the **urinary pole** of the renal corpuscle is the **proximal convoluted tubule (pars convoluta)**, whose lumen is continuous with Bowman's space (Figure 16-7). The epithelium is simple cuboidal with a brush border and a prominent basal lamina, demonstrable with a PAS stain. In most paraffin preparations, the lumen is closed. Juxtamedullary nephrons have two parts to the proximal tubule: the tortuous proximal convoluted tubule in the cortex, and the **proximal straight tubule (pars recta)**[1] in medullary rays. Up to 80% of the sodium, chloride, and water is reabsorbed from the ultrafiltrate in the proximal tubule and returned to the blood, as are all the glucose and amino acids.

The **descending thin segment of Henle's loop** is a continuation of the proximal straight tubule (Figure 16-8). It passes into the medulla where it makes a hairpin turn called **Henle's loop**, and continues back to the cortex as the **ascending thin segment of Henle's loop**. All parts are lined with a simple squamous epithelium. The thin limbs resemble capillaries (which are also present—see page 213) except for the absence of red blood cells and their thicker epithelial cells with less-dense-staining nuclei. The ascending thin segment then becomes the **distal straight tubule**.

Henle's loop is involved in a **countercurrent multiplier mechanism** for concentration of the urine; it establishes the range of osmolarities for final urine concentration. This is accomplished, in part, by differences in permeability to water of the descending and ascending limbs, with the former being permeable and the latter being impermeable. Thus, the filtrate at the base of the loop is more concentrated than when it entered the PCT. In addition, the descending limb is relatively impermeable to sodium and chloride ions, whereas the ascending limb actively transports sodium and chloride ions into the interstitial fluid, making the filtrate more and more dilute as it passes upward toward the cortex. The overall workings of this countercurrent multiplier mechanism are beyond the scope of this book, but the bottom line is that the filtrate and interstitial fluid is most concentrated at the tip of Henle's loop, and this sets the maximum urine concentration that can be produced. For a complete description, the reader is referred to a general physiology text.

The distal tubule is composed of the **distal straight tubule**, or **pars recta**, the **macula densa**, and the **distal convoluted tubule**, or **pars convoluta**. A simple cuboidal epithelium lacking a brush border lines the distal tubule, which is in the cortex (Figure 16-9). The distal tubule passes between its own afferent and efferent arterioles. This portion is called the macula densa and is characterized by narrower cells. The distal convoluted tubule is less tortuous and shorter than its proximal counterpart (and therefore less abundant in sections of renal cortex). The cells are paler staining with round, apical nuclei and prominent nucleoli, and the lumen is typically open. The distal tubule is impermeable to water and urea, which contributes to the mechanism of urine concentration. In addition, a sodium-potassium pump reclaims sodium from the urine in response to the hormone aldosterone from the adrenal cortex, and excess hydrogen and potassium ions are pumped into the lumen.

The **juxtaglomerular (JG) apparatus** (Figure 16-10) is formed from the macula densa, **juxtaglomerular (JG) cells** in the tunica media of the afferent arteriole (and sometimes the efferent arteriole), and the extraglomerular mesangial cells. The basal lamina is absent from the macula densa cells, so they are in direct contact with the JG cells. The JG apparatus is involved in maintaining blood pressure via two separate mechanisms. First, if the macula densa cells detect a low sodium concentration in the filtrate, they cause dilation of

---

[1] Terminology for the loop of Henle is potentially confusing. Some authors refer to its parts as the thick and thin segments of the descending limb and the thin and thick segments of the ascending limb. Other authors refer to the thick segments as the proximal straight tubule and distal straight tubule, respectively.

the afferent arteriole, which increases intraglomerular pressure. Second, they stimulate the JG cells to release **renin** into the blood. Renin activates the **angiotensin system**, which causes vasoconstriction and increases blood pressure. It also stimulates the adrenal cortex to release **aldosterone**, resulting in greater sodium resorption and an increase in blood volume, which also increases blood pressure.

The distal convoluted tubules of several nephrons empty into a **collecting duct**, which is not considered part of the nephron. **Cortical collecting ducts** have a simple cuboidal epithelium and are located in the medullary rays (Figure 16-11). They are involved in acid-base homeostasis through secretion of hydrogen ions. Cortical collecting ducts join to form **medullary collecting ducts**, which also have a simple cuboidal epithelium but are located in the pyramids. These join and form papillary ducts (of Bellini) (Figure 16-12) that empty into a minor calyx at the renal papilla and have a simple columnar epithelium. All collecting ducts are impermeable to water, but their permeability is increased in the presence of antidiuretic hormone (ADH, also known as vasopressin); the more ADH, the more water is resorbed from the tubule, and the more concentrated the urine becomes.

Renal Circulation and the Renal Interstitium

Normally, gross circulation is not in the domain of histology, but often the following blood vessels are identifiable in kidney sections. The kidneys receive approximately one-fourth of the cardiac output, a disproportionate amount considering their size, but consistent with their function as blood filters. Blood enters the kidney through the **renal artery** at the hilus. The renal artery branches into **segmental arteries, lobar arteries, interlobar arteries** (found next to the pyramids), **arcuate arteries** (found along the base of pyramids), and **interlobular arteries** (which go into the cortex between medullary rays). Several afferent arterioles branch off the interlobular arteries and empty into the glomeruli, which are drained by the efferent arterioles. **Peritubular capillaries** (associated with cortical nephrons) and **vasa recta** (associated with juxtaglomerular nephrons) arise from the efferent arteriole and form a plexus around the convoluted tubules and loop of Henle, respectively (Figure 16-13). These extensive capillary networks pick up materials that have left the renal tubule as a result of active transport, osmosis, or diffusion. Thus, useful materials that left the blood as ultrafiltrate are returned to the blood.

Arcuate veins drain the capillary networks. The veins leading out of the kidney follow the arteries coming in, and have the same names (with the exception of lobar and segmental veins, which are absent).

All blood vessels in the kidney are found in the **renal interstitium**, the region between the tubules. It is composed of a small amount of fibrous connective tissue with fibroblasts, macrophages, and interstitial cells.

Calyces and Renal Pelvis

Each renal papilla projects into a minor calyx. Minor calyces combine to form three or four major calyces, which in turn empty into the renal pelvis. All are lined with a transitional epithelium and lamina propria. A thin, smooth muscle layer is deep to the lamina propria and is responsible for moving urine toward the ureters.

Ureters

The ureters are 25 to 30 cm long and 4 mm in diameter. They are retroperitoneal, passing along the dorsal body wall until they enter the posterior and inferior aspect of the urinary bladder. Each is composed of three layers: mucosa, muscularis, and adventitia (Figure 16-14).

The **mucosa** is made of a transitional epithelium and a moderately dense irregular connective tissue in the **lamina propria**. Deep to this is the **muscularis** made up of two smooth muscle layers: an inner **longitudinal layer** and an **outer circular layer**. Note that the arrangement is just the opposite of the muscularis layers in the digestive tube, but the function is the same, that is, peristalsis. In the distal third of the ureter, an additional layer of longitudinal muscle is added on the surface of the circular layer. The outermost layer is the fibrous **adventitia**, which blends with the renal capsule and the adventitia of the urinary bladder.

Urinary Bladder

The **urinary bladder** stores urine until micturition. A smooth, triangular region called the **trigone** is formed where the two ureters enter and the urethra leaves.

There are three layers in the urinary bladder wall (Figure 16-15). These are the mucosa, muscularis, and adventitia or serosa. The **mucosa** consists of a transitional epithelium and a connective tissue **lamina propria,** which are seen as two distinct layers with the more superficial being more dense. The epithelium is an osmotic barrier, preventing water from the bladder's wall entering the hyperosmotic urine. In the empty bladder, the mucosa demonstrates nonpermanent folds called **rugae** (except at the trigone). These flatten as the bladder fills.

Three loosely organized layers of smooth muscle form the **muscularis (detrusor muscle)**. These correspond to the layers seen in the distal ureter. That is, an **inner longitudinal layer, middle circular layer,** and an **outer longitudinal layer,** but these are often difficult to identify. The circular layer is thicker at the **internal urethral orifice** where it forms the **internal urinary sphincter**. A dense irregular connective tissue comprises the **adventitia**, which covers most of the organ. The superior aspect of the bladder is covered with a **serosa,** the parietal peritoneum.

Urethra

The **urethra** carries urine from the bladder to the external environment. As the urethra penetrates the **urogenital diaphragm** a ring of skeletal muscle acts as the voluntary **external urinary sphincter**.

The **female urethra** (Figure 16-16) is about 3 to 5 cm long and 6 mm in diameter and the **external urethral orifice** opens into the **vestibule of the vagina**. The **mucosa** presents longitudinal folds and is mostly lined with nonkeratinized stratified squamous epithelium with transitional epithelium at the proximal end and occasional patches of pseudostratified columnar epithelium. **Paraurethral glands (of Littré)**, found in the **lamina propria**, secrete mucus to lubricate the mucosa. An **inner longitudinal layer** and an **outer circular layer** of smooth muscle comprise the **muscularis**. The muscularis is surrounded by skeletal muscle at the external urinary sphincter.

The **male urethra** (Figure 16-17) is longer than the female urethra, being up to 20 cm in length. It is divided into three segments based on location. These are the prostatic urethra, membranous urethra, and spongy (penile) urethra.

The **prostatic urethra**, lined with transitional epithelium, passes through the prostate gland. The microscopic prostatic ducts and the two ejaculatory ducts empty into it. The **membranous urethra** passes through the urogenital diaphragm. Its epithelium is stratified columnar with occasional regions of pseudostratified columnar. This segment is the site of the external urinary sphincter. The **spongy (penile) urethra** passes through the **corpus spongiosum** of the penis and leads to the **external urethral orifice** at the end of the **glans penis**. Most of its length is lined with stratified or pseudostratified columnar epithelium with stratified squamous at the orifice.

Glands of Littré are present in the lamina propria of this segment.

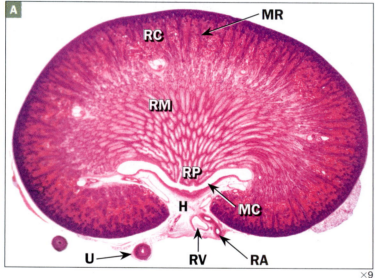

×9

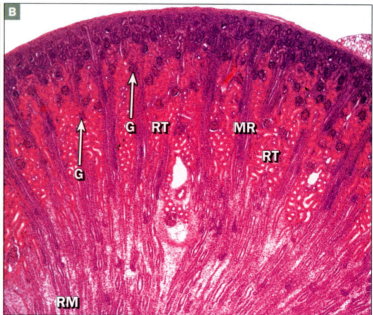

×40

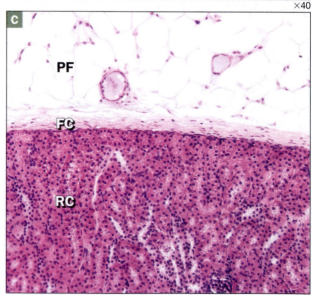

×100

16-2 **Kidney Panorama** ■ **(A)** Shown is an entire kidney from a small mammal. The renal cortex (RC), medullary rays (MR), and renal medulla (RM), composed of a single renal pyramid (humans have between 6 and 18), are visible. With only one pyramid, there is only one renal papilla (RP), which projects into the equivalent of a minor calyx (MC). Also visible at the hilus (H) are a renal vein (RV), renal arteries (RA), and the ureter (U). In a different plane of section, the ureter would show continuity with the calyx. (×9) **(B)** In this higher magnification of the specimen shown in **(A)**, glomeruli (G), and proximal and distal renal tubules (RT) are visible in the cortex. Tubules of the medullary rays and the medulla (pyramid) are seen more clearly. (×40) **(C)** Shown in this specimen is a portion of renal cortex. External to the cortex is the fibrous capsule (FC) and perirenal fat (PF), which packs around each kidney and, along with renal fascia, helps keep the kidneys in position. (×100)

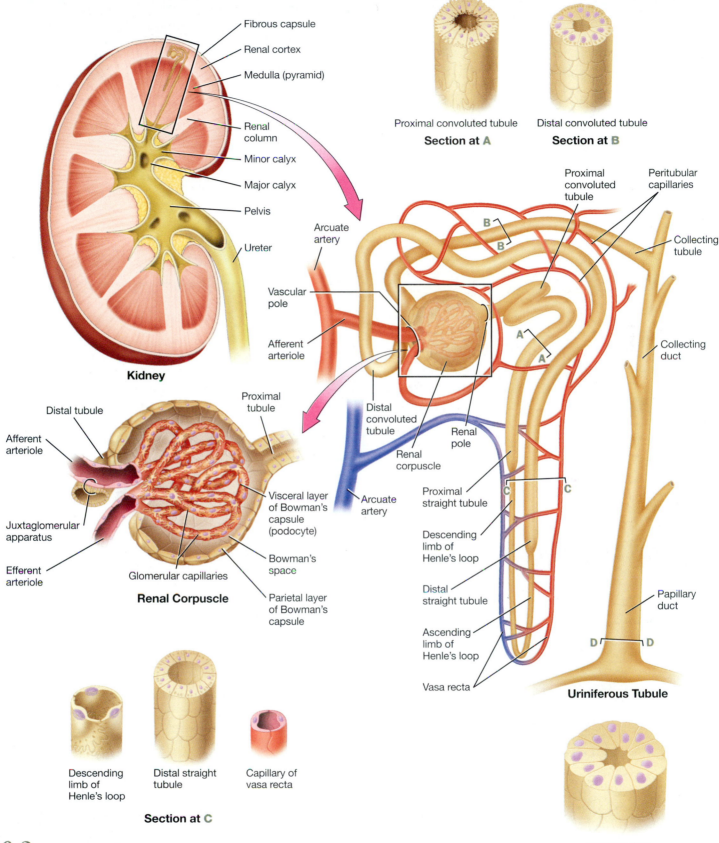

Fibrous capsule
Renal cortex
Medulla (pyramid)
Renal column
Minor calyx
Major calyx
Pelvis
Ureter

Kidney

Proximal convoluted tubule
Section at A

Distal convoluted tubule
Section at B

Proximal convoluted tubule
Peritubular capillaries
Collecting tubule
Collecting duct

Arcuate artery
Vascular pole
Afferent arteriole
Distal convoluted tubule
Renal pole
Renal corpuscle
Proximal straight tubule
Descending limb of Henle's loop
Distal straight tubule
Ascending limb of Henle's loop
Vasa recta
Papillary duct

Uriniferous Tubule

Distal tubule
Proximal tubule
Afferent arteriole
Visceral layer of Bowman's capsule (podocyte)
Juxtaglomerular apparatus
Bowman's space
Efferent arteriole
Glomerular capillaries
Parietal layer of Bowman's capsule
Arcuate artery

Renal Corpuscle

Descending limb of Henle's loop
Distal straight tubule
Capillary of vasa recta

Section at C

Papillary duct
Section at D

16-3 Gross and Microscopic Anatomy of the Kidney ◼ The two kidneys occupy a retroperitoneal position inferior to the diaphragm. Microscopically, the kidneys are made of uriniferous tubules, each of which consists of a nephron and a collecting tubule (shared by many nephrons). There are over one million nephrons in each human kidney. Glomeruli, and proximal and distal convoluted tubules are found in the cortex, whereas the loops of Henle and collecting tubules are found in the medulla (pyramids and rays).

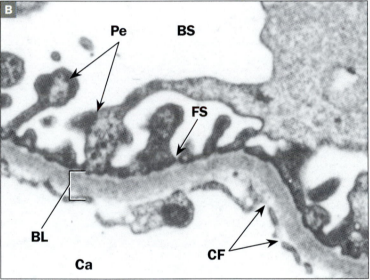

16-4 **Renal Corpuscle** ■ Renal corpuscles consist of a glomerulus (G) surrounded by a Bowman's capsule. The parietal layer of Bowman's capsule (BC) is a simple squamous epithelium and lines Bowman's space (BS). The glomerular capillaries (C), podocytes (P), and mesangial cells (M) can be difficult to sort out in some preparations, but are visible in this thin section. (×530)

×530

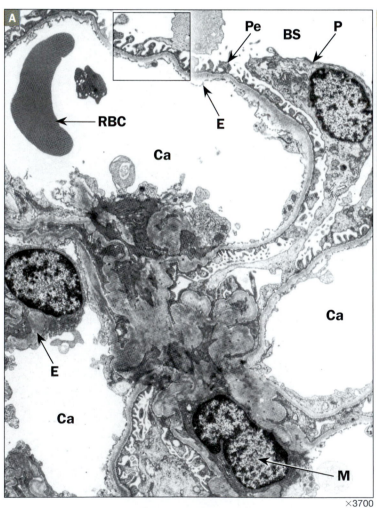

×3700

×18,500

16-5 **Electron Micrograph of a Glomerulus** ■ (**A**) Visible in this micrograph is a podocyte (P) with pedicels (Pe) on the endothelium (E) of a glomerular capillary (Ca). An RBC, a mesangial cell (M), and Bowman's space (BS) are also visible. (×3700) (**B**) This is an enlargement of the boxed area in (**A**). Capillary fenestrations (CF) and one filtration slit (FS) are visible, as is the three-layered basal lamina (BL). (×18,500)

(Courtesy of UCSD Medical Center)

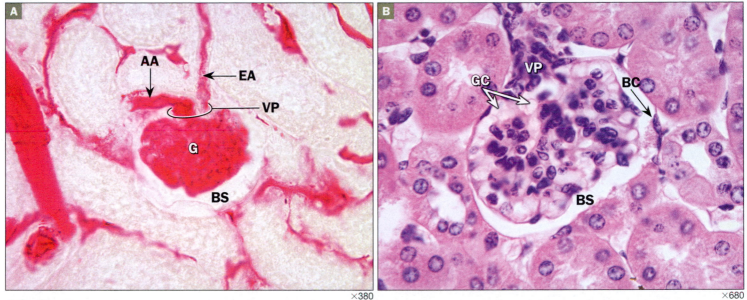

×380

×680

16-6 **Afferent and Efferent Arterioles** ▪ (**A**) In this micrograph, the blood vessels have been injected with a red dye, and the elements of a renal corpuscle vascular pole (VP) are seen. Notice the afferent arteriole (AA) has a larger diameter than the efferent arteriole (EA) emerging from the glomerulus (G). Bowman's space (BS) is also visible although the details of Bowman's capsule are not. (×380) (**B**) In standard sections, the vascular pole (VP) of the renal corpuscle is often visible, but it is difficult to distinguish between the afferent and efferent arterioles. Glomerular capillaries (GC) with blood cells and the parietal layer of Bowman's capsule (BC) are visible, however. (×680)

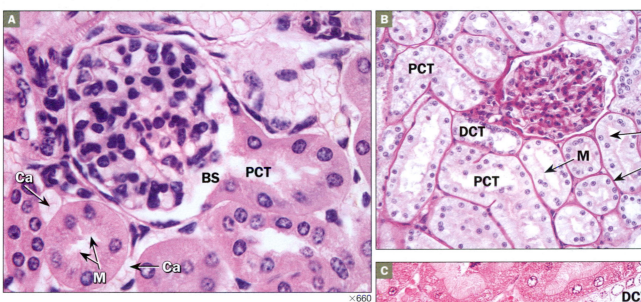

×660

×260

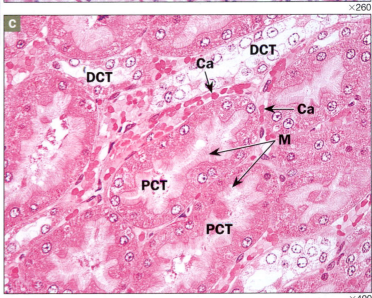

×400

16-7 **Proximal Convoluted Tubule** ▪ (**A**) The lumen of a proximal convoluted tubule (PCT) is continuous with Bowman's space (BS) at the urinary pole. Proximal tubules have a simple cuboidal epithelium with microvilli (M) (also called a brush border), barely discernible in this specimen. All the tubules in this field are proximal convoluted tubules. Note the abundant capillaries (Ca) surrounding the tubules. (×660) (**B**) In this PAS plus hematoxylin preparation, the basement membranes (BM) are prominently shown as magenta lines, as are the microvilli lining the proximal convoluted tubules. Most tubules in the cortex are proximal tubules, but a couple of distal convoluted tubules (DCT) are also identifiable in this specimen by their open lumen and lack of microvilli. (×260) (**C**) The microvilli of proximal convoluted tubules are seen in this thin section micrograph, as are capillaries and a distal convoluted tubule. Compare these to Figure 16-9. (×400)

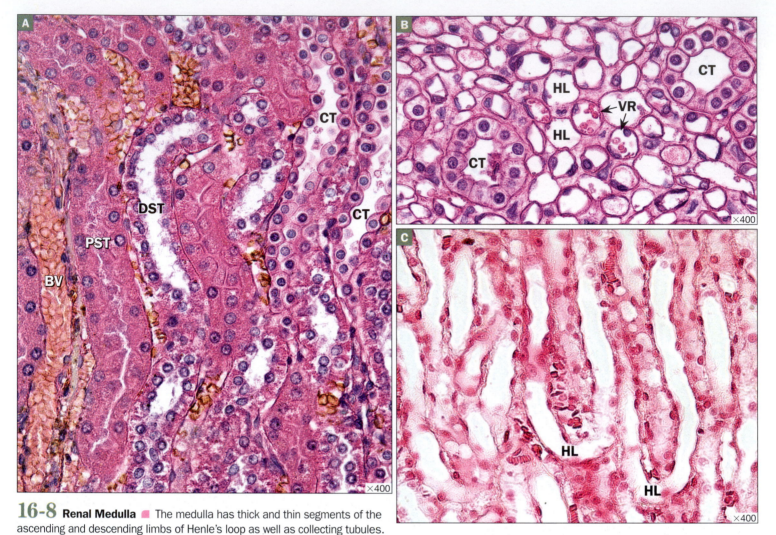

16-8 **Renal Medulla** 🟥 The medulla has thick and thin segments of the ascending and descending limbs of Henle's loop as well as collecting tubules. (Recall that thick segments of Henle's loops are also known as proximal and distal straight tubules.) Depending on where the section is made or viewed, that is, its proximity to the cortex or to the papilla or somewhere in the middle, you will see different tubules. (**A**) This is a section through the medulla near the cortex. Distal straight tubules (DST) have an open lumen with nuclei often protruding into it. Proximal straight tubules (PST) are fewer in number and their lumen is smaller because of the brush border. Don't overlook the obvious straightness of these tubules in comparison to how they look in the cortex! Least abundant are the collecting tubules (CT), which have well-defined cell boundaries and are generally lighter staining than the straight tubules. Also note the abundance of blood vessels (BV). (×400) (**B**) This is a section deeper in the medulla (closer to the papilla). Visible are collecting tubules (CT), vasa recta (VR) with RBCs, and thin segments of Henle's loops (HL). (×400) (**C**) This micrograph shows two Henle's loops (HL) in longitudinal section. Filtrate concentration is at its highest in this region of the medulla. (×400)

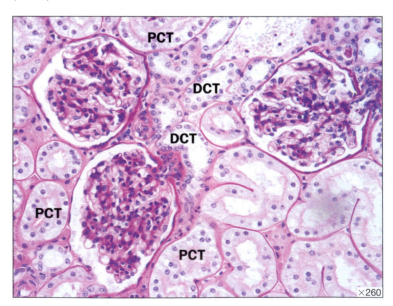

16-9 **Distal Convoluted Tubule** 🟥 Distal convoluted tubules (DCT) are shorter than proximal tubules (PCT), and so are seen less frequently in renal cortex sections. Their lumen is more open and they lack microvilli (a brush border). Compare this micrograph to Figure 16-7. (×260)

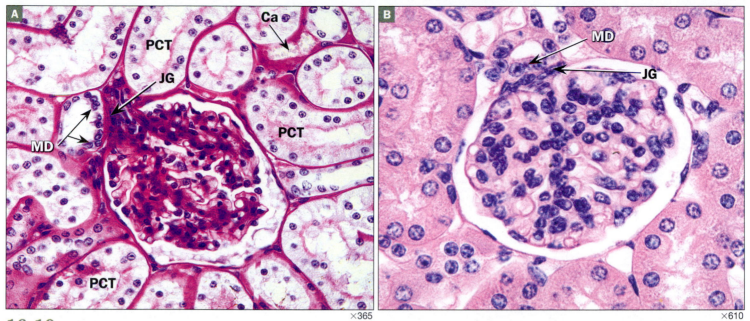

16-10 **Juxtaglomerular Apparatus** ■ The distal convoluted tubule contacts the afferent (and sometimes the efferent) arteriole at the vascular pole of its renal corpuscle to form the juxtaglomerular apparatus. The arteriole contributes juxtaglomerular cells (JG), whereas the distal tubule cells form the macula densa (MD). The macula densa cells are taller and narrower with darker-staining nuclei than the other cells of the distal tubule. (**A**) Note the abundance of proximal tubules (PCT) and the relative scarcity of distal tubules in this specimen. Also notice the capillary (Ca). (×365) (**B**) The macula densa and juxtaglomerular cells are clearly evident in this micrograph. Note that the distal tubule of the JG apparatus is the only one in the field. (×610)

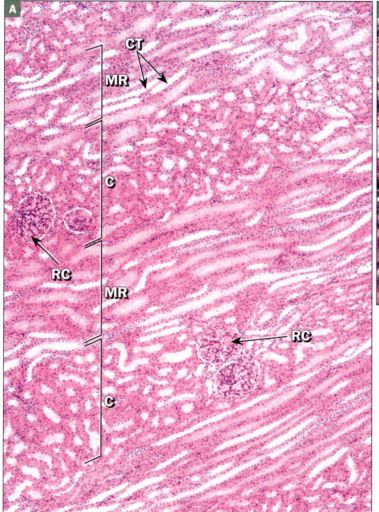

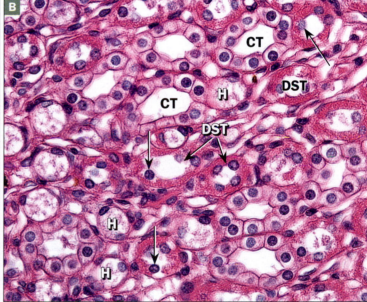

16-11 **Medullary Ray** ■ (**A**) Medullary tissue is found in the subcapsular cortex as medullary rays (MR). They are easily distinguished from the cortex (C) by the absence of renal corpuscles (RC). The rays contain cortical collecting tubules (CT), which are generally easily identified because of their distinct cell margins. (×80) (**B**) Medullary rays contain collecting tubules (CT), and proximal and distal straight tubules (DST). The straight tubules are also known as the thick segments of Henle's loop, with the PST and the DST synonymous with the descending and ascending thick segments, respectively. Nuclei of DST cells are apical in position and often protrude into the lumen (arrows). The PST are shorter than the DST and are not seen in this cross section through the medullary ray. At the level of this section, they have become descending thin segments of Henle's loops (H). (×100)

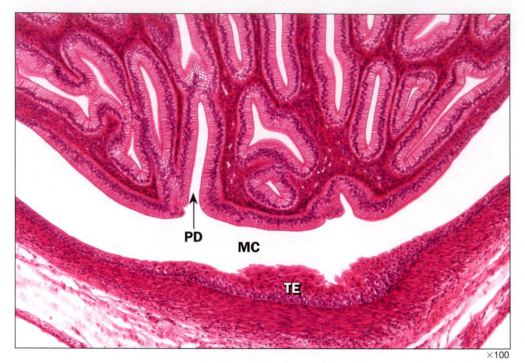

16-12 **Renal Papilla** 🟥 The medullary collecting tubules converge at the renal papilla to form papillary ducts of Bellini (PD), which are lined with simple columnar epithelium. The papilla projects into the minor calyx (MC), which is lined with transitional epithelium (TE). (×100)

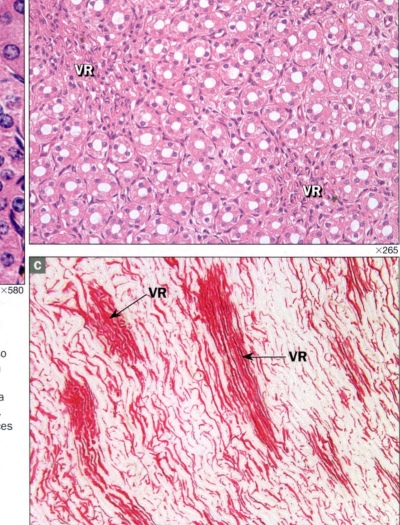

16-13 **Blood Vessels Associated with the Nephron** 🟥 (A) Peritubular capillaries (P) are found in the interstitium around proximal and distal convoluted tubules. Endothelial cell nuclei (E), the macula densa (MD), and juxtaglomerular cells (JG) of the JG apparatus are also seen in this specimen. (×580) (B) The vasa recta (VR) of the medulla near the cortex are often in bundles and are surrounded by collecting tubules, and proximal and distal straight tubules. (×265) (C) The vasa recta near the cortex are seen longitudinally in this injected specimen. The various tubule cells are not stained well, but occupy the light spaces between the injected vessels. (×65)

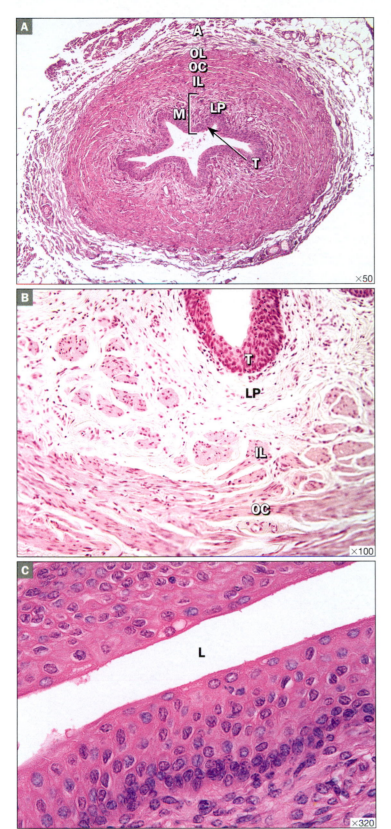

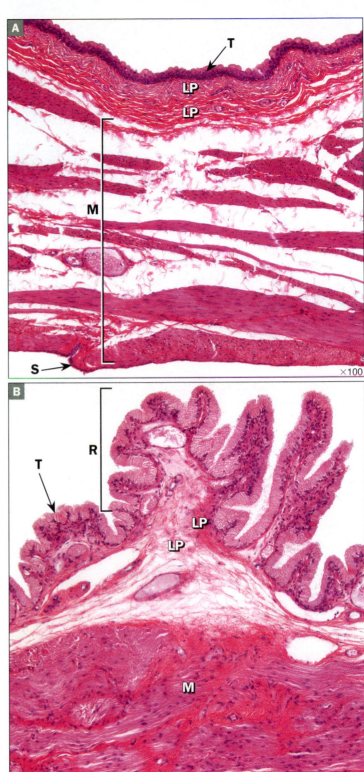

16-14 **Ureter** ■ The ureter wall consists of a mucosa (M) made of transitional epithelium (T) and a dense connective tissue lamina propria (LP). Inner longitudinal (IL) and outer circular (OC) layers of smooth muscle comprise the muscularis. On the outer surface is a fibrous adventitia (A). (**A**) In the distal third of the ureter, an outermost longitudinal (OL) layer of smooth muscle is present. (×50) (**B**) This specimen was magnified ×100. (**C**) The transitional epithelium lining the ureter's lumen (L) is clearly seen in this longitudinal section. (×320)

16-15 **Urinary Bladder** ■ Transitional epithelium (T) and a connective tissue lamina propria (LP) comprise the mucosa of the urinary bladder. In both micrographs, two layers of the lamina propria are visible, with the more superficial layer being denser. The mucosa has nonpermanent folds called rugae (R) that allow the bladder to accommodate filling with urine, as seen in (**B**). The muscularis (M) has three irregularly arranged layers of smooth muscle—called the detrusor muscle. On the outer surface is a fibrous adventitia or a serosa (S). Both micrographs are ×100.

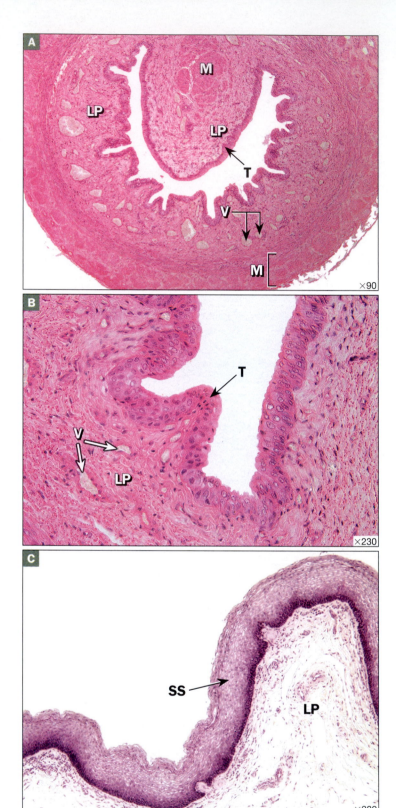

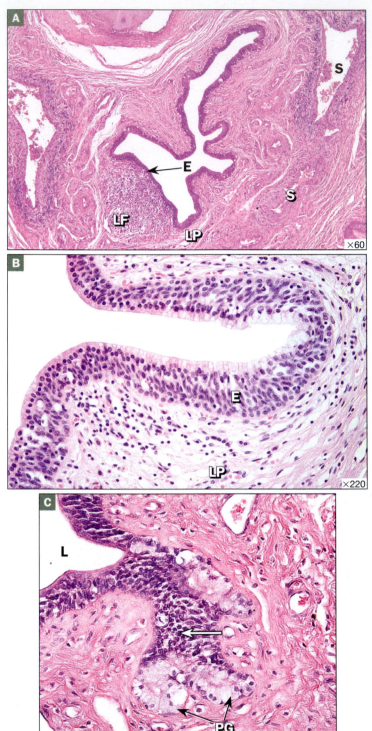

16-16 **Female Urethra** ◼ The female urethra is lined by a transitional epithelium (T) in the proximal segment and a nonkeratinized stratified squamous (SS) in the distal part. The mucosa is folded due to a highly elastic lamina propria (LP). Thin-walled veins (V) form erectile tissue similar to the corpus spongiosum of the male. Inner longitudinal and outer circular smooth muscle layers comprise the muscularis (M). (**A**) In this panoramic view, the longitudinal mucosal folds and the venous sinuses are prominent. (×90) (**B**) The transitional epithelium indicates that this section is from the proximal urethra. (×230) (**C**) This specimen illustrates the stratified squamous epithelium of the distal female urethra as well as a mucosal fold. (×280)

16-17 **Male Urethra** ◼ The male urethra consists of three segments: prostatic, membranous, and spongy. The epithelium of the prostatic urethra is transitional, but it is either stratified or pseudostratified columnar in the other two segments. These micrographs show the longest portion: the spongy urethra. A fibroelastic lamina propria (LP) and blood sinusoids (S) of the corpus spongiosum surround it. (**A**) This is a section through the penis showing the spongy urethra. A couple of lymph follicles (LF) are also visible. (×60) (**B**) The stratified columnar epithelium is shown in this section. (×220) (**C**) Small mucus paraurethral glands (PG) of Littré can be found in the lamina propria. In a different plane of section, there would be a space separating the two stratified columnar epithelial layers into which the two glands would empty their secretion (arrow). That space would also be continous with the lumen (L) in the upper left. Also see Figures 17-9 and 17-11. (×200)

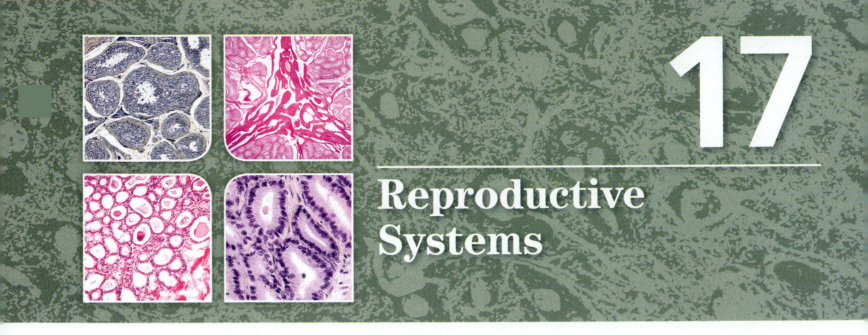

17

Reproductive Systems

:: Introduction to the Reproductive Systems

The male and female reproductive systems (Figure 17-1) are responsible for producing **gametes** (sex cells), a process known by the general term **gametogenesis**. Ova, the female gametes, are produced by **oogenesis**; whereas the male gametes, sperm, are produced by **spermatogenesis**. The organs responsible for gametogenesis are called **gonads**—ovaries in the female and testes in the male. In addition to gametogenesis, the gonads also produce sex hormones, which are necessary for reproduction as well as establishment of **morphological sex** in the male

and **secondary sex characteristics** in both males and females. Other reproductive organs include the **penis** and **vagina** for **copulation**, the **uterus** to house the developing embryo/fetus, **mammary glands** to nourish the newborn child, and a variety of **accessory glands**.

:: Male Reproductive System

The organs of the male reproductive system include the testes, epididymis, ductus (vas) deferens, ejaculatory duct, and urethra. Accessory glands include the prostate gland, seminal vesicles, and the bulbourethral glands.

Testes

The **testes** are the primary sex organs, or gonads, of the male. They develop in the abdominal cavity in utero, and then descend into the **scrotum** about the 28th week of development. In the adult, they are about 4 cm by 3 cm with a thickness of about 2.5 cm.

Each testis is almost completely covered by a double layer of peritoneum called the **tunica vaginalis** obtained from the abdominal cavity during its descent into the scrotum. As with all serous membranes, there is an outer **parietal layer** and a **visceral layer** in contact with the testicular surface. The space between is lubricated by serous fluid. Deep to the tunica vaginalis is a tough, thick, fibrous covering called the **tunica albuginea** (Figure 17-2). Deep to the tunica albuginea is a layer of vascular loose connective tissue called the **tunica vasculosa**. Fibrous extensions of the tunica albuginea form **septa** and divide each testis into about 250 **lobules**. Each testicular lobule contains up to four **seminiferous tubules**, which are responsible for spermatogenesis. The seminiferous tubules empty into the **rete testis**, a network of tubules that leads to the **ductuli efferentes**, which carry sperm to the **epididymis**, located on the posterior of the testis.

The interior of the testis is composed of seminiferous tubules and the **testosterone**-producing **interstitial cells** (of

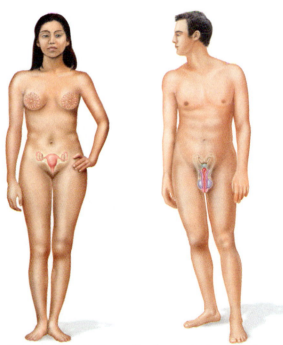

17-1 **Male and Female Reproductive Systems** ■ The gonads, ovaries in females and testes in males, are the primary sex organs in that they produce reproductive cells or gametes—eggs and sperm—necessary for creating a new individual. Other organs of the reproductive systems are involved in successful fertilization of the egg by the sperm and subsequent successful development of the fertilized egg. They include a variety of exocrine and endocrine glands, the copulatory organs, and the uterus.

Leydig), that occupy the vascular connective tissue (derived from the tunica vasculosa) between the seminiferous tubules.

Each **seminiferous tubule** is up to 70 cm long and is composed of a thin connective tissue covering called the **tunica propria** and the relatively thick **germinal (seminiferous) epithelium** with its basal lamina. Three to five layers of contractile **myoid cells** are present in the tunica propria. In addition to assisting sperm movement through the tubule, they produce the collagen fibers of the tunica propria, because fibroblasts are absent. Several layers of spermatogenic cells in various stages of meiosis, which reduces the diploid chromosome number to the haploid number, and the taller **Sertoli cells** comprise the germinal epithelium. Spermatogenesis is under either the direct or indirect control of several hormones, with **follicle stimulating hormone (FSH)** and **testosterone** being the most commonly discussed. These are summarized in Table 17.1.

Table 17-1	Hormones of Male Reproduction	
Hormone	**Source**	**Effect**
Gonadotropic releasing hormone (GnRH)	Hypothalamus	Stimulates anterior pituitary to release luteinizing hormone and follicle stimulating hormone
Luteinizing hormone (LH); also known as interstitial cell stimulating hormone in males (ICSH)	Anterior pituitary gland	Stimulates Leydig cells to produce testosterone
Follicle stimulating hormone (FSH)	Anterior pituitary gland	Stimulates Sertoli cell activity
Testosterone	Testicular interstitial (Leydig) cells	Stimulates development of male embryo. It is also responsible for development of male secondary sex characteristics, normal sperm development, and stimulation of Sertoli cells. It inhibits secretion of GnRH and LH.
Inhibin	Sertoli cells	Inhibits FSH secretion

Spermatogenic cells are the most abundant cells in the germinal epithelium (Figure 17-3). **Spermatogonial cells** are the least differentiated and are located on the basal lamina. Three subpopulations are recognized. **Type A dark spermatogonia** have a dark-staining (basophilic) nucleus with uniformly fine chromatin. Mitotic division of these cells either produces two more Type A dark cells or two **Type A pale spermatogonial cells**, which have a lighter-staining nucleus and are destined to develop into sperm cells. When Type A pale spermatogonia divide, they either produce two of the same cells, or they produce two **Type B spermatogonia**. These latter cells have a nucleolus and regions of condensed chromatin (heterochromatin) at the periphery of their nuclei. They divide mitotically to produce **primary spermatocytes**, which are pushed closer to the lumen. These are identifiable by their abundant cytoplasm and condensed chromatin in the nucleus. Primary spermatocytes undergo the first meiotic division to produce **secondary spermatocytes**, which are difficult to find because they immediately undergo the second meiotic division and produce haploid **spermatids.**

Younger spermatids are round cells with relatively light-staining, round nuclei. They nestle into pockets of Sertoli cells, which support them in their conversion into sperm cells. During **spermiogenesis**, the process of conversion to typical sperm cell morphology, the most dramatic changes in spermatids are formation of the acrosome (see below), loss of most of their cytoplasm (called a **residual body**, which is phagocytosed by the Sertoli cell), and development of a flagellum (which projects into the lumen). Mature spermatids have an elongated, dark, uniformly staining nucleus (Figure 17-3b). It takes approximately 74 days for a human spermatogonium to go through the spermatogenic process and be released into the lumen of the seminiferous tubule. Further maturation occurs in the epididymis (see page 225). Then, sperm must undergo the chemical process of **capacitation** in the female reproductive tract in order to fertilize an ovum.

Sperm cells (Figure 17-4) are composed of a **head**, a short **neck** with centrioles, a **midpiece** with mitochondria for ATP synthesis, and a **tail**, which is a flagellum. The pointed, flattened head carries the haploid nucleus and the membranous **acrosome**, which surrounds the anterior portion of the nucleus. It holds a variety of enzymes necessary for penetrating the cellular (**corona radiata**) and the noncellular (**zona pellucida**) layers surrounding the ovum. Overall, a mature sperm is approximately 60 μm long, with about 45 μm of that length being the flagellum.

Sertoli (sustentacular) cells (Figure 17-3) are columnar epithelial cells of the germinal epithelium's basal layer. They have a complex shape, with cytoplasmic extensions that course between the spermatogenic cells, but these are difficult to see with the light microscope. Most visible are their ovoid to irregularly shaped nuclei with a prominent nucleolus. Sertoli cell nuclei may be found at almost any level of the germinal epithelium.

Sertoli cells have many and varied functions, and their activities are regulated by FSH and testosterone. As stated above, Sertoli cells are responsible for nourishing spermatids during their development. They also produce a number of endocrine and exocrine secretions. One exocrine secretion delivered to the tubule's lumen is **androgen-binding protein (ABP)**, which sequesters testosterone to maintain an environment favorable to sperm development. They also secrete a nourishing fluid in which the not yet motile sperm are suspended as they leave the testes. One hormone they secrete is **inhibin**, which inhibits FSH secretion by the anterior pituitary gland. Finally, because of tight junctions between Sertoli cells, a **blood-testis barrier** is formed that prevents antibodies from entering the tubule's lumen and attacking the antigenically unique sperm cells. The barrier also prevents those same antigens from entering circulation and contacting the immune system.

A round nucleus with dispersed chromatin and one or two nucleoli, and an eosinophilic cytoplasm with lipid vacuoles characterize the **interstitial cells** (Figure 17-5). They occupy the region between seminiferous tubules and are surrounded by numerous capillaries and lymphatics, into which they secrete the male sex hormone testosterone. It is necessary for embryonic development into a male, development of secondary sex characteristics, and normal sperm development. Interstitial cell activity is under the control of **luteinizing hormone (LH)** from the anterior pituitary.

Genital Ducts

When released into the lumen by the germinal epithelium of the seminiferous tubule, sperm are not motile. They are suspended in fluid secreted by Sertoli cells and are propelled through the seminiferous tubules by contraction of the myoid cells. Eventually, they reach the short **straight tubules (tubuli recti)** and then the **rete testis**, both of which are of the same embryonic origin as the seminiferous tubules and reside within the testis. They are, therefore, referred to as **intratesticular ducts** (Figure 17-6). The straight tubules are extensions of the seminiferous tubules and are lined with Sertoli cells over most of their length, but this is replaced with simple cuboidal epithelium in their distal portion. No spermatogenic cells are present. The rete testis is located along the posterior of the testis in the **mediastinum region** and is composed of a network of tubules lined with simple cuboidal (to simple squamous) epithelium. The cells have sparse microvilli and each has a single cilium that propels the sperm and fluid. Surrounding the tubules is a vascular connective tissue.

Extratesticular genital ducts are found outside the testis and include **efferent ductules (ductuli efferentes)** and the **epididymis** (Figure 17-7). Fifteen to 20 efferent ductules receive sperm from the rete testis and deliver them to the head of the epididymis. The efferent ductules are lined by a simple ciliated columnar epithelium alternating with a simple nonciliated cuboidal epithelium, giving the surface a characteristic scalloped, or sawtooth, appearance. The ciliated cells assist the sperm in moving, whereas the nonciliated cells function to absorb the majority of fluid secreted by the seminiferous tubules. A thin, circular layer of smooth muscle also assists sperm movement.

An **epididymis** is located on the posterior of each testis. Grossly, it consists of a **head** (superior), **body**, and **tail** (inferior). Microscopically, the efferent ductules enter the head and deliver sperm to the **duct of the epididymis**, a coiled tube

up to 5 m long that occupies the body and tail. The duct is lined with a pseudostratified epithelium composed of short **basal (stem) cells** and taller **principal cells**. These columnar cells have long, branched **stereocilia** that increase surface area and continue fluid absorption begun in the efferent ductules. The circular, smooth muscle layer thickens from the head to the tail, at which point a longitudinal layer is added. The gaps between coils of the duct are filled with a connective tissue capsule, blood vessels, and lymphatics, and give the organ its gross shape. The main functions of the epididymis are storage and maturation of sperm cells. It is in the epididymis that sperm develop the ability to swim and to fertilize an ovum, though the latter becomes inhibited until capacitation.

The **ductus (vas) deferens** (Figure 17-8) is a muscular tube that carries sperm from each epididymis to the urethra. Its terminal portion, the **ampulla,** is dilated and joins with the seminal vesicle to form the **ejaculatory duct** within the prostate gland. The ejaculatory ducts empty into the prostatic urethra. The **mucosa** is folded longitudinally and is lined with a pseudostratified columnar epithelium with occasional stereocilia resting on a thin, elastic **lamina propria**. The thick **muscularis** is composed of three smooth muscle layers: **inner longitudinal, middle circular,** and **outer longitudinal**. These produce peristaltic contractions during ejaculation. Covering its surface is a loose connective tissue **adventitia.**

The **male urethra** (Figures 16-17 and 17-9) is between 15 and 20 cm long. Three segments are identifiable based on location. These are the prostatic urethra, membranous urethra, and spongy (penile) urethra. The **prostatic urethra** passes through the prostate gland and is lined with transitional epithelium. The microscopic prostatic ducts and the two ejaculatory ducts empty into it. The **membranous urethra,** lined with stratified columnar epithelium, passes through the urogenital diaphragm. This segment is the site of the **external urinary sphincter.** The **spongy (penile) urethra** is found within the **corpus spongiosum** of the penis. It is lined with stratified or pseudostratified columnar epithelium with stratified squamous at the **external urethral orifice.** Mucous glands of Littré empty into the spongy urethra.

Penis

The **penis** is a cylindrical organ that functions in urine elimination and as the male copulatory organ. It is covered with skin, which is hairless at the distal end, but has coarse hairs proximally. A loose hypodermis is also present.

Internally, three cylindrical bodies of erectile tissue run its length (Figure 17-9). These are the two dorsal **corpora cavernosa** and the ventral **corpus spongiosum,** which surrounds the **spongy urethra** and forms the glans penis, distally. A fibrous connective tissue layer called the **tunica albuginea** surrounds each cavernous body. The erectile tissue is composed of vascular spaces lined with endothelium and separated by connective tissue trabeculae. These spaces fill with blood from dilated **helicine arteries** during erection. As the cavernous bodies fill, they compress the veins draining them against the surrounding tunica albuginea and they become tumescent (swollen). Constriction of helicine arteries allows the veins to drain blood from the cavernous bodies and the penis returns to its flaccid state.

Accessory Glands

The **seminal vesicles** (Figure 17-10) are tubular glands that produce a secretion rich in fructose (the major source of energy for the sperm), prostaglandins, and other materials. The mucosa is highly folded and lined with a pseudostratified epithelium supported by a thin lamina propria. The secretory cells are tall, and shorter basal cells act as stem cells. A **muscularis** consisting of an inner circular layer and an outer longitudinal layer of smooth muscle surrounds each seminal vesicle and creates peristaltic contractions during ejaculation and forces the secretion into the ejaculatory duct. A connective tissue adventitia covers the surface. Proper functioning of the seminal vesicles is testosterone dependent.

Prostate Gland

The **prostate gland** (Figure 17-11) is about 4 cm long and 3 cm wide and is found inferior to the urinary bladder. It surrounds the proximal (prostatic) urethra and also surrounds the ejaculatory ducts. Its alkaline secretion is rich in many chemicals such as citric acid, lipids, and proteolytic enzymes, including prostate-specific antigen (PSA), which if found in elevated amounts in the blood is a good indicator of prostate cancer. Prostate function is also testosterone dependent.

A vascular dense irregular connective tissue **capsule** containing smooth muscle cells surrounds the prostate and penetrates into the gland as the **stroma**. Up to 50 tubuloalveolar glands are arranged in concentric layers around the urethra. The **mucosal glands** are found in the transitional zone, the layer next to the urethra. These are surrounded by the **submucosal glands** in the central zone and the **main glands** in the peripheral zone, which is the thickest layer. A simple to pseudostratified columnar epithelium lines them. **Prostatic concretions** (**corpora amylacea**) are often found inside the glands. They are made of calcified prostatic secretions and are of unknown function, but they do increase with age.

Semen

Semen contains only about 5% sperm cells by volume. The seminal vesicles (70%), prostate gland (25%), and bulbourethral glands (minimal) contribute the remainder of seminal fluid.

▪▪ Female Reproductive System

Female reproductive organs include the ovaries, uterus and Fallopian tubes, vagina, and breasts with mammary glands. In addition, the placenta and umbilical cord are organs of pregnancy. As with the male, the female reproductive system is under the control of many hormones. These are listed and their actions summarized in Table 17-2.

Table 17-2 Hormones of Female Reproduction		
Hormone	**Source**	**Effect**
Gonadotropic releasing hormone (GnRH)	Hypothalamus	Stimulates anterior pituitary to release luteinizing hormone and follicle stimulating hormone
Luteinizing hormone (LH)	Anterior pituitary gland	Stimulates ovulation and is necessary for growth and development of the corpus luteum. Stimulates theca lutein cells to produce an estrogen precursor and progesterone, and granulosa lutein cells to produce estrogen from the androgen precursor.
Follicle stimulating hormone (FSH)	Anterior pituitary gland	Simulates growth and development of the ovarian follicles, including promoting the conversion of androgen precursors from the theca interna cells into estrogen by the granulosa cells
Prolactin	Anterior pituitary gland	Promotes mammary gland development and milk secretion in pregnancy. Maintains corpus luteum of pregnancy.
Estrogens	Granulosa cells of ovarian follicle, granulosa lutein cells of corpus luteum, and the placenta	Stimulates growth and development of primary and secondary female sex organs. Promotes development of endometrium in proliferative phase and inhibits FSH secretion. Also involved in mammary gland development during pregnancy.
Inhibin	Follicular granulosa cells	Inhibits FSH secretion
Progesterone	Theca interna cells of ovarian follicle, theca lutein cells of corpus luteum, and the placenta	Stimulates development of the endometrium, especially in the secretory phase, and prepares mammary glands for lactation. Along with estrogen, promotes development of decidua cells of endometrium. High levels in pregnancy maintain endometrium, promote mammary gland development, and inhibit FSH.
Human chorionic gonadotropin	Syncytiotrophoblast	Maintains corpus luteum during pregnancy
Oxytocin	Posterior pituitary gland	Causes contraction of myoepithelial cells of mammary glands resulting in milk ejection; also causes contraction of uterine smooth muscle during parturition

A Photographic Atlas of Histology

Ovary

Ovaries are the female gonads (Figure 17-12). Like the testes, the ovaries have a gametogenic and an endocrine function. **Simple cuboidal germinal epithelium**, which is continuous with the mesothelium of parietal peritoneum, covers each ovary. Deep to it is the thin, dense irregular connective tissue **tunica albuginea.** The bulk of the ovary is divided into a cellular **cortex** and a loose connective tissue **medulla**, although the boundary between them is not sharp.

The **ovarian medulla** (Figure 17-12a) consists of a loose, fibrous connective tissue with large blood vessels, lymphatics, and nerves. The main cells are fibroblasts and the epithelioid **hilus cells**, which produce androgens.

Within the ovarian cortex (Figure 17-13) are developing **ovarian follicles** surrounded by a connective tissue **stroma.** The embryonic ovarian cortex becomes populated by **primordial germ cells** from the yolk sac, which then divide to become **oogonial cells.** Of the 5 million to 7 million original oogonial cells, only about 1 million become surrounded by follicle cells to form **primordial follicles** and survive to the female child's birth. The remaining cells die in a process called **atresia.** The cells derived from oogonia are called **primary oocytes** and they are suspended in prophase of meiosis I until they continue development just prior to ovulation. Only about 400,000 primordial follicles (estimates vary greatly) survive to the beginning of puberty; the remainder become atretic. Of these, most undergo atresia with only about 450 reaching full maturity during a woman's reproductive years at a rate of one per month.

Beginning with puberty and approximately every 28 days thereafter until menopause, a number of primordial follicles resume their development under the influence of follicle stimulating hormone (FSH) from the anterior pituitary. The process begins with a single layer of flat follicle cells enclosed within a basal lamina, which surrounds the primary oocyte, and ends with a mature **Graafian follicle**, though normally only one will complete the process.

The primary oocyte has a large, eccentric nucleus with one nucleolus and is approximately 25 μm in diameter. As it resumes development, it enlarges to about 100 μm and the follicle cells, now called **granulosa cells** (that form the **membrana granulosa**, also known as the **stratum granulosum**), become cuboidal and stratified to form a **multilaminar primary follicle.** The granulosa cells do not form a blood-follicle barrier analogous to the one formed by Sertoli cells in the testes. The **zona pellucida**, an amorphous glycoprotein layer, forms between the primary oocyte and the granulosa cells. In addition, the stroma immediately external to the basal lamina forms an inner vascular and cellular layer called the **theca interna**, and an outer fibrous layer called the **theca externa.** The theca externa also contains smooth muscle cells that contract during ovulation. Under the influence of FSH, the theca interna and granulosa cells produce the hormone estrogen (from an androgen precursor).

Development of a primary follicle into a **secondary follicle** involves continued proliferation of the granulosa cells and the formation of small intercellular spaces that coalesce to form the **antrum. Follicular fluid (liquor folliculi)** accumulates in the antrum. Some granulosa cells multiply and form a mound called the **cumulus oophorus.** Further development results in the layer of cells next to the zona pellucida retracting from the oocyte but remaining attached via thin cytoplasmic threads. The layer of cells surrounding the oocyte, which will be ovulated with it, is called the **corona radiata.**

Of the many secondary follicles that form each month, only one continues development into a mature Graafian follicle, which attains a size of 2.5 cm and bulges from the ovary's surface. In response to FSH and LH, the primary oocyte and the corona radiata detach and float free in the follicular fluid until ovulation. The primary oocyte completes the first meiotic division and forms a **secondary oocyte** and the **first polar body.** Most of the cytoplasm ends up in the secondary oocyte; the polar body serves its purpose by carrying the second haploid nucleus produced by meiosis I. Then, the secondary oocyte begins the second meiotic division and stops at metaphase II unless fertilized.

Ovulation is a complex process, but basically is associated with the spike of luteinizing hormone (LH), which leads to three events: increased internal pressure due to follicular fluid accumulation, enzymatic weakening and rupture of the follicle's granulosa cells near the ovarian surface, and contraction of smooth muscle fibers in the theca externa. The secondary oocyte enters the **infundibulum** of its **Fallopian tube** (see page 228) and begins its journey toward the uterus and perhaps fertilization. If fertilization does not occur within about 24 hours after ovulation, the secondary oocyte degenerates.

Meanwhile, under the influence of LH, the follicle cells remaining in the ovary fold inward on themselves and the antrum fills with blood to form a **corpus hemorrhagicum**, which then develops into a highly vascularized **corpus luteum** (Figure 17-14). The majority of corpus luteum cells are derived from the granulosa cells. These **granulosa lutein cells** are large and pale staining, and secrete progesterone, estrogens, and inhibin. As in the male, inhibin inhibits FSH production and secretion by the anterior pituitary gland. Cells derived from the theca interna cells are at the periphery and in folds of the granulosa lutein cell layer. They are smaller, fewer in number, and darker staining than the granulosa cells. They are called **theca lutein cells** and also produce progesterone and an estrogen precursor converted to estrogen by the granulosa lutein cells. Failing fertilization, this **corpus luteum of menstruation** dies and becomes replaced with fibroblasts that form scar tissue called the **corpus albicans** (Figure 17-15).

If fertilization does occur, then under the influence of human chorionic gonadotropin (HCG), the corpus luteum continues enlarging to a size of 5 cm and forms a **corpus luteum of pregnancy** (Figure 17-16), which supplies estrogen and progesterone necessary to maintain the pregnancy. The placenta assumes this function after about four to five months, but the corpus luteum continues to contribute for several months into the pregnancy.

Uterine (Fallopian) Tube

The **uterine (Fallopian) tubes** are lateral extensions from the superior portion of the uterus. There are four segments to each. These are the infundibulum, ampulla, isthmus, and intramural region. The **infundibulum** is the funnel-shaped, open end that receives the ovulated secondary oocyte from the ovary. It has fingerlike projections called **fimbriae** extending from its margin. The **ampulla** is the longest portion of the Fallopian tubes and is the usual site of fertilization. Where the ampulla becomes more constricted, it forms the **isthmus**, which leads to the **intramural region** within the uterine wall.

There are three layers in the uterine tubes (Figure 7-17). These are the mucosa, muscularis, and serosa. The **mucosa** forms longitudinal folds, which are branched in the ampulla, and is lined with a simple columnar epithelium. **Ciliated cells** sweep the oocyte and fluid formed by **nonciliated secretory (peg) cells** toward the uterus. The secretion nourishes the sperm and oocyte and assists in capacitation of the sperm, in which their membrane becomes capable of binding to the zona pellucida. Further, their flagella become more active, among many other chemical changes. Deep to the epithelium is an unremarkable **lamina propria** made of a loose connective tissue. Movement of the oocyte is also assisted by peristaltic waves produced by an **inner circular** and a thinner **outer longitudinal layer of smooth muscle**. The entire uterine tube is covered with peritoneum, which forms the **serosa**.

Uterus

The **uterus** is a pear-shaped organ, 7 cm by 4 cm, located in the pelvic cavity. There are three regions of the uterus. These are the body, fundus, and cervix. The **uterine body** is the major portion of the organ. The uterine tubes enter the superior portion of the body. The **fundus** is located superior to the entry of the uterine tubes. The **cervix** is the cylindrical portion that projects into the vagina.

The uterine wall is composed of three major layers (Figure 17-18). These are the endometrium, myometrium, and perimetrium. The **endometrium** is the uterine mucosa and is the site of **blastocyst** (the multicellular derivative of the fertilized ovum after about one week of development) implantation during pregnancy. It is lined with a simple columnar epithelium overlying a vascular **stroma** (lamina propria). Glycogen-secreting simple tubular **uterine glands** are the most distinctive feature of the endometrium. During the **proliferative (follicular) phase** of the menstrual cycle, these glands elongate and become coiled under the influence of ovarian estrogen. Coincident with this, the stroma gets thicker and more vascular. Glycogen secretion and the vascularity of the stroma both serve to support the implanted

blastocyst until the placenta forms. The **secretory (luteal) phase** begins after ovulation. During this phase the endometrium is maintained by progesterone from the corpus luteum. If no fertilization and implantation occur, progesterone levels decrease as a result of the corpus luteum dying, and the stratum functionalis (see below) is shed during menstruation.

The cyclic growth, death, and repair of the endometrium during the menstrual cycle have resulted in the recognition of three layers in it (Figures 17-19 and 17-20). The **stratum basalis** is next to the myometrium (there is no submucosa) and is relatively unchanged during the cycle. It serves as the source of new endometrium after menstruation. The thickest layer, characterized by a spongy-looking stroma, is the **stratum spongiosum**. On the surface is the thin **stratum compactum**, characterized by a denser stroma. Together, the stratum spongiosum and compactum undergo the most change during the menstrual cycle and are collectively referred to as the **stratum functionalis**. During the menstrual cycle, the endometrium varies in thickness from 1 to 6 mm.

Straight arteries and **spiral arteries** supply the endometrium. The former provide blood to the stratum basalis, whereas the latter supply the stratum functionalis. Both layers are generously supplied with capillaries and thin-walled, dilated vessels called **lacunae**. The spiral arteries constrict in the absence of progesterone (due to corpus luteum degeneration), which makes the stratum functionalis ischemic, resulting in its death and loss.

The **myometrium** (Figure 17-21) forms a continuous muscle layer with the uterine tubes and vagina. It is composed of smooth muscle in three poorly defined layers. There are inner and outer longitudinal layers with a thick circular (spiral) layer between. Muscle fibers of the nonpregnant uterus are approximately 50 μm long. During pregnancy the uterus enlarges, the wall (mostly myometrium) becomes thinner, and the muscle cells become elongated by tenfold or more.

The outer surface of the fundus and posterior body is covered with a **serosa (parietal peritoneum)**. The remainder is covered with a fibrous **adventitia**.

The **cervix** (Figure 17-22) is divided into an **endocervical canal** and an **ectocervix**, which protrudes into the vagina. The mucosa of the endocervical canal is lined by a mucous-secreting simple columnar epithelium, which also lines depressions called **endocervical glands**. While the cervical mucosa remains relatively unchanged during the menstrual cycle, the same is not true of the glands. Their mucus production increases manifold as ovulation approaches and the mucus is of a thinner consistency, which makes passage of sperm cells easier. In other parts of the cycle, the mucus is less abundant and stickier. The ectocervix resembles the vagina in that it is lined with a stratified squamous epithelium. The myometrium is mostly replaced with elastic connective tissue as an adaptation to the stretching necessary during childbirth. Lymphocytes may be seen in this layer near the surface.

A Photographic Atlas of Histology

Vagina

The **vagina** (Figure 17-23) is the female copulatory organ and serves as the birth canal. It is about 9 cm long and is lined with a **mucosa** composed of **nonkeratinized stratified squamous epithelium** and a dense, elastic **lamina propria**. Neutrophils and lymphocytes are abundant in the lamina propria. The mucosa folds when relaxed and the lumen is closed. There are no vaginal glands; cervical mucus is primarily responsible for its lubrication. Deep to the mucosa is a **muscularis** composed of an **inner circular** and a thicker **outer longitudinal layer** of smooth muscle, although they are not well defined and the fibers mix. Deep to the muscularis is a dense fibrous **adventitia**, which becomes less dense and blends in with the adventitial layers of the urinary bladder and rectum.

Breast

The **breasts** contain **mammary glands** and are responsible for producing milk (Figure 17-24). Mammary glands are present in both sexes, but under the influence of estrogen, progesterone, and prolactin (from the anterior pituitary gland) in the female, the glands develop further. The 15 to 25 **lobes** in each breast are made of independent **compound tubuloacinar glands**. A **lactiferous duct** drains the gland to a **lactiferous sinus,** which leads to the **nipple**. The glands are surrounded by adipose tissue and are separated by fibrous **septa**. The skin covering the nipple has sebaceous glands not associated with hair follicles.

During pregnancy, the mammary glands branch and grow into **alveoli**, composed of a **simple columnar epithelium** and surrounded by **myoepithelial cells**. Release of milk is under the influence of the hormone oxytocin from the posterior pituitary gland. Initially the glands produce a viscous, protein-rich substance called colostrum; within a few days after the child is born, they produce true milk.

Placenta

If fertilization occurs, the zygote undergoes mitotic cell divisions without growth between (called **cleavage divisions**) to form a solid ball of cells—the **morula**—by the third day. By this time, the morula has reached the uterine cavity. Over the next couple of days, divisions continue and produce a hollow ball of cells called a **blastocyst** composed of an outer layer of cells called the **trophoblast** and an inner mass of cells destined to become the embryo called the **embryoblast**. It is in this state between 6 and 10 days after fertilization that the blastocyst implants into the endometrium.

The **placenta** (Figures 17-25 and 17-26) is a complex organ that connects the embryo/fetus with the mother's endometrium. The fully formed placenta serves as the fetus' kidneys, lungs, and intestines. That is, it absorbs oxygen and nutrients from maternal blood and transfers metabolic wastes into it. Under normal circumstances, there is no mixing of maternal and fetal blood; no blood cells cross the **placental barrier** (see below). Maternal antibodies, however, do enter fetal circulation.

The placenta is constructed from embryonic and maternal tissues. The trophoblast next to the embryoblast becomes the embryo's contribution to the placenta, while the endometrium in this vicinity differentiates to become the **decidua basalis**, the maternal contribution. Beginning with the third month, **chorionic villi** anchor the developing embryo to the decidua basalis. In the mature placenta, the villi are branched and are not attached. Thus, **free villi** outnumber **anchoring villi**. Both types are covered with a cellular layer composed of **syncytial trophoblasts**, whose nuclei are seen to form clusters called **syncytial knots**. The core of each villus contains **fetal capillaries** (and sometimes larger vessels) and embryonic **mesoderm**. Open spaces in the decidua called **lacunae**, or **intervillous spaces**, surround the villi and contain maternal blood. Thus, the villi are bathed in maternal blood, but the syncytial trophoblasts and connective tissue form the placental barrier and prevent mixing with fetal blood.

Umbilical Cord

The **umbilical cord** (Figure 17-27) is derived from the early connecting stalk that attaches the embryo to the trophoblast layer. When fully formed, it is covered by **amniotic membrane** and is filled with a ground substance called **Wharton's jelly**, which contains mesenchymal cells. The two **umbilical arteries**, which carry oxygen-poor blood to the chorionic villi, and the single **umbilical vein**, which brings oxygen-rich blood to the fetus, are also present.

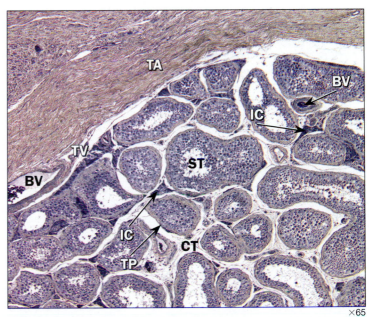

×65

17-2 **Testis** ■ In this micrograph, the fibrous tunica albuginea (TA) of the testis and a portion of a lobule are visible. Also seen are seminiferous tubules (ST) with developing sperm cells and covered with tunica propria (TP), intestinal cells (IC), loose connective tissue (CT), and a blood vessel (BV) in the tunica vasculosa (TV). (×65)

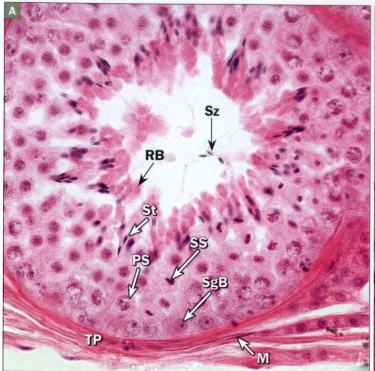

×400

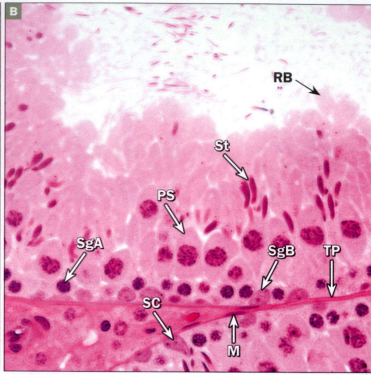

×400

17-3 **Seminiferous Tubules** ◾ Each seminiferous tubule is surrounded by a connective tissue tunica propria (TP) with contractile myoid cells (M). The seminiferous tubules are the site of sperm production (spermatogenesis), and the majority of cells in the wall are at different stages of sperm development, with the least developed cells being located at the basement lamina. As cells mature, they are pushed toward the luminal surface and are eventually released as fully formed spermatozoa, a process that takes approximately 74 days in humans. The developmental sequence of sperm cells is as follows: spermatogonia, primary spermatocytes (PS), secondary spermatocytes (SS), spermatids (St), and mature spermatozoa (Sz). Three types of spermatogonia have been described: two Type A spermatogonia (SgA), each with finely granular chromatin, and Type B spermatogonia (SgB), with distinct nucleoli and peripheral heterochromatin. Primary spermatocytes are large cells with condensed chromatin, usually in some portion of prophase I. Secondary spermatocytes are not seen in all tubules all the time because they divide and form spermatids almost immediately upon their formation. However, cells in metaphase II or anaphase II of meiosis may provisionally be identified by the meiotic figure, their location closer to the lumen, and a smaller size than primary spermatocytes. Spermatids undergo a great degree of modification as they are converted from more-or-less spherical cells into spermatozoa with a head, acrosome, midpiece, and tail projecting into the lumen. Look for the nuclei to become more darkly staining and elongated as they develop, as well as the obvious presence of the tail. As these changes occur, the cytoplasm is extruded from the spermatid to form a

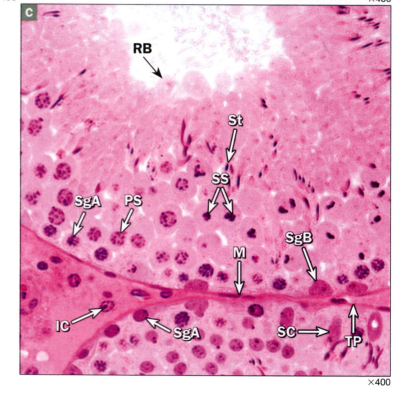

×400

residual body (RB), which is phagocytosed by the Sertoli cell (SC) that has been supporting the sperm through much of the developmental process. Sertoli cells are large and are readily recognizable by their prominent nucleoli. Interstitial cells of Leydig (IC) are located in the spaces between the tubules, as are blood vessels and lymphatics. (**A**) This is a cross section of one seminiferous tubule stained with H&E. Note how the most mature spermatids are seen in groups. This is a consequence of all cells derived from a single spermatogonium retaining cytoplasmic connections that are only broken when they are released into the tubule's lumen. (×400) (**B**) and (**C**) are thin H&E sections showing two tubules at different stages of spermatogenesis. Notice the spermatid nuclei in (**B**) are larger and don't stain as intensely as the more developed spermatid nuclei in (**C**). Also note the groupings due to cytoplasmic connections. Both are ×400. Also see Figure 17-5.

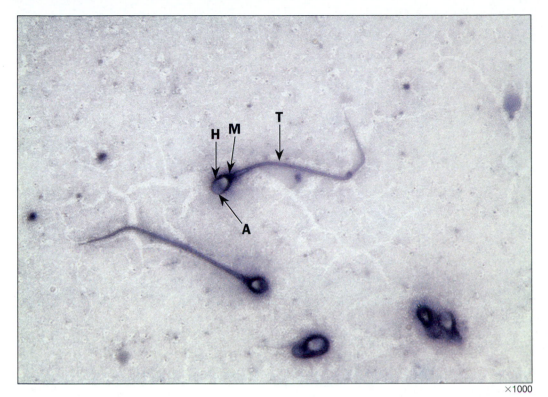

17-4 Sperm Cells ◾ The head (H), midpiece (M), and tail (T) are visible in these sperm cells. The acrosome (A) is visible in some. (×1000)

×1000

×400

×400

17-5 Interstitial Cells of Leydig ◾ Interstitial cells (IC) are found in the vascular connective tissue (CT) located between seminiferous tubules (ST) and constitute the main endocrine portion of the testis. (**A**) Interstitial cells secrete testosterone and are identified by their location between seminiferous tubules and their nuclei with prominent nucleoli. In many preparations, cytoplasmic lipid vacuoles (LV) typical of steroid-secreting cells are clearly visible. Some seminiferous tubule cells are also identifiable in this micrograph: M = myoid cell, SgA and SgB = spermatogonial cell, PS = primary spermatocyte, St = spermatid, and SC = Sertoli cell. (Iron hematoxylin stain, ×400) (**B**) This is an H&E stain of a thin section showing parts of three seminiferous tubules surrounding interstitial connective tissue with interstitial cells. The distinctive interstitial cell nuclei are present, but the cytoplasmic lipid vacuoles are more difficult to see in this preparation. Note the capillaries (Ca) in the connective tissue. Seminiferous tubule cells are labeled as in (**A**). (×400)

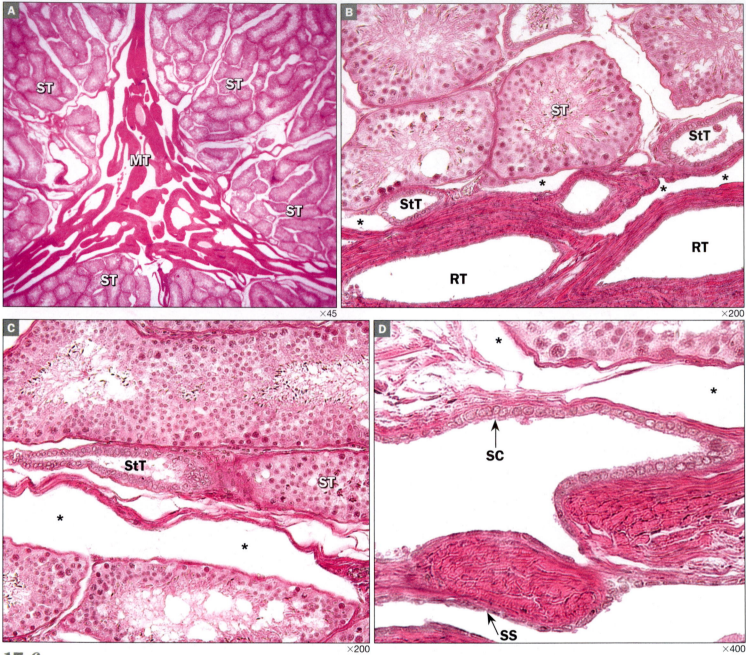

17-6 Intratesticular Genital Ducts ▮ Emerging from each seminiferous tubule (ST) is a short, straight tubule (StT) composed of Sertoli cells and no germinal cells. This leads into a network of tubules called the rete testis (RT) located on the posterior of each testis in a region known as the mediastinum testis (MT). These are lined with a simple epithelium ranging in height from squamous to short columnar. (**A**) The mediastinum testis is the darker region in the center of this micrograph. Seminiferous tubules comprise the rest of the field. (×45) (**B**) In this micrograph seminiferous tubules, straight tubules (lined with simple columnar epithelium), and rete testis (with the thick connective covering) are visible. Just because a microscope slide is labeled "Testis" or "Seminiferous Tubules" doesn't mean other structures aren't there! Scan the slide and see if these other tubules are present. Note: The asterisks (*) are where the specimen separated during preparation and are artifacts, not real spaces. (×200) (**C**) In this micrograph taken from a different region of the same slide used in (**B**) we are fortunate to see a seminiferous tubule changing into a straight tubule in longitudinal section. (×200) (**D**) In this higher magnification, the varying shapes of the epithelium lining the rete testis are apparent. It ranges from simple squamous (SS) to simple cuboidal (SC) epithelium. (×400)

A Photographic Atlas of Histology

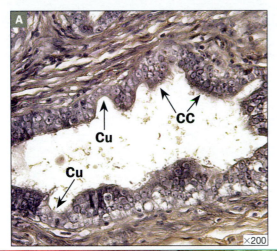

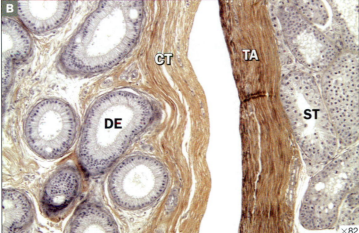

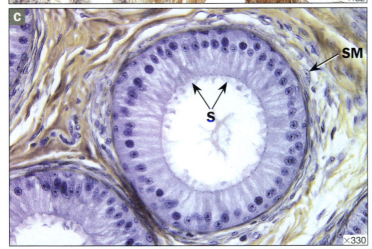

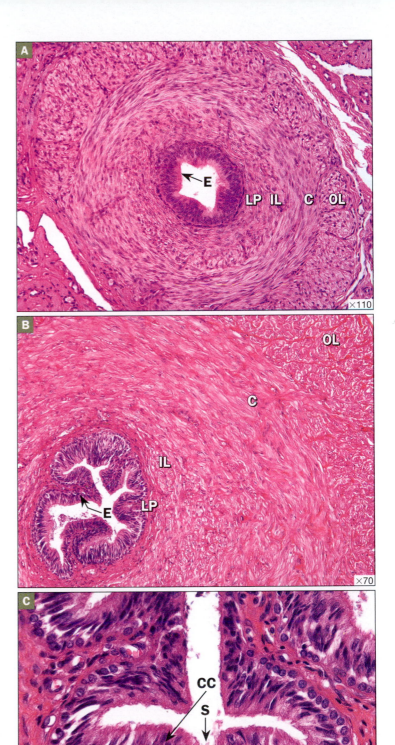

17-7 **Extratesticular Genital Ducts** 🔲 The rete testis empties into 15–20 efferent ductules at the head of the epididymis, which in turn empty into a single duct of the epididymis. (**A**) This efferent ductule is in the head of the epididymis. Patches of ciliated columnar cells (CC) interrupted by nonciliated cuboidal (Cu) cells give the epithelium an uneven, "scalloped" surface. (×200) (**B**) An epididymis is located on the posterior of each testis. Shown is a portion of the epididymis on the left and the testis on the right. Note the coiled duct of the epididymis (DE) and its connective tissue capsule (CT), and the tunica albuginea (TA) and seminiferous tubules (ST) of the testis. (×82) (**C**) The duct of the epididymis is lined with pseudostratified columnar epithelium. The tallest cells have long, branched stereocilia (S), which are responsible for fluid absorption. Smooth muscle (SM) is also found in the duct's wall. It becomes thicker toward the tail of the epididymis. (×330)

17-8 **Ductus (Vas) Deferens** 🔲 The longitudinally folded mucosa of the ductus (vas) deferens consists of a pseudostratified epithelium (E) and a connective tissue lamina propria (LP). The very muscular wall is composed of inner (IL) and outer (OL) longitudinal smooth muscle layers, with a circular (C) layer between. Note the distinctly different basal cells (BC) and columnar epithelial cells (CC) with stereocilia (S) in (**C**). (**A**) ×110 (**B**) ×70 (**C**) ×300

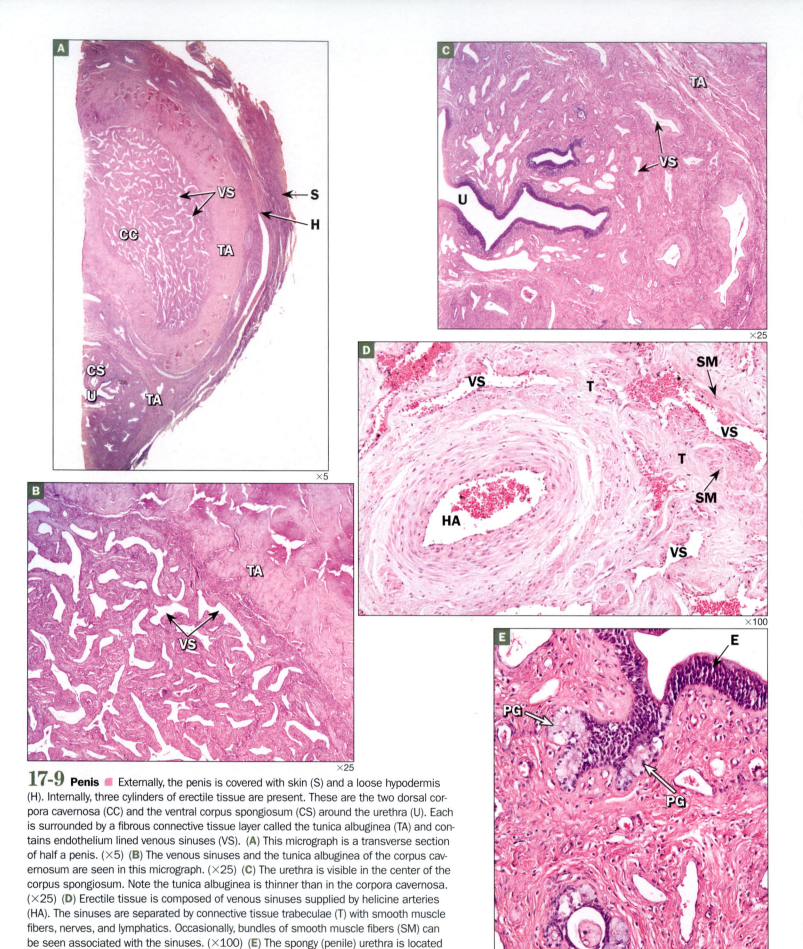

17-9 **Penis** ▥ Externally, the penis is covered with skin (S) and a loose hypodermis (H). Internally, three cylinders of erectile tissue are present. These are the two dorsal corpora cavernosa (CC) and the ventral corpus spongiosum (CS) around the urethra (U). Each is surrounded by a fibrous connective tissue layer called the tunica albuginea (TA) and contains endothelium lined venous sinuses (VS). (**A**) This micrograph is a transverse section of half a penis. (×5) (**B**) The venous sinuses and the tunica albuginea of the corpus cavernosum are seen in this micrograph. (×25) (**C**) The urethra is visible in the center of the corpus spongiosum. Note the tunica albuginea is thinner than in the corpora cavernosa. (×25) (**D**) Erectile tissue is composed of venous sinuses supplied by helicine arteries (HA). The sinuses are separated by connective tissue trabeculae (T) with smooth muscle fibers, nerves, and lymphatics. Occasionally, bundles of smooth muscle fibers (SM) can be seen associated with the sinuses. (×100) (**E**) The spongy (penile) urethra is located within the corpus cavernosum and is lined with a stratified or pseudostratified columnar epithelium (E). Mucous paraurethral glands of Littré (PG) are also visible. (×140)

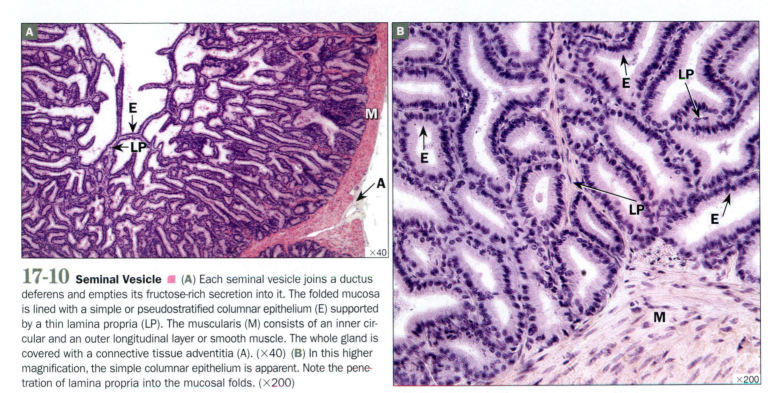

17-10 **Seminal Vesicle** 🔴 (**A**) Each seminal vesicle joins a ductus deferens and empties its fructose-rich secretion into it. The folded mucosa is lined with a simple or pseudostratified columnar epithelium (E) supported by a thin lamina propria (LP). The muscularis (M) consists of an inner circular and an outer longitudinal layer or smooth muscle. The whole gland is covered with a connective tissue adventitia (A). (×40) (**B**) In this higher magnification, the simple columnar epithelium is apparent. Note the penetration of lamina propria into the mucosal folds. (×200)

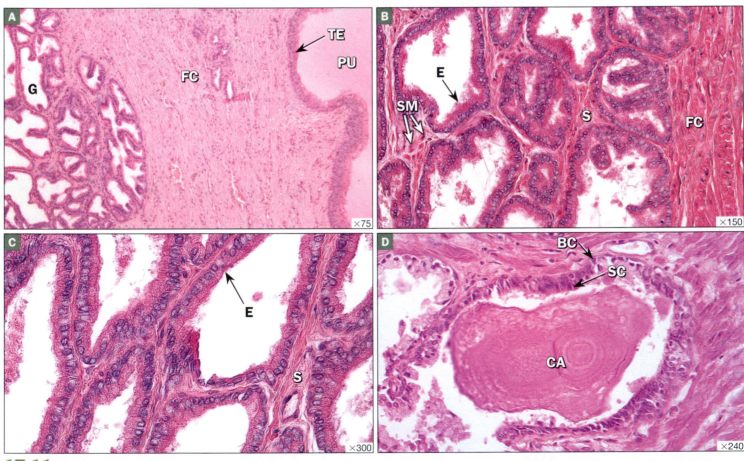

17-11 **Prostate Gland** 🔴 (**A**) The prostate gland is located inferior to the urinary bladder and surrounds the prostatic urethra. In this micrograph, the branched tubuloacinar glands (G) of the prostate are seen on the left and the prostatic urethra (PU) lined with transitional epithelium (TE) is seen on the right. The prostatic fibrous capsule (FC) is also visible. (×75) (**B**) The prostatic glands are branched and present an irregular surface when sectioned. The glandular epithelium (E) rests upon a vascular fibrous stroma (S) with scattered smooth muscle cells (SM). The stroma consists of extensions of the capsule into the gland. (×150) (**C**) The glandular epithelium is a simple columnar (as seen here) to a pseudostratified columnar with basal cells. (×300) (**D**) Corpora amylacea (CA) are calcified secretions unique to the prostate gland. They become more numerous with age. In this micrograph, the epithelium is pseudostratified, with basal cells (BC) and tall secretory cells (SC). (×240)

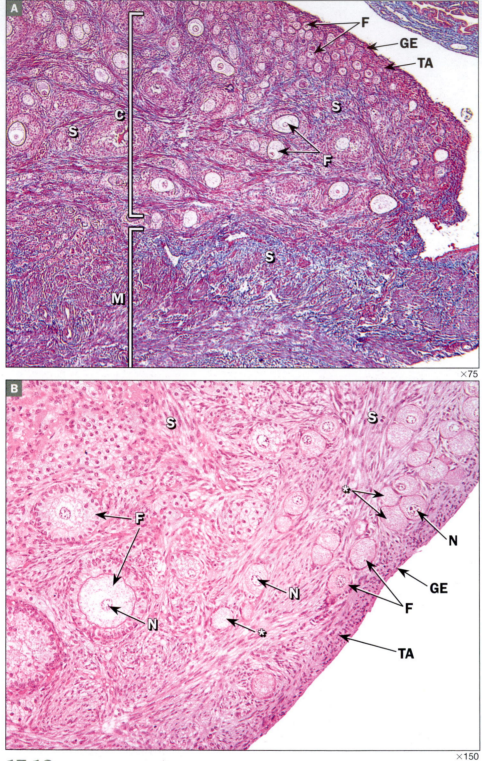

17-12 The Ovary ■ The ovary is covered with a germinal epithelium (GE) overlying a connective tissue tunica albuginea (TA). The bulk of the ovary is filled with connective tissue stroma (S), which is divided into a cortex (C) containing ovarian follicles (F) and a medulla (M) where follicles are absent. (**A**) Connective tissue fibers are stained blue in this section of cat ovary. (×75) (**B**) Shown in this micrograph is the ovarian cortex with follicles in various stages of development. Notice the chromatin in oocyte nuclei (N) is condensed, an indication that they have begun meiosis. In fact, the first meiotic division begins in utero and remains arrested in prophase I until postpubertal development (if any) resumes. Oocytes indicated by an asterisk (∗) have been sectioned in a plane that missed the nucleus. (×150)

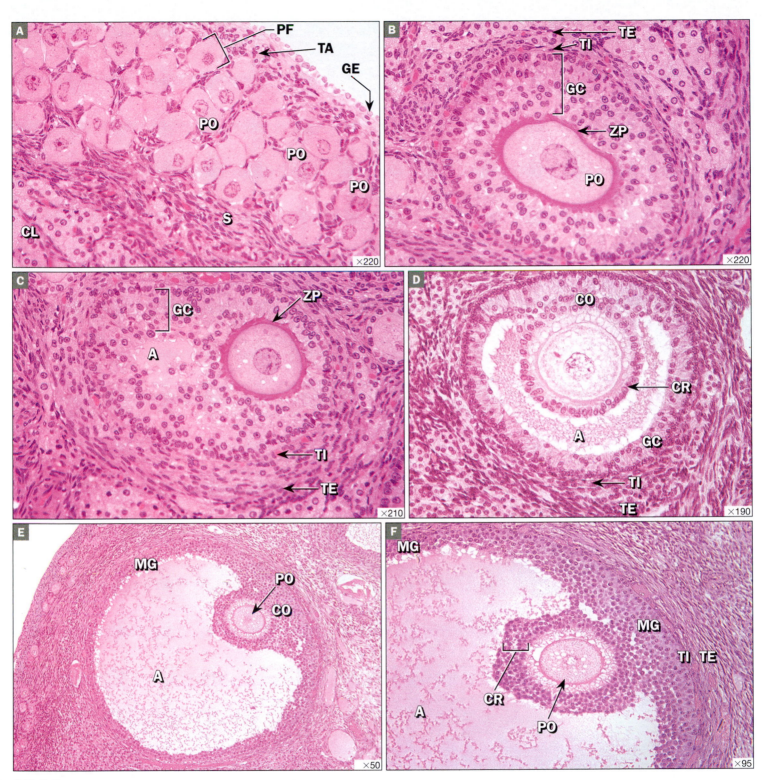

17-13 **Ovarian Follicle Development** ■ **(A)** A layer of primordial follicles (PF) is found deep to the tunica albuginea (TA) and germinal epithelium (GE) of the ovary. A single layer of flat cells surrounds each primary oocyte (PO). Note the prominent nucleolus and the condensed chromatin in the nucleus of the labeled primary oocytes. At this stage of development, primary oocytes are approximately 30 μm in diameter. A small part of a corpus luteum (CL) and the stroma (S) are also visible. (×220) **(B)** In this multilaminar primary follicle, there are several layers of cuboidal granulosa cells (GC) separated from the primary oocyte (PO) by the amorphous zona pellucida (ZP). A vascular and cellular theca interna (TI) and the fibrous theca externa (TE) have begun to develop in the stroma. (×220) **(C)** The antrum (A) has begun to develop in this secondary follicle and is filled with liquor folliculi, the diagnostic feature of a secondary follicle. By this time, the primary oocyte has reached its maximum size of approximately 125 μm. Notice the more advanced state of the theca interna (TI) and theca externa (TE). (×210) **(D)** In this secondary follicle, the cumulus oophorus (CO) is starting to develop. (×190) **(E)** This micrograph shows a mature Graafian follicle. At this point, the primary oocyte is about to complete the first meiotic division. Note the well-developed antrum and membrana granulosa (MG). (×50) **(F)** In this micrograph, the primary oocyte and corona radiata (CR) are starting to detach from the membrana granulosa/cumulus oophorus in preparation for ovulation. The theca interna and theca externa are also visible. (×95)

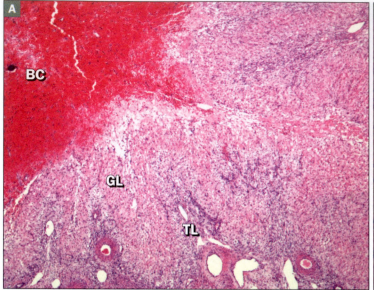

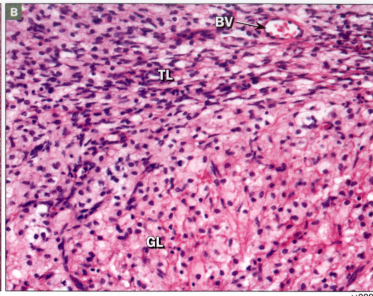

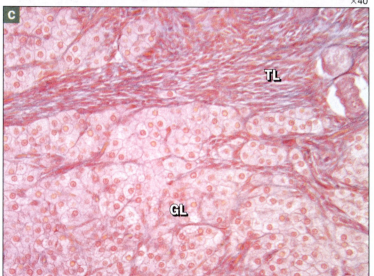

×40

×200

×210

17-14 **Corpus Luteum** ▪ After ovulation the remnants of the follicle collapse on the antrum and fold upon themselves to form a corpus luteum. Under the influence of LH, the follicular membrana granulosa cells develop into granulosa lutein (GL) cells, whereas the theca interna is the source of theca lutein (TL) cells, both of which have an endocrine function. Granulosa lutein cells are the larger and more abundant of the two and comprise the bulk of the corpus luteum. The less abundant and smaller theca lutein cells are found in the folds and on the surface of the corpus luteum. (**A**) In this panoramic view, a blood clot (BC) is seen in what was once the follicular antrum. It will be replaced with fibrous connective tissue as the corpus luteum continues to develop. Note the overall size and folded appearance of the corpus luteum. Layers of granulosa lutein and theca lutein cells are well defined at this magnification. (×40) (**B**) In this higher magnification, the granulosa lutein cells can be distinguished from the theca lutein cells by their larger size and lighter staining. Also note the blood vessel (BV). (×200) (**C**) Notice the characteristic folded appearance of the granulosa lutein cell layer. Granulosa lutein cells convert an estrogen precursor made in the theca lutein cells into estrogen. (×210)

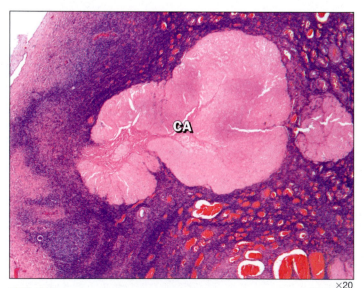

×20

17-15 **Corpus Albicans** ▪ After it has served its purpose, the corpus luteum is invaded by fibroblasts and macrophages, the luteal cells undergo autolysis, and a corpus albicans (CA) is formed. Notice that it still has the folded appearance. (×20)

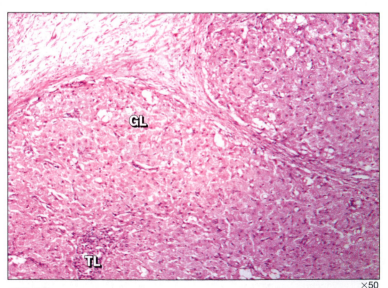

×50

17-16 **Corpus Luteum of Pregnancy** ▪ The corpus luteum of pregnancy continues to grow and develop. It remains functional for the first few months of pregnancy. In this micrograph, a portion of the corpus luteum is shown. Granulosa lutein cells (GL) and theca lutein cells (TL) are visible. (×50)

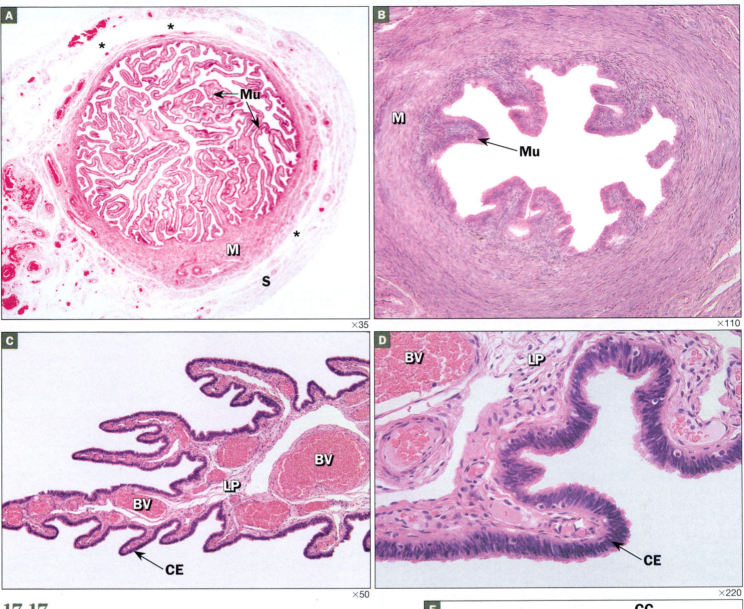

×35

×110

×50

×220

×400

17-17 **Uterine (Fallopian) Tubes** ◾ The uterine tubes are muscular structures extending laterally from the uterus. Their wall is made of a folded mucosa (Mu), a muscularis (M) consisting of poorly defined inner circular and outer longitudinal smooth muscle layers, and a serosa (S) made of visceral peritoneum. No submucosa is present. (**A**) This section is from the ampulla, the typical site of fertilization. Note how complex the mucosal folds are in this region. The continuation of the serosa to the left is part of the broad ligament, which is made of the two layers back-to-back. The broad ligament is a mesentery that carries blood vessels, nerves, and lymphatics to the ovaries, uterine tubes (as shown here), and uterus. The spaces indicated by asterisks (*) are artifacts of preparation. (×35) (**B**) This section is from the isthmus, which is narrower than the ampulla—compare the magnifications. Also compare the mucosal folding to that in the ampulla. (×110) (**C**) Shown are fimbriae, the fingerlike projections extending from the infundibulum that assist in capturing the ovum at ovulation. The ciliated epithelium (CE) sweeps into the uterine tube. Note the abundant blood vessels (BV) in the lamina propria (LP). (×50) (**D**) This micrograph is a higher magnification of the specimen shown in (**C**). Because they are mucosal folds, the muscularis is absent from the fimbriae. However, contraction of uterine tube smooth muscle positions the fimbriae over the ovary where ovulation will occur, assisting in capture of the secondary oocyte. (×220) (**E**) Uterine tube epithelium is made up of ciliated cells (CC) and secretory nonciliated peg cells (PC), which produce a secretion that nourishes the ovum and sperm, and assists in sperm capacitation. The proportion of peg cells and ciliated cells changes during the reproductive cycle, with ciliated cells being more abundant before ovulation (under the influence of estrogen) and peg cells dominating after ovulation (under the influence of progesterone). The thickness of the epithelium also changes during the cycle, reaching its maximum at ovulation. Again, notice the absence of smooth muscle cells. (×400)

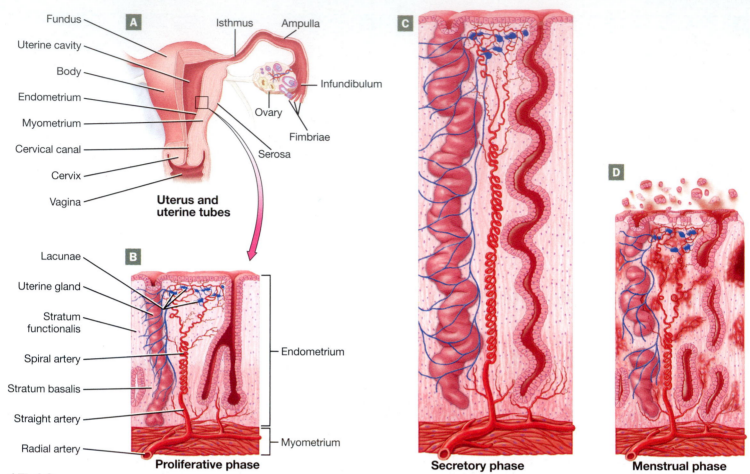

17-18 **Uterus** ■ (**A**) The uterus is a pear-shaped organ divided into the body, cervix, and above the entry point of the uterine tubes, the fundus. The uterine tubes open into the uterine cavity. The wall of the uterus is divided into a mucosal layer called endometrium. Deep to this is the muscular myometrium, which is covered by the serous membrane perimetrium over its posterior surface, with a fibrous adventitia covering most of the anterior surface. (**B**) The endometrium undergoes cyclic changes during the menstrual cycle. Prior to ovulation, the stratum basalis (the 1 mm thick portion of endometrium remaining after menstruation) grows to produce a thick superficial layer called the stratum functionalis. In this proliferative phase, uterine glands are relatively straight with narrow lumina, and the spiral arteries grow upward and supply the numerous capillaries in the stratum functionalis. The endometrium is about 3 mm thick at this point. The proliferative phase corresponds to the ovarian follicular phase and is influenced by the hormone estrogen. (**C**) Within a day after ovulation and under the influence of progesterone from the corpus luteum, the endometrium enters the secretory phase. The uterine glands become longer and coiled, their lumina fill with secretions rich in glycogen, and the endometrium achieves a thickness of up to 7 mm. (**D**) If implantation of the blastocyst doesn't occur, the corpus luteum dies and the progesterone levels drop below what is necessary to maintain the endometrium, and the stratum functionalis sheds during menstruation.

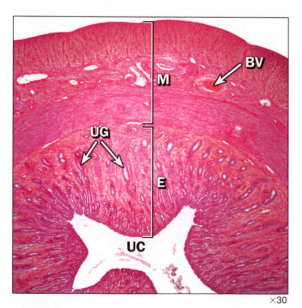

17-19 **Uterus in Transverse Section** ■ In this uterine transverse section, the endometrium (E) and myometrium (M) are easily seen, but the perimetrium is not. Uterine glands (UG) penetrate the endometrium and are relatively straight, indicating this uterus was probably in the proliferative phase. Note the prominent circular layer of muscle and the numerous blood vessels (BV) in the myometrium. The space in the center is the uterine cavity (UC). (×30)

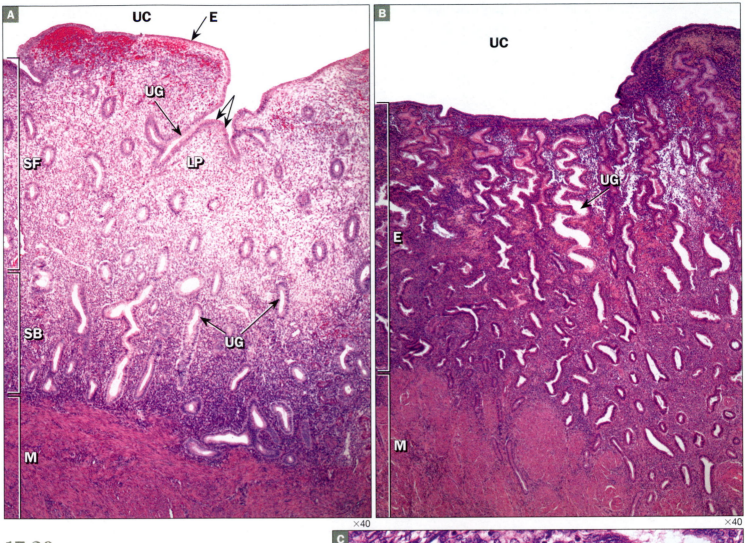

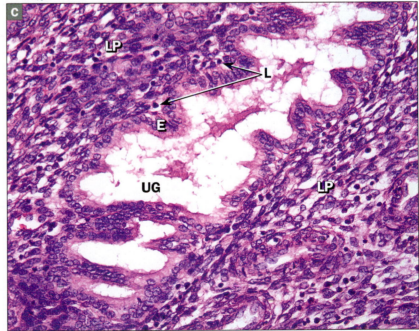

17-20 **Endometrium** ■ The endometrium is lined by a simple columnar epithelium (E) supported by a very cellular lamina propria (LP). Two endometrial layers are recognized. These are the basal stratum basalis (SB) and the more superficial stratum functionalis (SF). During the menstrual cycle, the endometrium grows thicker, becomes more vascular, and the glands become coiled. (A) This micrograph shows the endometrium in the proliferative (follicular) phase of the menstrual cycle. Note the few, straight glands (UG) and their continuity with the surface (arrows). The residual blood at the surface suggests this specimen was in early proliferative phase when the slide was prepared. The uterine cavity (UC) is at the top of the field and myometrium (M) is visible at the bottom. (×40) (B) The glands are more coiled in this micrograph of endometrium in the secretory (luteal) phase. (×40) (C) A coiled gland is shown in this micrograph. Note the secretion in the lumen, the cellular lamina propria, and the dark-staining lymphocytes (L). (×230) (Note: See Figure 17-18 for more detail.)

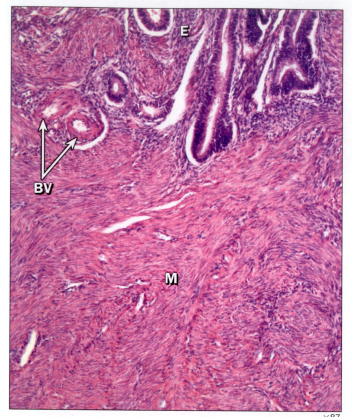

17-21 **Myometrium** ■ The smooth muscle of the myometrium (M) is arranged into poorly defined inner and outer longitudinal layers, separated by a vascular middle circular layer. This micrograph of a human uterus shows muscle fibers in multiple orientations. Endometrium (E) is visible at the top as are two blood vessels (BV). (×87)

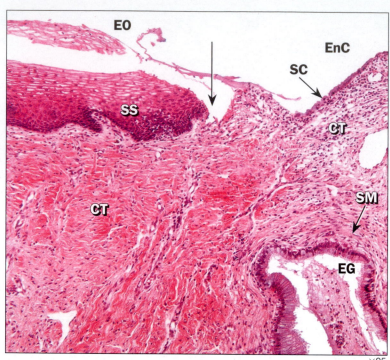

×95

17-22 **Cervix** ■ This is a longitudinal section of one side of the cervix and canal. The endocervical canal (EnC) is lined by a simple columnar epithelium (SC) that changes to a nonkeratinized stratified squamous epithelium (SS) where it projects into the vagina as the ectocervix (left of the arrow). The opening of the canal into the vagina beyond this point is called the external os (EO). Highly branched mucus-secreting endocervical glands (EG) are present in the endocervix, but only a portion of one is visible in this preparation. Deep to the epithelium is a dense elastic connective tissue layer (CT) with a few smooth muscle (SM) cells and numerous lymphocytes (tiny dark dots in endocervix). (×95)

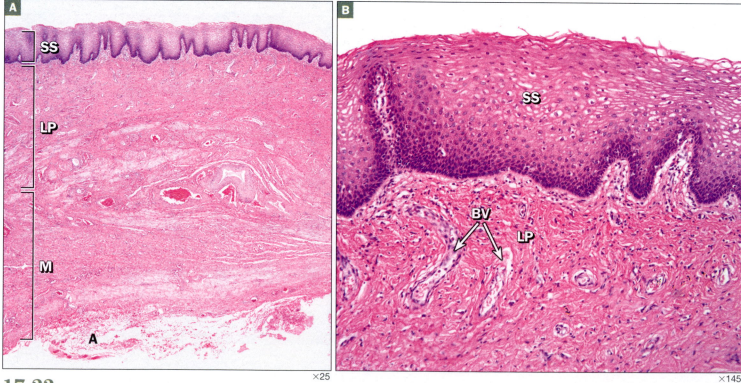

17-23 **Vagina** ■ The vagina consists of a mucosa, muscularis, and an adventitia. The mucosa is made of a nonkeratinized stratified squamous epithelium (SS) and is supported by a thick, vascular (note the blood vessels [BV]), fibrous, elastic lamina propria (LP). Longitudinal and circular smooth muscle fibers comprise the muscularis (M), but the layers are not well defined. An outer fibrous adventitia (A) blends with surrounding structures. **(A)** ×25 **(B)** ×145

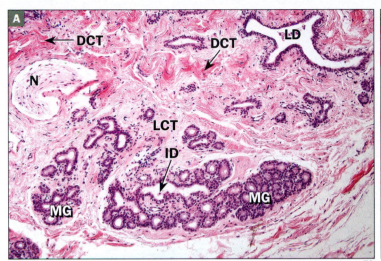

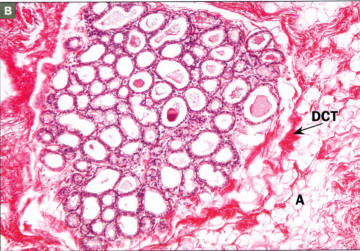

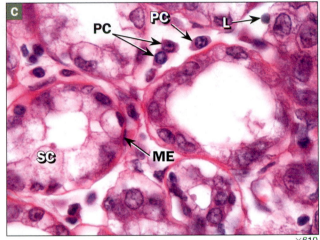

17-24 Breast ▪ The mammary glands are compound tubuloalveolar glands occupying the approximately 15 to 25 lobes in each breast. (**A**) Mammary glands are present even in nonlactating breasts. Shown here are two lobules of inactive mammary glands (MG) surrounded by a loose connective tissue (LCT) stroma. Farther from the lobules, a denser connective tissue (DCT) stroma is seen. Each gland is drained by an intralobular duct (ID), which in turn drains into a lactiferous duct (LD) and opens at the nipple. In the inactive gland, the "alveoli" are more tubular and are lined by nonfunctional secretory cells. Because they are hard to differentiate from the actual interlobular ducts, some authors refer to them as terminal ductules. Note the nerve (N), but no adipose tissue is visible in this micrograph, though the open region at the bottom may have been prior to slide preparation. (×72) (**B**) Shown is an active mammary gland. Note that the alveoli are more numerous and have displaced the loose connective tissue stroma. The lobule is surrounded by dense connective tissue and adipose tissue (A). (×72) (**C**) In this micrograph we see secretory alveoli. Secretory cells (SC) appear vacuolated because the milk fat was removed during slide preparation. Myoepithelial cells (ME) surround the alveoli and propel milk out the ducts. Lymphocytes (L) and plasma cells (PC) are visible in the region between alveoli. Lymphocytes are small cells with dark-staining nuclei, whereas plasma cells are larger, elongated, and have dark-staining heterochromatin. Plasma cells are responsible for secreting antibodies into the milk. (×610)

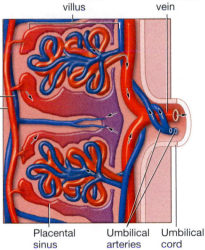

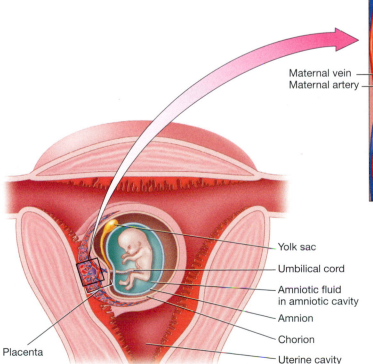

17-25 Placenta ▪ The embryonic trophoblast and the decidua cells of the endometrium form the placenta. Fetal blood is carried to the chorionic villi by the umbilical arteries and returned to the fetus through the umbilical vein. Maternal blood enters placental sinuses (intervillous spaces) between the chorionic villi. As shown in this illustration, fetal and maternal blood do not mix; rather, each stays in its own compartment. However, oxygen, nutrients, and antibodies are able to pass from maternal blood to the fetal capillaries in the chorionic villi. Carbon dioxide and other wastes pass from fetal capillaries into maternal blood in the intervillous spaces.

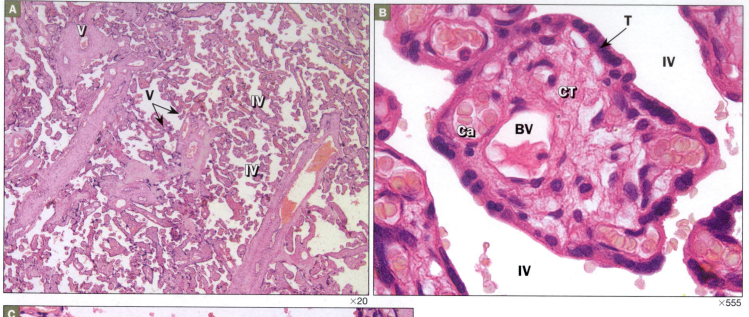

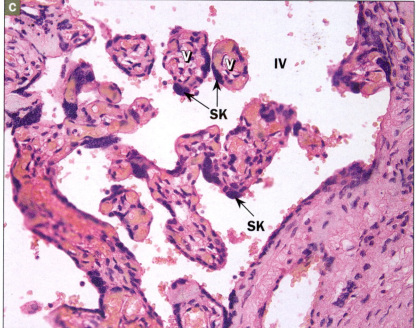

17-26 **Placenta** 🔴 (A) This micrograph is a panoramic view of a fully formed placenta. Large and small chorionic villi (V) and intervillous spaces (IV) are visible. Note the branching of the smallest villi. (×20) (B) In this cross section of a villus, the trophoblast layer (T), connective tissue (CT), fetal blood vessels (BV), and smaller capillaries (Ca) are seen. Maternal blood is found in the intervillous space (IV). (×555) (C) In the third trimester, syncytial trophoblast nuclei frequently form clusters called syncytial knots (SK). (×245)

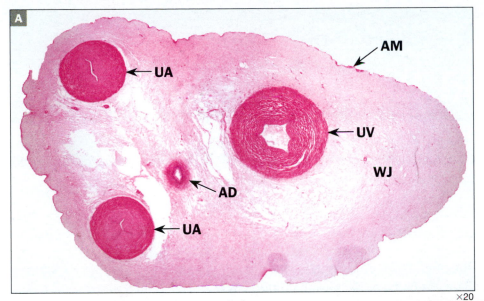

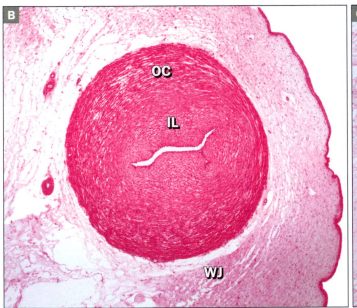

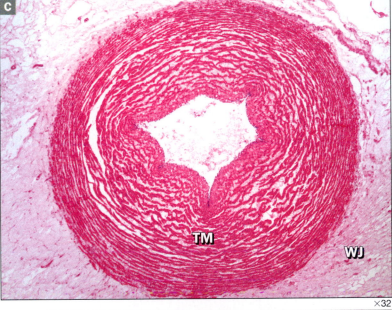

17-27 **Umbilical Cord** ■ The umbilical cord carries the blood vessels that connect fetal circulation with the placenta. (**A**) This umbilical cord has been cut in cross section. The two umbilical arteries (UA) and the single umbilical vein (UV) are surrounded by mesenchymal tissue called Wharton's jelly (WJ). Also visible is the allantoic duct (AD), a membranous structure that leads from different parts of the fetus at different times during development, but ultimately becomes an outgrowth of the fetal urinary bladder, and then degenerates. The outer surface of the umbilical cord is covered with amniotic membrane (AM). (×20) (**B**) The two umbilical arteries carry relatively oxygen-poor blood from fetal internal iliac arteries to the placenta at low pressure, so no internal elastic lamina is present. The lumen is frequently star shaped, as in the lower artery of the umbilical cord in (**A**), and the tunica media is composed of an inner longitudinal (IL) and an outer circular (OC) layer of smooth muscle. Outside of the tunica media is Wharton's jelly; there is no tunica adventitia. (×32) (**C**) The single umbilical vein carries oxygen-rich, nutrient-rich blood from the placenta to the fetal liver or to the inferior vena cava through the ductus venosus. Its tunica media (TM) is composed primarily of circularly arranged smooth muscle fibers. No valves are present. (×32) (**D**) The relationship between the allantoic duct and the urinary bladder is revealed by the presence of transitional epithelium (TE) lining its inner surface. The duct is only found in umbilical cord sections made near the embryo before the second month because the extraembryonic portion has degenerated by then. (×90)

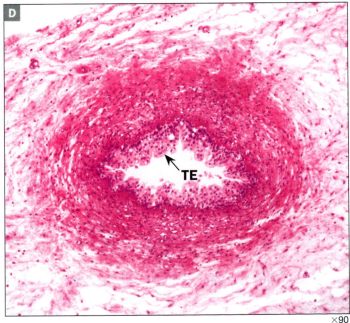

Selected Readings

▪ Anderson, Shauna C. and Keila B. Poulsen. 2013. *Anderson's Atlas of Hematology, 2nd Ed*. Lippincott Williams & Wilkins. Baltimore, MD.

▪ Barrett, Kim E., Susan M. Barman, Scott Boitano, and Heddwen L. Brooks. 2012. *Ganong's Review of Medical Physiology, 24th Ed*. McGraw Hill Lange. New York, NY.

▪ Cui, Dongmei. 2011. *Atlas of Histology with Functional & Clinical Correlations*. Lippincott Williams & Wilkins. Baltimore, MD.

▪ Eroschenko, Victor P. 2013. *diFiore's Atlas of Histology: with Functional Correlations, 12th Ed*. Lippincott Williams & Wilkins. Baltimore, MD.

▪ Gartner, Leslie and James L. Hiatt. 2014. *Color Atlas and Text of Histology, 6th Ed*. Lippincott Williams & Wilkins. Baltimore, MD.

▪ Harmening, Denise M. 2008. *Clinical Hematology and Fundamentals of Hemostasis, 5th Ed*. F.A. Davis Company. Philadelphia, PA.

▪ Martini, Frederic H., Michael J. Timmons, and Robert B. Tallitsch. 2012. *Human Anatomy, 7th Ed*. Pearson Benjamin Cummings. San Francisco, CA.

▪ Mescher, Anthony L. 2013. *Junqueira's Basic Histology Text and Atlas, 13th Ed*. McGraw Hill Lange. New York, NY.

▪ Moore, Keith L., T.V.N. Persaud, and Mark G. Torchia. 2013. *The Developing Human: Clinically Oriented Embryology, 9th Ed*. Saunders Elsevier. Philadelphia, PA.

▪ Netter, Frank H., MD. 2011. *Atlas of Human Anatomy, 5th Ed*. Saunders Elsevier. Philadelphia, PA.

▪ Ovalle, William K. and Patrick C. Nahirney. Illustrations by Frank H. Netter, MD. 2008. *Netter's Essential Histology*. Saunders Elsevier. Philadelphia, PA.

▪ Reece, Jane B., Lisa A. Urry, Michael L. Cain, Steven A. Wasserman, Peter V. Minorsky, and Robert B. Jackson. 2011. *Campbell Biology, 9th Ed*. Pearson Benjamin Cummings. San Francisco, CA.

▪ Ross, Michael H. and Wojciech Pawlina. 2011. *Histology: A Text and Atlas with Correlated Cell and Molecular Biology, 6th Ed*. Lippincott Williams & Wilkins. Baltimore, MD.

▪ Young, Barbara, Phillip Woodford, and Geraldine O'Dowd. 2013. *Wheater's Functional Histology: A Text and Colour Atlas, 6th Ed*. Churchill Livingstone. London, UK.